NSCA's Guide to Sport and Exercise Nutrition

National Strength and Conditioning Association

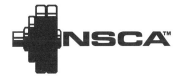

Bill I. Campbell, PhD, CSCS, FISSN
University of South Florida, Tampa

Marie A. Spano, MS, RD, LD, CSCS, CSSD, FISSN
Spano Sports Nutrition Consulting

EDITORS

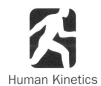

Human Kinetics

Library of Congress Cataloging-in-Publication Data

National Strength & Conditioning Association (U.S.)
  NSCA's guide to sport and exercise nutrition / National Strength and
Conditioning Association ; Bill I. Campbell, Marie A. Spano, editors.
      p. ; cm. -- (Science of strength and conditioning series)
  Guide to sport and exercise nutrition
  Includes bibliographical references and index.
  ISBN-13: 978-0-7360-8349-2 (print)
  ISBN-10: 0-7360-8349-9 (print)
  1. Athletes--Nutrition. 2. Sports--Nutritional aspects. I. Campbell,
Bill I., 1975- II. Spano, Marie A., 1972- III. Title. IV. Title: Guide to sport
and exercise nutrition. V. Series: Science of strength and conditioning
series.
  [DNLM: 1. Nutritional Physiological Phenomena. 2. Dietary Supplements.
3. Exercise. 4. Nutrition Assessment. 5. Sports. QU 145]
  TX361.A8N38 2011
  613.2'024796--dc22
                                    2010037212
  ISBN-10: 0-7360-8349-9 (print)
  ISBN-13: 978-0-7360-8349-2 (print)

The Web addresses cited in this text were current as of August, 2010, unless otherwise noted.

Developmental Editor: Katherine Maurer; **Assistant Editor:** Steven Calderwood; **Copyeditor:** Joyce Sexton; **Indexer:** Michael Ferreira; **Permission Manager:** Dalene Reeder; **Graphic Designer:** Nancy Rasmus; **Graphic Artist:** Dawn Sills; **Cover Designer:** Keith Blomberg; **Photographer (interior):** © Human Kinetics; **Photo Production Manager:** Jason Allen; **Art Manager:** Kelly Hendren; **Associate Art Manager:** Alan L. Wilborn; **Art Style Development:** Jennifer Gibas; **Illustrator:** © Human Kinetics; **Printer:** Sheridan Books

Printed in the United States of America   10 9 8 7 6 5 4 3 2

The paper in this book is certified under a sustainable forestry program.

Human Kinetics
Web site: www.HumanKinetics.com

United States: Human Kinetics
P.O. Box 5076
Champaign, IL 61825-5076
800-747-4457
e-mail: humank@hkusa.com

Canada: Human Kinetics
475 Devonshire Road Unit 100
Windsor, ON N8Y 2L5
800-465-7301 (in Canada only)
e-mail: info@hkcanada.com

Europe: Human Kinetics
107 Bradford Road
Stanningley
Leeds LS28 6AT, United Kingdom
+44 (0) 113 255 5665
e-mail: hk@hkeurope.com

Australia: Human Kinetics
57A Price Avenue
Lower Mitcham, South Australia 5062
08 8372 0999
e-mail: info@hkaustralia.com

New Zealand: Human Kinetics
P.O. Box 80
Torrens Park, South Australia 5062
0800 222 062
e-mail: info@hknewzealand.com

E4829

Science of Strength and Conditioning Series

NSCA's Guide to Sport and Exercise Nutrition

NSCA's Guide to Tests and Assessments

NSCA's Guide to Program Design

National Strength and Conditioning Association

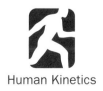

Human Kinetics

<u>Contents</u>

Introduction

What is sport nutrition? Ask 10 different people this question, and you are likely to receive 10 different answers. At its most basic level, sport nutrition is the practice of ingesting nutrients in the correct amounts at specific times to improve exercise or sport performance. But while improving sport performance is a goal for some, many individuals are not competitive in their activities but rather are concerned with improving their body composition, 5K time, or maximum bench press, for example. An intriguing aspect of sport nutrition is that the same principles apply to the elite athlete as to the individual who has hired a personal trainer for the first time. One of the primary objectives of this book is to relay practical, scientific information to this diverse range of fitness enthusiasts and competitive athletes.

Scientific inquiry into the domain of sport nutrition has steadily increased over the past few decades. In fact, since 1990, the number of scholarly, peer-reviewed publications in the realm of sport nutrition has exponentially increased. It appears that almost each issue of every scientific journal in the fields of exercise science and nutrition includes at least one study or comprehensive review related to sport nutrition. Even though this research is answering a number of questions, many unanswered questions and divided opinions on fundamental aspects of nutrition intake, supplementation, and exercise performance remain. Examples include the amount of protein ingestion that will maximize training adaptations, the safety of creatine supplementation, and the best combinations of supplements to use to improve performance. It is these unanswered questions and differing opinions that drive the progression and growth of sport nutrition research. This research is pertinent to many populations, from mothers of teenagers playing multiple sports to Olympic athletes specializing in one particular movement pattern.

This book discusses how food and sport supplements interact with the body's biological functions. Pertinent research is cited to highlight specific nutrient intakes that have been shown to improve exercise and sport performance. Chapters also present information on assessing an athlete's nutritional status and developing a plan based on this assessment. As a whole, the book will give readers a better understanding of how ingested food is metabolized, stored, and oxidized for energy. The research presented demonstrates how the proper selection of these nutrients can improve performance.

This book is divided into 12 chapters. The first chapter overviews how nutrition affects training and performance. The next several chapters discuss the macronutrients (carbohydrate, protein, and fat), specifically how these nutrients are metabolized, stored, and oxidized for energy, and presents scientifically based recommendations for ingesting these macronutrients to improve aerobic, anaerobic, and strength training performance. Chapter 5 discusses fluids, including the fluid needs of aerobic endurance and strength athletes, and outlines common problems resulting from an inadequacy or overabundance of ingested fluids. Chapter 6 considers micronutrients and their role in metabolism and exercise. The next several chapters discuss specific nutrition techniques and nutritional ergogenic aids that have been shown to improve aerobic endurance, strength, and power performance, as well as nutrition techniques and nutritional ergogenic aids that may help improve body composition. The final two chapters provide important information on assessing nutrition status and developing a comprehensive plan based on the assessment.

Sport nutrition is an umbrella term that can encompass a great deal of information. It is our hope that through this book the reader will gain an enhanced understanding of how food, sport supplements, and their inter-actions with the body's biological systems can enhance exercise and sport performance.

Acknowledgments

We would like to thank everyone who has paved the path and opened doors in the field of sport nutrition. Your hard work, dedication, and knowledge have created opportunities for those of us who have come after you. We would especially like to acknowledge Richard Kreider, PhD, Jose Antonio, PhD, and Jeff Stout, PhD, for your mentorship, leadership, and extensive work in the field of sport nutrition.

Foods and Fluids for Training and Sport Performance

Bill I. Campbell, PhD, CSCS, FISSN

Marie A. Spano, MS, RD, LD, CSCS, CSSD, FISSN

Many modifiable factors contribute to an athlete's success. The most important ones are a sound strength and conditioning program, sport psychology, sport-specific training, nutrition, supplementation, rest, and recovery. Not only do these factors affect long-term training and subsequent performance, but they can also play a major role in just one competition.

The science of nutrition and performance (and also of nutrition and physique changes) is growing by leaps and bounds. As this body of research expands and scientists scrutinize ever more closely the factors that can affect an athlete's performance and physique, the need for sport nutrition practitioners is also growing. At both the college and professional level, sport nutritionists use scientific research to make sound recommendations to athletes. They often work with coaches, strength and conditioning professionals, and trainers as part of a comprehensive team whose primary goal is to assist the athletes. Sport nutritionists help athletes make sound changes to their dietary intake, apply nutrient timing techniques, alter their supplementation regimen, and make sense of all the information related to supplements. Sport nutritionists also develop healthy training tables, measure body composition and bone density, help athletes navigate the grocery store, teach them the basics of preparing healthy meals, and work with a team of professionals to develop a treatment plan for athletes with eating disorders.

New Developments in Nutrition Research

What are some of the hottest areas of research relevant to an athlete's diet? From macronutrients to electrolyte balance to supplements that mitigate fatigue, sport nutrition incorporates a multifaceted body of research. When it comes to macronutrients, the timing of consumption is just as important as the specific macronutrient consumed. **Nutrient timing**, the practice of consuming a specific nutrient in a given time period within proximity to training or performance, affects physique changes, glycogen replenishment, muscle protein synthesis, and performance.

> ➤ nutrient timing—The practice of consuming a specific nutrient in a given time period within proximity to training or performance to achieve a desired outcome.

Carbohydrate consumption is an area of nutrient timing that has a great impact on many athletes. Twenty years ago, carbohydrate research largely focused on aerobic endurance athletes. However, studies since then have examined the importance of pre- and postexercise carbohydrate consumption for resistance training as a means of restoring glycogen losses (Robergs et al. 1991; Tesch et al. 1998), altering hormone secretion, and influencing muscle protein synthesis (Volek 2004). In addition, the types of carbohydrate ingested play a critical role, with a glucose plus fructose beverage possibly the best means of staying hydrated (Jeukendrup and Moseley 2010) and potentially sparing endogenous carbohydrate during exercise (Currell and Jeukendrup 2008). And a unique, high molecular weight starch-based carbohydrate made from barley amylopectin may be preferable to low molecular weight carbohydrates such as monosaccharides and disaccharides for expediting glycogen replenishment (Stephens et al. 2008).

Protein research has evolved from studies of the amino acid profiles (**PDCAAS,** protein digestibility–corrected amino acid score) of various sources of protein to research on nutrient timing and on types of protein (i.e., whey) that may play a role in weight loss (Lockwood et al. 2008). In addition, researchers have determined when and how branched-chain amino acids (BCAAs) and to what extent essential amino acids (EAAs) increase muscle protein synthesis (Borsheim et al. 2002; Norton and Layman 2006; Shimomura et al. 2006; Tipton et al. 1999). The final macronutrient, fat, may play an important role in overall health, while some types of fat, such as conjugated linoleic acid (CLA) and medium-chain triglycerides, continue to spark interest for their potential role in improving exercise performance and enhancing weight loss.

> ➤ PDCAAS (protein digestibility–corrected amino acid score)—A method of evaluating protein quality based on the amino acid requirements of humans and ease of digestion; 100% is often used as the highest value (values above 100 are truncated) and 0 is the lowest (Schaafsma 2000).

Though the ingestion of **micronutrients** above and beyond the Recommended Dietary Intake (RDI) has not been shown to enhance performance, population-based studies are uncovering that many people do not consume the RDI of certain nutrients and that some individuals are deficient in one or more micronutrients. And, making up for a dietary deficiency by consuming a micronutrient may directly or indirectly enhance performance. For instance, taking extra iron even if you have enough in your diet will not help performance. However, individuals who are iron deficient should notice an improvement in their levels of fatigue and their athletic performance if they correct this deficiency through supplementation. When it comes to specific micronutrients, certain groups of people are more likely to experience a deficiency than others (women are more likely to be deficient in calcium and iron, for example, than men). In some cases, correcting micronutrient deficiencies may directly enhance performance (iron deficiency anemia, for example); and in others it may benefit overall health, help prevent injuries and illness (vitamin D, for example), or quicken the recovery process (sodium for enhancing thirst and therefore rehydration). Chapter 6 presents an in-depth analysis of the various micronutrients and their importance to exercise performance.

➤ micronutrient—A substance needed in small amounts by the body. All vitamins and minerals are micronutrients.

Possibly the hottest topic among athletes is supplements. In a society fascinated with finding "magic bullets," athletes are also in search of anything that will help them get stronger, faster, and leaner and possibly even concentrate better. Consequently, a wide variety of sport supplements fill up store shelves and the cabinets of physically active individuals. Fortunately, there is scientific research to substantiate marketing claims for some of these purported ergogenic aids. Creatine, protein, caffeine, amino acids, electrolyte replacement sport beverages, beta-alanine, and high molecular weight starch-based carbohydrates are among the most widely researched supplements to date (these are explored in more depth in chapters 7 and 8).

Topics in Nutrition and Performance

In research on an athlete's diet, three of the top areas sport nutritionists hone in on are macronutrients, hydration, and ergogenic aids. The type and amount of macronutrients, as well as the timing of consumption, can have a major impact on performance, recovery, and overall health. And changing the variables related to macronutrient intake, including the type of macronutrient consumed, when it is consumed, and the amount consumed, can often have an immediate impact on how an athlete feels. Hydration encompasses more than just cooling the body. Hydration also affects electrolyte status and nutrient delivery. Finally, ergogenic aids are very popular among athletes looking for an edge on their competition. Ergogenic aids are a very large category of supplements and range from ineffective to effective, as well as from dangerous to very safe for intended use.

Macronutrients

Macronutrient (carbohydrate, protein, and fat) ingestion is essential for a multitude of life-sustaining activities, including preservation of the structural and functional integrity of the human body. In the realm of sport nutrition, the macronutrients are often discussed in terms of energy production and their role in building skeletal muscle that can subsequently be trained or stimulated to enhance force production (table 1.1). Specifically, carbohydrate and fat are the primary nutrients used for energy production; protein contributes only a small amount of the total energy used (Lemon and Nagle 1981; van Loon et al. 1999).

> ➤ macronutrient—Substances required by the body in large amounts. Carbohydrate, protein, and fat are all macronutrients.

Adenosine triphosphate (ATP), the energy currency of the cell, allows the conversion of chemical energy into mechanical energy. The energy in food (chemical energy) does not transfer directly to the cells for biologic work. Rather, "macronutrient energy" funnels through the energy-rich ATP compound (McArdle, Katch, and Katch 2008). This process can be summarized in two basic steps: (1) the extraction of chemical energy from macronutrients and its transfer to the bonds of ATP; (2) the extraction and transfer of the chemical energy in ATP to fuel biologic work such as skeletal muscle contraction (McArdle, Katch, and Katch 2008). All three macronutrients are oxidized for energy during exercise. Several factors regulate the extent to which each of the macronutrients is oxidized, including nutrition status, exercise intensity, and training status. The following is a brief discussion of the major roles of the macronutrients in terms of fueling activity and their ability to build lean body mass.

Fuels for Aerobic and Anaerobic Exercise

Carbohydrate and fat (in the form of fatty acids) are the two primary substrates oxidized by skeletal muscle to provide energy during prolonged exercise. As the exercise intensity increases, a greater percentage of fuel

TABLE 1.1 Primary Roles of Macronutrients Relative to Exercise Performance

Macronutrient	Role
Carbohydrate	Energy production (high intensity)
Fat	Energy production (low intensity)
Protein	Lean tissue accretion and maintenance

used is from carbohydrate. As people near 100% of $\dot{V}O_2$max, they progressively use more carbohydrate and less fat (Mittendorfer and Klein 2003; van Loon et al. 1999). However, as exercise duration increases, fat metabolism is increased and carbohydrate metabolism decreased (Jeukendrup 2003). The main carbohydrate sources are muscle and liver glycogen, liver gluconeogenesis (the production of carbohydrate from noncarbohydrate sources), and ingested carbohydrate. Even though carbohydrate and fat are the major energy sources during aerobic exercise, athletes who consistently train aerobically alter the amounts of energy contribution from these macronutrients. Whole-body calorimetry measurements have clearly shown that aerobic endurance training leads to an increase in total fat oxidation and a decrease in total carbohydrate oxidation during exercise at a given intensity (Coggan et al. 1990; Friedlander et al. 1997; Hurley et al. 1986). Although amino acids are not a major contributor to energy production, several clinical investigations have demonstrated that their contribution to aerobic exercise energy production is linearly related to exercise intensity (Brooks 1987; Lemon and Nagle 1981; Wagenmakers 1998).

The energy to perform short-term, high-intensity anaerobic exercise comes from existing ATP-PC (ATP phosphocreatine) stores and carbohydrate oxidation via glycolysis (refer to chapter 2 for an in-depth discussion of carbohydrate metabolism and glycolysis) (Maughan et al. 1997). In fact, anaerobic energy transfer from the macronutrients occurs only from carbohydrate breakdown during glycolytic reactions (McArdle, Katch, and Katch 2008). Also, carbohydrate catabolism, or breakdown, is the fastest source of ATP resynthesis. Due to its rate and quantity of oxidation, carbohydrate is the main source for ATP resynthesis during maximal exercise tasks lasting approximately 7 seconds to 1 minute (Balsom et al. 1999; Mougios 2006).

Protein for Building Lean Body Mass

The contribution of amino acid oxidation to the total energy production is negligible during short-term, high-intensity exercise. It likely accounts for 3% to 6% but has been reported to be as high as 10% of the total ATP supplied during prolonged exercise (Hargreaves and Spriet 2006; Phillips et al. 1993; Brooks 1987). The role that protein plays as a substrate during exercise is principally dependent on the availability of branched-chain amino acids and the amino acid alanine (Lemon and Nagle 1981). Protein has a limited role in energy production; its primary function is to increase and maintain lean body mass. One needs to consider many factors when determining an optimal amount of dietary protein for exercising individuals. These factors include protein quality, energy intake, carbohydrate intake, mode and intensity of exercise, and the timing of the protein intake (Lemon 2000). For an in-depth discussion of the various types of protein and specific protein intake recommendations, refer to chapter 3. A protein intake of 1.5 to 2.0 g/kg per day for physically active individuals not only is safe but also may improve the adaptations to exercise training (Campbell et al. 2007).

Hydration

Hydration is not limited to the replenishment of body fluids but is also a vehicle for delivering electrolytes, sugar, and amino acids. Dehydration and hyponatremia (low blood sodium, often due to overhydration in the absence of sodium) still affect "weekend warriors" and experienced athletes alike. Further, dehydration can result in a dangerous increase in core body temperature leading to heat illness (Greenleaf and Castle 1971). However, even mild dehydration, which is more common, can lead to decreases in both strength and aerobic endurance and subsequently to impaired athletic performance (Bigard et al. 2001; Schoffstall et al. 2001; Walsh et al. 1994). The young and the elderly are the two groups at greatest risk for heat-related illness, including heat cramps, heat exhaustion, and heatstroke (Wexler 2002). Two major factors put young athletes at risk: (1) They do not sweat as much as adults (sweat helps dissipate heat); and (2) they have a greater surface area relative to their body mass, which increases their heat gain from the environment when ambient temperatures are elevated (Delamarche et al. 1990; Drinkwater et al. 1977).

In the elderly, age-related changes in thirst and thermoregulation contribute to dehydration. Elderly individuals experience a decreased thirst sensation in response to drops in blood volume, a reduction in renal water conservation capacity, and disturbances in fluid and electrolyte balance (Kenney and Chiu 2001). Some prescription medicines, as well as cardiovascular disease (still the number one cause of death in the United States), can impair fluid homeostasis (Naitoh and Burrell 1998).

The quest for enhanced hydration has led to the examination of hyperhydrating agents such as glycerol. In addition, nutrition scientists have investigated the effects of adding amino acids to sport beverages and regular electrolyte replacement beverages to improve hydration and mitigate muscle damage. Fortunately, beverage companies are continuing to sponsor research on the effectiveness of their products, which indicates a continued focus on hydration and its effects on health and performance. Companies that conduct studies on their products should hire independent labs with no financial interest in the company itself to conduct unbiased, well-designed clinical trials.

Ergogenic Aids

Modern-day Olympic athletes are no different from high school athletes attempting to make their junior varsity basketball team—both groups are seeking to improve their athletic performance. Naturally, any athlete attempting to improve performance will continually manipulate his training regimen. Along with this focus on training methodology is often an equal attention on the use of ergogenic aids to improve performance. **Ergogenic aids** are nutritional, physical, mechanical, psychologic, or pharmacologic procedures or devices intended to improve exercise or sport performance. Since by definition, ergogenic aids are work-enhancing substances or devices believed to increase performance (McNaughton 1986), they may range from caffeine for the aerobic endurance athlete to eyewear for a skier or snowboarder. Nutritional ergogenic aids receive a lot of attention from athletes and others in the sport performance industry. They may directly influence the physiological capacity of a particular body system and thereby improve performance, or they may increase the speed of recovery from training and competition.

> ➤ ergogenic aid—A work-enhancing substance or device believed to increase performance. Examples include nutritional, physical, mechanical, psychologic, or pharmacologic procedures or aids to improve exercise or sport performance.

Macronutrients and Sport Supplements

Nutritional ergogenic aids can be categorized into two broad categories: macronutrient intake manipulations (carbohydrate loading, increasing protein intake during a hypertrophic resistance training phase, etc.) and the ingestion of dietary supplements. Dietary supplements, products intended to make the diet more complete, contain one or more of the following ingredients: a vitamin, mineral, amino acid, herb, or other botanical; a dietary substance intended to supplement the diet by increasing the total dietary intake of certain macronutrients or total calories; a concentrate, metabolite, constituent, extract, or combination of any of the ingredients already mentioned and intended for ingestion in the form of a liquid, capsule, powder, softgel or gelcap, and not represented as a conventional food or as a sole item of a meal or the diet (Antonio and Stout 2001; U.S. Food and Drug Administration [FDA] 1994). Commonly used supplements such as vitamins and minerals are considered ergogenic aids only if the athlete is correcting a deficiency. Other ergogenic aids are not taken specifically to correct a deficiency but instead for a very specific benefit. For instance, a hockey player taking a time-released beta-alanine supplement for four to six weeks prior to preseason practice is doing so to zone in on one very specific component of training and recovery: buffering fatigue. Sport supplements and nutritional ergogenic aids are classified under the umbrella of dietary supplements. Often, sport supplements provide a substance that is a component of a normal physiological or biochemical process (creatine monohydrate, alpha ketoglutarate, etc.). Other nutritional ergogenic aids augment physiological or bioenergetic pathways to enhance energy production (e.g., creatine monohydrate, caffeine) or skeletal muscle mass (creatine monohydrate, leucine, etc.). Table 1.2 lists common sport supplements and their proposed benefits in relation to health and performance.

TABLE 1.2   Proposed Benefits of Popular Sport Supplements

Sport supplement	Proposed benefits
BCAAs (branched-chain amino acids)	Increase rates of protein synthesis
Caffeine	Improve aerobic endurance performance, mental alertness
Creatine	Increase strength and muscle mass
EFAs (essential fatty acids)	General health, weight loss
Energy drinks	Increase alertness and metabolism
Glycerol	Hyperhydration
HMB (β-hydroxy-β-methylbuteric acid)	Increase strength and muscle mass; anticatabolic
Hydration drinks	Improve aerobic endurance performance, improve hydration
Medium Chain Triglycerides	Improve aerobic endurance exercise performance
Multivitamins and multiminerals	General health
Nitric oxide boosters	Increase blood flow to active musculature
Protein	Increase strength and muscle mass; recovery
Patented, highly branched high molecular weight (HMW) glucose polymer solution	Increase aerobic endurance performance; recovery

Prevalence of Ergogenic Aid Use

Throughout history, athletes have experimented with nutritional ergogenic aids to improve performance. The ancient Greeks may have been
the first to ponder how to gain a competitive edge through proper diet and
supplementation (Antonio and Stout 2001). Greek warriors from the fifth
century B.C. reportedly used such things as hallucinogenic mushrooms and
deer liver for ergogenic purposes (Applegate and Grivetti 1997; McArdle,
Katch, and Katch 2008). For a comprehensive review on the history of
dietary practices of ancient athletes, refer to Grivetti and Applegate 1997
and Grandjean 1997.

A look at past practices of nutritional supplementation suggests that
elite athletes in various civilizations ingested nutritional ergogenic aids.
Modern times have seen a shift in the prevalence and types of individuals
who consume nutritional ergogenic aids. Statistics on high school athletes
are a sign of this shift (Hoffman et al. 2008). A self-report survey asking
about dietary supplement intake was administered to approximately 3,000
students (with an approximately equal gender distribution) representing
grades 8 through 12 in the United States. The results revealed that 71.2% of
the adolescents reported use of at least one supplement. The most popular

supplements used were multivitamins and high-energy drinks. The use of supplements to increase body mass and strength (e.g., creatine, protein powder, weight gain formulations) increased across grades and was more prevalent in males than females. The authors concluded, not surprisingly, that reliance on nutritional supplements and ergogenic aids increases during adolescence. Other survey-based investigations have yielded similar results (Bell et al. 2004; O'Dea 2003).

As greater numbers of adolescents and high school athletes ingest nutritional ergogenic aids, their coaches, athletic trainers, personal trainers, physicians, and parents need an increased knowledge base. Weekend warriors, mothers interested in the long-term effects of creatine on their high school children, and fitness enthusiasts striving to obtain a leaner physique—all must have a working knowledge of nutrition and ergogenic aids and how they affect the physiology of the human body. Given the increase in sport nutrition research, this information is becoming more available.

Professional Applications

The need for accurate nutrition and supplement information among athletes, coaches, strength and conditioning professionals, strength coaches, athletic trainers, and support staff is clear. Various surveys, including the General Nutrition Knowledge Questionnaire (GNKQ) and Eating Attitude Test (EAT-26), have been used to assess athletes' nutrition knowledge (Raymond-Barker, Petroczi, and Quested 2007). Most of these surveys reflect limitations in athletes' knowledge. Studies have found that formal education in nutrition or closely related subjects does not influence nutrition knowledge (Raymond-Barker, Petroczi, and Quested 2007). In addition, nutrition knowledge does not necessarily impact eating attitudes in females at risk for the female athlete triad (Raymond-Barker, Petroczi, and Quested 2007); adolescent females may have nutrition misconceptions (Cupisti 2002); and college athletes in general cannot identify the recommended intake for all macronutrients, and also many do not know what roles vitamins play in the body (Jacobson, Sobonya, and Ransone 2001). In addition, coaches often have a low level of knowledge of sport nutrition (Zinn, Schofield, and Wall 2006).

Filling the sport nutrition knowledge gap requires testing and education. After testing an athlete's body composition and bone density and analyzing food records and subjective data (how the athlete feels, energy levels, etc.), practitioners can use the results as a starting place for education. In addition, one-on-one consultations with athletes provide a great opportunity for each athlete to ask pertinent questions. A sport nutritionist's knowledge of the current research and how it can be applied to athletes is essential to helping athletes meet their goal of improved performance. Sport nutritionists use this knowledge to develop plans and progress charts for athletes, make sound recommendations, and help design the treatment plan for those with eating disorders.

SUMMARY POINTS

- Sport nutritionists are an integral part of the athletic training team that also includes coaches, strength and conditioning specialists, athletic trainers, sport psychologists, team physicians, and physical therapists.

- Carbohydrate and fat are the two nutrients that provide athletes with energy.

- The main carbohydrate sources are muscle and liver glycogen, liver gluconeogenesis (the production of carbohydrate from noncarbohydrate sources), and ingested carbohydrate.

- Aerobic endurance training leads to an increase in total fat oxidation and a decrease in total carbohydrate oxidation during exercise at a given intensity.

- Due to its rate and quantity of oxidation, carbohydrate is the main source for ATP resynthesis during maximal exercise tasks lasting approximately 7 seconds to 1 minute.

- Protein's primary function is to increase and maintain lean body mass.

- A protein intake of 1.5 to 2.0 g/kg per day for physically active individuals not only is safe but also may improve the adaptations to exercise training.

- Dehydration can result in a dangerous increase in core body temperature leading to heat illness. Even mild dehydration, which is more common, can lead to decreases in both strength and aerobic endurance and subsequently to impaired athletic performance.

- The young and the elderly are the two groups at greatest risk for heat-related illness, including heat cramps, heat exhaustion, and heatstroke.

- Though the ingestion of micronutrients above and beyond the RDI has not been shown to enhance performance, population-based studies reveal that many people do not consume the RDI of certain nutrients. In addition, many people are deficient in certain micronutrients. And, making up for low levels of a nutrient or a true deficiency may directly or indirectly impact performance.

- Creatine, protein, caffeine, amino acids, electrolyte replacement sport beverages, beta-alanine, and high molecular weight starch-based carbohydrates are among the most widely researched supplements to date (these are explored in more depth in chapters 7 and 8).

Carbohydrate

Donovan L. Fogt, PhD

Carbohydrates are compounds consisting of three types of atoms: carbon, hydrogen, and oxygen. As an example, the chemical formula for glucose (the sugar present in the blood as blood sugar) is $C_6H_{12}O_6$. The majority of human carbohydrate is provided by dietary plant sources. However, some dietary carbohydrate is found in animal products, and the liver can make carbohydrate using certain amino acids and components of fats such as glycerol.

Carbohydrates are used throughout the body in myriad functions. When it comes to energy metabolism and exercise performance, carbohydrates serve four important functions in various tissues:

- They are a metabolic energy fuel source for nerve cells and red blood cells.
- They are a metabolic energy fuel source for skeletal muscle, especially exercising muscle.
- As carbohydrates are metabolized, they serve as a carbon primer for fat entry into the Krebs cycle.
- They spare protein from use as an energy source during exercise and intense training.

The primary role of carbohydrates is as a metabolic fuel for nerve cells and red blood cells. Nerve tissues can use alternative fuel sources in very limited quantities, but red blood cells use only glucose. Under normal conditions, the brain uses the blood sugar *glucose* almost exclusively, and the body works to maintain the level of blood glucose within narrow limits to serve this function. Even though nerve and red blood cells provide the anatomic and physiological infrastructure for proper cardiovascular functions, muscle recruitment, and oxygen delivery, their carbohydrate requirements are not typically considered in the context of exercise metabolism. The secondary role of carbohydrate in the body is as an energy fuel for contracting skeletal muscle. Energy derived from the catabolism, or breakdown, of carbohydrate ultimately powers the contractile elements of the muscle, as well as other biological processes. Thus, skeletal muscle's reliance on carbohydrate fuel increases from rest to high-intensity exercise (discussed later in this chapter). Carbohydrate is also oxidized in contracting smooth muscle. The third role of carbohydrate oxidation (the breakdown of carbohydrate) is to serve as a carbon primer for fat entry into the Krebs cycle (also known as the tricarboxylic acid cycle). Fatty acid–derived two-carbon *acetyl-CoA* (acetyl-coenzyme A) units combine with carbohydrate derivatives in the Krebs cycle, leading to fat oxidation. Without adequate Krebs cycle primers, optimal fat metabolism is not possible. Finally, carbohydrate fuel metabolism helps spare energy provision of adenosine triphosphate (ATP) from protein, leaving protein to its primary role in tissue structure maintenance, repair, and growth.

Types of Carbohydrate

Not all types of carbohydrate have the same form, function, and impact on exercise and sport performance. The basic, single-molecule unit of all carbohydrates is the monosaccharide. The dietary monosaccharides absorbed by humans all have six carbons; while they vary only slightly in chemical configuration, these subtle variations account for important metabolic differences. The number of monosaccharides bonded together provides the basis for classifying carbohydrates and enhances the functionality of carbohydrates in the body. The term "sugar" is commonly used to refer to both monosaccharides and disaccharides such as sucrose (also known as table sugar). The terms "complex carbohydrate" and "starch" are widely used to refer to longer chains, or polymers, of monosaccharides in plants and plant-derived foods like grains, breads, cereals, vegetables, and rice. The following sections discuss the terminology for these and other types of sugar in the diet. It is important for athletes to understand the different types of carbohydrate and how they function in the body—which types quickly restore depleted muscle glycogen, which types maintain blood glucose levels during competition (essential for maintaining force production), and which types promote general health (i.e., cardiovascular health).

Monosaccharides

In humans, the three dietary monosaccharide sugar molecules have similar arrangements of the hexose (six-carbon) chemical formula, $C_6H_{12}O_6$. These sugars are glucose, fructose, and galactose (figure 2.1). Glucose, also known as dextrose or blood sugar, is the most important monosaccharide in humans and the primary one used by human cells. This monosaccharide is readily absorbed from the diet, synthesized in the body from the digestion and

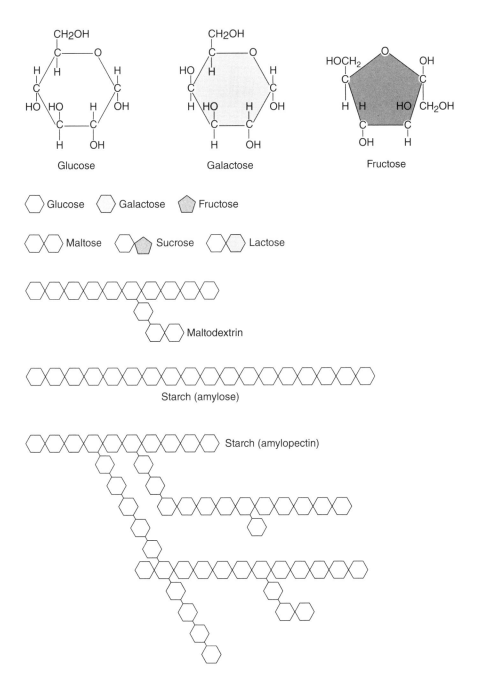

FIGURE 2.1 Chemical structure of carbohydrate molecules. Glucose, galactose, and fructose are monosaccharides. Pairs of monosaccharides form disaccharides such as maltose, sucrose, and lactose; and longer chains form complex polysaccharide molecules such as maltodextrin, amylose, and amylopectin.

conversion of the other monosaccharides, or liberated from more complex carbohydrate molecules called polysaccharides such as starch or glycogen. In addition, the process of **gluconeogenesis** creates glucose in the liver from carbon residues of other compounds such as amino acids, glycerol, pyruvate, and lactate.

➤   gluconeogenesis—The formation of glucose from noncarbohydrate sources.

After digestion, dietary glucose is absorbed from the small intestine into the blood to serve as an energy source for cellular metabolism, for intercellular storage as glycogen (primarily in the liver and skeletal muscle), or for limited conversion to fat in the liver. Fructose and galactose have slightly different carbon, hydrogen, and oxygen linkages than glucose. Fructose, also known as levulose or fruit sugar, is the sweetest-tasting sugar and is found in fruits and honey. Dietary fructose is absorbed from the small intestine into the blood and delivered to the liver for conversion to glucose. Galactose exists in nature only in combination with glucose, forming the disaccharide lactose, the milk sugar present only in the mammary glands of lactating humans and animals. As with fructose, the liver converts dietary galactose to glucose. Of the three monosaccharides, glucose is of primary importance, especially for physically active people or for athletes who are training. Once absorbed by the small intestine, fructose and galactose must enter the liver for conversion to glucose, which takes time. In contrast, ingested glucose is much more readily available to the working muscles.

Oligosaccharides

Oligosaccharides (from the Greek "oligo," meaning a few) are composed of 2 to 10 monosaccharides bonded together. Disaccharides, composed of two monosaccharides, are the major oligosaccharides found in nature. These "double sugars" form when a glucose molecule chemically binds with fructose to form sucrose, with galactose to form lactose, or with another glucose monosaccharide to form maltose. Sucrose, or "table sugar," is the most common dietary disaccharide, contributing to a quarter of the total calories consumed in the United States (Liebman 1998). Sucrose is abundant in most carbohydrate foods but is especially prevalent in highly processed foods. The milk sugar, lactose, is the least sweet disaccharide. Maltose, also called malt sugar, is found in grain products such as cereal and seed foods. Although maltose consists of two glucose monosaccharides, alone it contributes only a small percentage of dietary carbohydrate. Together, mono- and disaccharides are known as the *simple sugars*. These sugars are packaged commercially under a variety of terms. Brown sugar, corn syrup, fruit syrup, molasses, barley malt, invert sugar, honey, and natural sweeteners are all simple sugars. In the United States, many foods and beverages are sweetened with inexpensive and readily available high-fructose corn syrup. High-fructose corn syrup consists primarily of glucose but contains enough fructose to increase the product's "sweetness" to a level similar to that of sugar beet or sugar cane sucrose.

Polysaccharides

The term "polysaccharide" refers to a carbohydrate substance that consists of 10 to thousands of chemically linked simple sugar molecules. Both plant and animal sources contain these large sugar chains. Starch and fiber are the plant sources of polysaccharide, while glucose is stored in human and animal tissues as the polysaccharide glycogen.

Starch

Starch is the storage form of glucose in plants, occurring in high concentrations in seeds, corn, and various grains used to make bread, cereal, pasta, and pastries, as well as in vegetables such as peas, beans, potatoes, and roots. This polysaccharide accounts for 50% of the American dietary carbohydrate intake (Liebman 1998). Starch exists in two forms: (1) amylose, a long, straight chain of glucose units twisted into a helical coil, and (2) amylopectin, a highly branched monosaccharide macromolecule structure. The relative proportion of each form of starch in a particular plant food determines its dietary characteristics, including its "digestibility," or the percentage of an ingested food that is absorbed by the body. Starches with a relatively large amount of amylopectin digest well and readily absorb in the small intestine, whereas starch foods with high amylose content digest poorly, thereby slowing the rate at which liberated sugar appears in the blood. The term *complex carbohydrate* is commonly used to refer to dietary starch.

Fiber

Fiber is classified as a structural, nonstarch polysaccharide. The National Academy of Sciences uses three terms to refer to human fiber intakes (National Academy of Sciences 2002).

- Dietary fiber consists of nondigestible carbohydrate and lignin found in plants, including digestion-resistant starch.
- Functional fiber consists of isolated, nondigestible carbohydrate with beneficial effects in humans (intestinal bacteria can ferment a small portion of some water-soluble dietary fiber producing small-chain fatty acids that are absorbed and are used as fuel for intestinal epithelial cells or white blood cells) (D'Adamo 1990; Roediger 1989). Functional fiber is a recent, novel classification of fiber. The term *functional fiber* is used in reference to the health-enhancing effects of fiber. Functional fiber can include not only dietary, nondigestible plant sources but also commercially produced sources of carbohydrate.
- Total fiber is the sum of dietary fiber and functional fiber.

Fibers differ widely in physical and chemical characteristics and physiological action. The cell walls of leaves, stems, roots, seeds, and fruit coverings contain different kinds of carbohydrate fibers (cellulose, hemicellulose, and pectin). Cellulose is the most abundant organic (i.e., carbon containing) molecule on the earth. Dietary fiber sources are commonly referred to as water insoluble or water soluble, although some of these fiber types can be isolated and extracted from foods and marketed as functional fiber sources. Examples of water-insoluble fiber include cellulose and hemicellulose. Wheat bran is a commonly consumed cellulose-rich product. Examples of water-soluble fiber include psyllium seed husk, beta-glucan, pectin, and guar gum—present in oats, beans, brown rice, peas, carrots, corn husk, and many fruits. Dietary fiber provides bulk to the food residues passing through the intestinal tract because it holds a considerable amount of water. Water-insoluble fiber types appear to aid gastrointestinal function and gastrointestinal health by exerting a scraping action on the cells of the intestinal wall, while water-soluble fiber types shorten the transit time needed for food residues to pass through the digestive tract. The sidebar lists examples of soluble and insoluble fiber and food sources of each. The typical American diet contains about 12 to 15 g of fiber daily (Lupton and Trumbo 2006). This amount is well under the 38 g for men and 25 g for women (30 g and 21 g for men and women over age 50, respectively) recommended by the Food and Nutrition Board of the National Academy of Sciences (National Academy of Sciences 2002).

Types and Sources of Dietary Fiber

Water-Soluble Fiber

Psyllium	Pectin
Beta-glucan	Guar gum

Foods Rich in Water-Soluble Fiber

Oats	Vegetables
Brown rice	Fruits

Water-Insoluble Fiber

Cellulose	Lignin
Hemicellulose	Chitin

Foods Rich in Water-Insoluble Fiber

Wheat bran	Vegetables
Whole wheat flour	Whole grains

Fiber has received considerable attention from researchers and the lay press. Much of this interest originates from studies that link high fiber intake, particularly whole-grain cereal fibers, with a lower occurrence of heart and peripheral artery disease, hyperlipidemia (elevated blood lipids), obesity, diabetes, and digestive disorders including cancers of the gastrointestinal tract (Marlett, McBurney, and Slavin 2002).

Adequate intake of fiber does not directly affect athletic performance but rather supports general health and chronic disease prevention.

Glycogen

Glycogen, a large, branched polymer of glucose units, serves as the body's storage form of carbohydrate. This irregularly shaped, highly branched polysaccharide polymer consists of hundreds to thousands of glucose units linked together into dense granules. The glycogen macromolecule also contains the enzymes that are responsible for, or catalyze, the synthesis and degradation of glycogen and some of the enzymes regulating these processes. The presence of glycogen greatly increases the amount of carbohydrate that is immediately available between meals and during muscular contraction.

The two major sites of glycogen storage are liver and skeletal muscles. The concentration of glycogen is higher in the liver; but due to its much greater mass, skeletal muscle stores more total glycogen (approximately 400 g of glycogen [70 mmol/kg muscle or 12 g/kg muscle]) (Essen and Henriksson 1974). Glycogen metabolism in skeletal muscle plays a major role in the control of blood glucose homeostasis by the pancreatic hormone **insulin**, the most important regulator of blood glucose levels. Insulin promotes skeletal muscle blood flow and stimulates glucose uptake, glycolysis, and glycogen synthesis in skeletal muscle. Glycolysis describes the process in which carbohydrate (glucose) is broken down to produce ATP. Maximizing glycogen stores is very important for not only aerobic endurance athletes but also for athletes involved in high-intensity training. Chapter 9 explores some nutritional practices that maximize glycogen resynthesis after exhaustive exercise.

> ➤ insulin—Hormone released from the pancreas in response to elevated blood glucose and amino acid concentrations; it increases tissue uptake of both.

Glycemic Index

The glycemic index (GI) of a carbohydrate source specifies the rate at which glucose levels rise in the blood after consumption of 50 g of that food (Burke, Collier, and Hargreaves 1998). The glycemic score for a food is largely determined by how quickly ingested carbohydrate is available to enzymes in the small intestine for hydrolysis and subsequent absorption. In turn, gastric emptying and the physical availability of a sugar or starch to intestinal enzymes determine a food's intestinal digestion rate.

Foods such as brown rice, whole-grain pasta, and multigrain breads have slow absorption rates and a low GI. High-GI foods such as refined table sugar (sucrose) included in many sport drinks and nondiet soft drinks, refined white rice, pasta, and mashed potatoes promote a pronounced, though transient, rise in both blood glucose and insulin production. Complex carbohydrate foods do not always have a lower glycemic response than simple sugar foods because cooking alters the integrity of a starch granule, creating a higher glycemic index. Similar considerations must be given to predicting the glycemic indexes of liquid versus solid carbohydrate sources (Coleman 1994).

Because dietary carbohydrate is a vital component of exercise preparation, performance, and recovery, the carbohydrate requirement for many athletes is increased due to the repetitive nature of their training (Costill 1988). During periods of intense physical training, an athlete's daily carbohydrate intake requirement may exceed 10 g/kg body weight. Athletes can take advantage of both high- and lower-glycemic carbohydrate foods to optimize performance. For instance, consumption of high-glycemic carbohydrate sources is paramount to maintenance of blood glucose levels during prolonged aerobic endurance exercise (Jeukendrup and Jentjens 2000; Jeukendrup 2004) and for rapid recovery of muscle glycogen immediately after an exercise bout. However, people can eat more slowly absorbed, unrefined, complex carbohydrate to optimize muscle carbohydrate storage between exercise bouts (Ivy 2001). Ingestion of lower-GI carbohydrate prevents dramatic fluctuations in blood glucose while maintaining an extended, low-level blood glucose exposure to the previously exercised muscle during prolonged recovery.

The next section discusses the regulation of carbohydrate in the body, including the maintenance of blood glucose and glycogen synthesis and degradation, as well as aerobic and anaerobic glycolysis.

Carbohydrate Regulation in the Body

Carbohydrate serves as an essential, but limited, fuel source in the body. In the resting state, the liver, pancreas, and other organs help keep blood glucose levels within a narrow range to match the carbohydrate energy needs of the various body tissues. Because the limited stored glycogen in skeletal muscle is a vital energy source during muscle contraction, this carbohydrate source is used sparingly at rest. After a meal, the body stores as much carbohydrate in the form of glycogen as possible while stimulating carbohydrate fuel use to help return the blood glucose level to normal. When in a fasted state, the body mobilizes glucose precursors for gluconeogenesis in the liver (hepatic gluconeogenesis) while promoting fat oxidation for energy to preserve carbohydrate fuel.

During exercise and performance, the body increases use of both carbohydrate and fat while the liver increases the rate of gluconeogenesis in an effort to maintain the blood glucose level. The levels of carbohydrate and fat use during exercise depend on a number of factors, but the primary factor is the nature of the exercise itself (e.g., total muscle mass used and intensity of muscle contractions).

Maintenance of Blood Glucose

The total blood volume of an average adult human is roughly 5 L. Of this total blood volume, adult human blood contains approximately 5 g of glucose. Carbohydrate from food, the breakdown of liver glycogen (hepatic glycogenolysis), and gluconeogenesis all help maintain blood glucose levels. During fasting, the latter processes contribute more to blood glucose levels. In this rested state, muscle glucose and glycogen utilization is very low. The balance of the plasma hormones glucagon and insulin has the strongest regulatory effects on blood glucose and tissue glycogen use at rest. When blood sugar falls below normal, the pancreatic alpha cells secrete glucagon, a carbohydrate-mobilizing hormone. Glucagon stimulates gluconeogenesis and glycogenolysis pathways in the liver to bring blood glucose levels back to normal (figure 2.2). When blood glucose levels rise above normal after a meal, the pancreatic beta cells secrete insulin. Insulin removes glucose from the blood by increasing blood flow to insulin-sensitive tissues (primarily skeletal muscle and adipose tissue) and by stimulating diffusion of the sugar molecule into these cell types. Insulin also stimulates cellular energy metabolism from carbohydrate, promotes glucose's storage as glycogen, and inhibits hepatic and skeletal muscle glycogenolysis and hepatic gluconeogenesis. From a practical standpoint, it is important that these systems work properly to maintain blood glucose levels because aerobic endurance performance declines as blood glucose levels decrease.

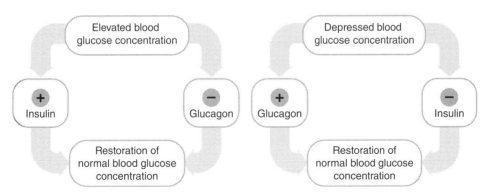

FIGURE 2.2   The roles of the pancreatic hormones insulin and glucagon in the maintenance of blood glucose.

Glycogen Synthesis

Glycogen is stored in both skeletal muscle and the liver. Muscle glycogen is very important for fueling intense anaerobic or aerobic exercise. Liver glycogen is degraded into glucose, which is then transported to the blood; this helps to maintain blood glucose levels during aerobic endurance exercise. This section explains how glycogen is synthesized.

In the synthesis of glycogen, intracellular glucose undergoes several modifications to generate uridine diphosphate (UDP)-glucose (Leloir 1971). This reaction takes place in three steps:

1. Intracellular glucose is **phosphorylated** by hexokinase as it enters the cell to generate glucose-6-phosphate.
2. Glucose-6-phosphate is then converted to glucose-1-phosphate (via phosphoglucomutase).
3. UDP-glucose is synthesized from glucose-1-phosphate and uridine triphosphate in a reaction catalyzed by UDP-glucose pyrophosphorylase.

The UDP-glucose that is formed is added to the growing glycogen molecule. This reaction is catalyzed by the enzyme glycogen synthase, which can add glucose residues only if the polysaccharide chain already contains more than four residues. Glycogen is not simply a long string of repeated glucose compounds; it is a highly branched polymer. Branching is important because it increases the solubility of glycogen. Branching also facilitates rapid glycogen synthesis and degradation (essential for providing glucose that can enter glycolysis for energy production during high-intensity exercise).

➤ phosphorylation—The process of attaching a phosphate group to another molecule. Phosphorylation turns many protein enzymes on and off.

Glycogen Breakdown

When glycogen is undergoing degradation during exercise, this indicates that the body needs **ATP** to fuel skeletal muscle contraction. The goal of glycogen breakdown is to release glucose (specifically, glucose-1-phosphate) compounds so that they can enter the glycolytic pathway, which yields quick ATP production.

➤ ATP—The high-energy phosphate compound synthesized and used by cells to release energy for cellular work.

In the complex process of glycogen breakdown, individual glucose compounds are cleaved from glycogen to form glucose-1-phosphate (catalyzed by the enzyme glycogen phosphorylase). Phosphorylase catalyzes the sequential removal of glycosyl residues from the nonreducing end of the glycogen molecule. The glucose-1-phosphate formed in the phosphorolytic cleavage of glycogen is converted into glucose-6-phosphate by phosphoglucomutase. In skeletal muscle, the glycogen-liberated glucose-6-phosphate joins glucose-6-phosphate, derived from glucose that enters the cell from the blood, for metabolic fuel processing by the glycolytic enzymes. The liver, and to a limited extent the kidney, either can process the glycogen-liberated glucose-6-phosphate through glycolysis or can dephosphorylate the glycogen-liberated glucose-6-phosphate and release the glucose into the blood. In cellular glucose metabolism (i.e., glycogen synthesis and glycogen breakdown), the intermediate glucose-6-phosphate plays a central role in the various conversions between glucose storage and glucose oxidation (figure 2.3).

Glycolysis

During exercise, intense training, and sport performance, ATP is needed quickly for energy production. One of the fastest processes by which ATP can be generated is glycolysis. In general, glycolysis is the breakdown of carbohydrate (i.e., glucose) to produce ATP. Glycolysis occurs in the cytoplasm of the muscle fiber. The key physiological outcome of glycolysis is

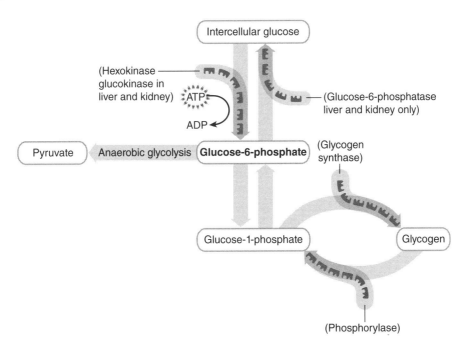

FIGURE 2.3 Central role of intercellular glucose-6-phosphate in glycolysis, glycogen storage, and glycogenolysis in skeletal muscle, liver, and kidney.

relatively quick ATP production to be used for muscle contraction. As can be seen in figure 2.4, glycolysis is a series of 10 enzymatically controlled chemical reactions that starts with one six-carbon glucose and ends with two three-carbon pyruvate molecules.

The pyruvate that is produced at the end of glycolysis has two possible fates: It can be converted to lactate, or it can enter the **mitochondria**. The next section describes the production of lactic acid. Before pyruvate enters the mitochondria, it is converted to acetyl-CoA and then enters what is known as the Krebs cycle. The Krebs cycle further metabolizes the pyruvate–acetyl-CoA compounds in a series of enzyme-catalyzed chemical reactions. Ultimately, these reactions in the Krebs cycle generate NADH and $FADH_2$ compounds; these carry electrons that are taken up by the electron transport chain in the mitochondria. The electron transport chain facilitates the production of more ATP to fuel skeletal muscle contraction, but this ATP production occurs at a slower rate as compared to glycolytic ATP production. It is important to understand that glycolysis produces ATP at a fast rate, needed during high-intensity training or exercise. This ATP is primarily generated by the oxidation (breakdown) of glucose, so it is easy to appreciate the importance of adequate carbohydrate in the diet to fuel intense exercise during training or competition.

> ➤   mitochondria—The part of a cell responsible for the production of ATP with oxygen; it contains the enzymes for the Krebs cycle, electron transport chain, and the fatty acid cycle.

Lactic Acid Production and Clearance

As already noted, the glycolysis end product is pyruvate. Pyruvate can be converted to acetyl-CoA and enter the Krebs cycle in the mitochondria, or it can be converted to lactic acid. When pyruvate is converted to lactic acid, the process is referred to as anaerobic glycolysis. Once produced inside the cell, lactic acid rapidly ionizes by releasing a hydrogen ion, lowering **sarcoplasmic** pH. The remaining ionized molecule is lactate. As lactic acid production increases, the decrease in cellular pH has deleterious effects on numerous metabolic and contractile processes. Therefore, the acid must be buffered immediately inside the cell or expelled from the cell for extracellular buffering. At rest and during low-intensity exercise, a small amount of lactic acid is produced; most of the acid is easily buffered inside the cell, and some is transported outside of the cell where it is quickly rendered harmless. The plasma hemoglobin protein plays the most prominent extracellular buffering role; plasma bicarbonate also provides effective extracellular chemical buffering. The muscle pain or "burning" sensation during sustained, high-intensity muscle contraction is primarily due to irritation of free nerve endings outside the muscle cells by the lower pH. The remaining three-carbon

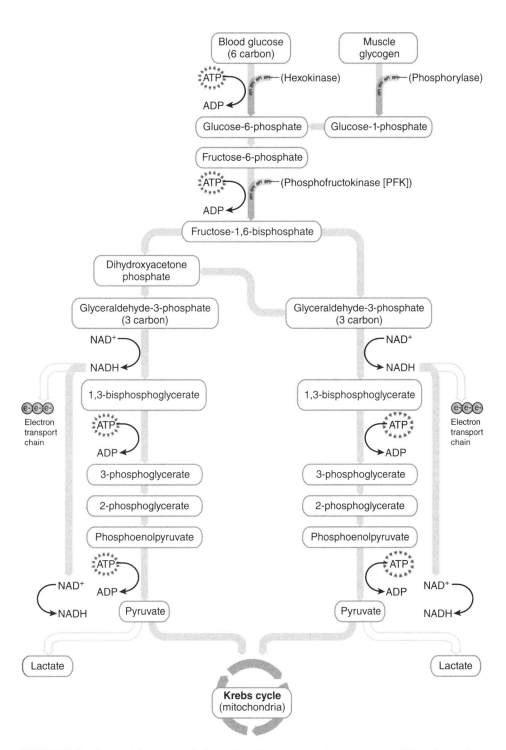

FIGURE 2.4 Anaerobic glycolysis from blood glucose or glycogen uses ATP and requires the coenzyme NAD. The products of anaerobic glycolysis include ATP, water, pyruvate or lactic acid, and NADH.

Reprinted, by permission, from NSCA, 2008, Bioenergy of exercise and training, by J.T. Cramer. In *Essentials of strength training and conditioning*, 3rd ed., edited by T.R Baechle and R.W. Earle (Champaign, IL: Human Kinetics), 25.

lactate molecule can be used as a potential fuel source for nonexercising muscle, for the heart, and even for the exercising muscle itself (Van Hall 2000). During moderate- to high-intensity exercise corresponding to the **anaerobic threshold**, lactate production outpaces the intracellular buffering capacity, and therefore excess lactate is transported out of the cell. As the exercise intensity increases, blood levels of lactate rise in an exponential fashion. The pronounced lactic acid production during higher-intensity exercise has detrimental effects on muscle performance. However, the formation of this metabolic by-product helps facilitate accelerated anaerobic ATP production from carbohydrate for a short period of time.

➤ sarcoplasm—The cytoplasm of a muscle fiber.

➤ anaerobic threshold—A term commonly used to refer to the level of oxygen consumption at which there is a rapid and systematic increase in blood lactate concentration.

Fatigue, as defined by an inability to maintain a desired power output or exercise intensity during short-term, high-intensity anaerobic exercise, is in part due to accumulation of lactic acid in working muscles (leading to a drop in pH). Sustained, higher-intensity contractions can rapidly deplete exercising muscle glycogen. The decreasing intercellular glycolytic **substrate** and the limited rate of blood glucose availability quickly precipitate muscle fatigue as the anaerobic system's ability to sustain rapid ATP resynthesis is compromised. Muscle contractions may continue but at a lower intensity as aerobic ATP is contributing more to the total muscle exercise ATP needs.

➤ substrate—A molecule upon which an enzyme acts.

While lactate accumulation is correlated to fatigue, there are no nutritional practices that can help to decrease lactate production during intense exercise. Rather, proper conditioning enables an athlete to work at a higher intensity with lower associated lactate levels. Broadly speaking, it is important that athletes include optimal amounts of carbohydrate in the diet to enable them to perform high-intensity training, which will result in adaptations that promote energy production from oxidative (i.e., fat) sources of energy.

Carbohydrate availability in the body controls its use for energy. The concentration of blood glucose provides feedback regulation of the liver's glucose output, with an increase in blood glucose inhibiting hepatic glucose release during exercise. Carbohydrate availability may also help limit fat metabolism by decreasing both fatty acid mobilization and oxidation in the cell (Spriet 1998). Intuitively, this makes metabolic sense as the fatty acid oxidation is far too slow to contribute significantly to the ATP requirements and would act only to congest the mitochondrial NADH and acetyl-

CoA concentrations, necessitating further lactic acid production to sustain anaerobic glycolysis.

Carbohydrate and Performance

The following sections describe the role of carbohydrate in various types of exercise training and sport performance. Some athletes are primarily aerobic athletes; others engage in primarily anaerobic activities in their training and competition. Regardless of the type of athlete, all athletes and physically active individuals can improve their performance by engaging in resistance exercise. Therefore, the discussion addresses the role of carbohydrate in strength training as well as considerations related to aerobic and anaerobic exercise and performance.

Aerobic Exercise

At rest and during exercise, the liver produces glucose to maintain a blood glucose concentration of 100 mg/dl (5.5 mmol/L) (Kjaer 1998). Blood glucose may account for 30% of the total energy fuel required by exercising muscles, with the remaining carbohydrate fuel derived from stored muscle glycogen (Coyle 1995). In prolonged, intense exercise, blood glucose concentration eventually falls below normal levels because of liver glycogen depletion while active skeletal muscle continues to utilize the available blood glucose.

An hour of high-intensity aerobic exercise decreases liver glycogen by about 55%, while a 2-hour bout of intense aerobic exercise may almost entirely deplete glycogen in the liver as well as in working muscle. Depletion is of particular concern during exercise after a prolonged period without food, for example early in the morning or after an exercise warm-up period, with the result that the athlete would begin a training session or competition with suboptimal glycogen levels. Individuals starting a carbohydrate-deficient diet rapidly compromise liver glycogen stores and nearly deplete skeletal muscle glycogen levels. This type of diet would likely negatively affect performance in all but the lowest of exercise intensities. While the lower caloric intake that normally accompanies low-carbohydrate dietary practices would theoretically promote fat loss, it also makes regular moderate-intensity, longer-duration aerobic exercise very difficult.

A decline in exercising muscle glycogen levels late in exercise results in an increased reliance on blood glucose as the exercising muscle carbohydrate source. Without ingestion of carbohydrate, hypoglycemia (<45 mg/dl; 2.5 mmol/L) can quickly ensue after liver and working muscle glycogen depletion (Shulman and Rothman 2001; Tsintzas and Williams 1998). This ultimately impairs exercise performance and can contribute to central nervous system fatigue associated with prolonged exercise.

Fatigue during prolonged aerobic-type exercise is caused primarily from depleted carbohydrate stores in the exercising muscle (Rauch et al. 2005). This occurs despite a sufficient oxygen supply to the muscle and almost unlimited stored energy available from fat. Aerobic endurance athletes commonly refer to this type of fatigue as "hitting the wall." Symptoms of significantly reduced blood glucose include weakness, dizziness, and decreased motivation. The decline in muscle glycogen results in perception of fatigue, and further decline and depletion necessitate termination of exercise or a significant reduction in exercise intensity (Ahlborg et al. 1967; Bergström et al. 1967). Thus, it should not be surprising that optimal aerobic endurance performance is directly related to the initial muscle glycogen stores (Ahlborg et al. 1967; Hultman 1967).

Optimizing preexercise muscle glycogen stores (i.e., >150 mmol/kg muscle) increases time to exhaustion by as much as 20% and increases aerobic endurance performance by reducing the time taken to complete a given workload (Hawley et al. 1997). The scientific literature suggests, however, that the exercise duration must be at least 90 minutes before exercise performance benefits are observed. Elevated carbohydrate stores are just one benefit of carefully planned dietary carbohydrate supplementation strategies. During exercise of 45 minutes or more, carbohydrate consumption (e.g., 0.5-2 g/minute or 30-120 g/hour) will help maintain exercise blood glucose levels and oxidation (Coyle et al. 1986) and has been demonstrated to improve aerobic endurance capacity and performance (Coyle et al. 1986; Jeukendrup et al. 1997). Whether or not this practice may promote glycogen synthesis during low-intensity exercise (Keizer, Kuipers, and van Kranenburg 1987) or offset some muscle glycogen use during exercise is debatable, with various studies demonstrating mixed results (Bosch, Dennis, and Noakes 1994; Coyle et al. 1986; Jeukendrup et al. 1999; Tsintzas et al. 1995). The rate of 0.5 to 2 g carbohydrate per minute during exercise matches the rate of carbohydrate oxidation during moderate-intensity aerobic-type exercise, as well as the rate of gastric emptying of dilute carbohydrate solutions (e.g., 6-8% carbohydrate sport drinks). After prolonged exercise, replenishment of muscle glycogen to within a normal range is an essential component of the recovery process (Hargreaves 2000). In essence, this postexercise recovery period can be considered the initial "preparation" for an upcoming exercise challenge (Ivy 2001).

The importance of beginning an exercise bout or training session with optimal muscle glycogen levels and rapidly replenishing glycogen after exercise before a subsequent performance should now be apparent. Chapter 8 outlines specific carbohydrate supplementation strategies for maximal performance. However, in general terms, an aerobic endurance athlete's carbohydrate consumption should account for approximately 55% to 65% of the total caloric intake (McArdle, Katch, and Katch 2009). The generally recommended carbohydrate intake for this type of training is not drastically different from that recommended for healthy individuals (45-65% of total calories). Keep in mind, however, that despite similar percentages, the absolute amount of recommended carbohydrate (in grams) will vary tremendously depending on the total dietary caloric intake.

Anaerobic Exercise

Skeletal muscle glycogen is a readily available energy source for the working muscle. Resting muscle glycogen levels are approximately 65 to 90 mmol/kg muscle. The rate at which glycogen is utilized is highly dependent on the exercise intensity. As the exercise intensity increases to high levels (i.e., above anaerobic threshold or >70-80% $\dot{V}O_2$max), the muscle energy requirements cannot be matched by accelerated mitochondrial oxidation of carbohydrate and fat. Muscle glycogen becomes the most important energy substrate, as anaerobic ATP production is required to match the rapid ATP utilization by the contractile machinery. Exercise-mediated depletion of muscle glycogen to <30 mmol/kg muscle will result in an increased reliance on the relatively slower process of blood glucose uptake as a carbohydrate fuel source. It is important to note that regardless of muscle glycogen content, fatigue during bouts of high-intensity exercise could likely result from the accompanying lactic acid production (leading to a decrease in pH) and accumulation in and around the working muscle fibers. Thus, the importance of muscle carbohydrate stores with respect to exercise performance is more relevant during prolonged (i.e., >2 minutes) and intermittent high-intensity exercise bouts (e.g., drills and wind sprints).

High-intensity intermittent exercise includes numerous activities performed in various types of exercise training sessions and in team sport competitions. In the short rest period between intermittent bouts, the muscle has time to clear or buffer some of the lactic acid (or do both), alleviating the potential detrimental effects of this by-product. Additionally, the performance of very high-intensity, short-duration (i.e., <10 seconds) exercise will depend primarily on the provision of ATP through the "immediate" or "creatine phosphate" energy system. During repetitions of these exercise "bursts," however, muscle glycogen would play an important role in maintaining the muscle ATP content over the course of a workout session consisting of many sets of high-intensity repetitions with short recovery periods.

Despite the importance of carbohydrate in anaerobic-type activities, the general carbohydrate recommendations for these athletes are slightly less than for an athlete performing more aerobic endurance exercise. Carbohydrate is important for both types of exercise, as the rate of carbohydrate utilization and thus glycogen depletion is directly related to the intensity of the exercise. During lower-intensity, aerobic-type exercise, glycogen depletion-related fatigue would occur later in the exercise session while the glycogen depletion-related fatigue associated with higher-intensity, anaerobic-type exercise would develop much earlier. Therefore, the optimization of preexercise muscle glycogen levels and rapid replenishment of glycogen in previously exercised muscle are just as important during anaerobic training and competition. Because preexercise muscle glycogen levels are similar in aerobic and anaerobic athletes, daily carbohydrate consumption should account for 55% to 65% of caloric intake for anaerobic athletes as well. Specifically, anaerobic athletes training or competing on a regular basis should ingest 5 to 7 g of carbohydrate per kilogram body weight a day.

Strength Training

Strength performance, as well as training to improve muscular strength, muscular endurance, and muscular power, consists of repetitive bouts of high-intensity work with relatively short rest intervals. Therefore, carbohydrate is the primary fuel source over the course of a resistance-type exercise session. As with anaerobic exercise, the intensity of the bout dictates the level of fast-twitch muscle fiber recruitment, which in large part determines the performance capabilities of a muscle or muscle group in resistance-type exercise. During high-intensity (i.e., >60% 1-repetition maximum [1RM]) resistance exercise, fast-twitch fibers are heavily recruited, and they quickly fatigue as their glycogen content is utilized. Not surprisingly, the recruitment of fast-twitch Type IIx fibers (formerly referred to as Type IIb) is increased during eccentric and high-speed contractions (Nardone, Romano, and Schieppati 1989; Tesch, Colliander, and Kaiser 1986). However, several studies have demonstrated that the faster-twitch fiber types are recruited at moderate- (i.e., 60% 1RM; Tesch et al. 1998) and even lower-intensity (i.e., 20-40% 1RM; Gollnick et al. 1974; Robergs et al. 1991) muscle contractions.

These findings suggest that the fatigue associated with muscular endurance-type exercise, such as that performed in many individual and team sport training sessions and competitions, could be limited by the initial glycogen content and rate of depletion in the recruited fast-twitch fibers. Because many strength and power athletes perform intense training several times a week, adequate carbohydrate intake is necessary to prevent a gradual depletion of glycogen in trained muscle over time. Further, the amount of glycogen used in their resistance training sessions also appears to be related to the total amount of work accomplished and the duration of the resistance training bout.

Because of the cumulative glycogen use in resistance-trained muscle during a workout or competition, including warm-up, stretching, and cool-down sessions, it has been suggested that consumption of higher levels of carbohydrate in the diet would improve muscle performance in these types of activities (Balsom et al. 1999; Casey et al. 1996; Maughan et al. 1997; Robergs et al. 1991; Rockwell, Rankin, and Dixon 2003; Tesch, Colliander, and Kaiser 1986). However, research studies have provided varied results with respect to specific nutritional carbohydrate practices and acute strength training performance (Haff et al. 1999, 2000; Kulik et al. 2008; Robergs et al. 1991).

Despite the lack of consensus about ingestion of a high-carbohydrate diet or ingestion of carbohydrate before weightlifting performance, it is clear that skeletal muscle carbohydrate sources facilitate overall resistance exercise performance by acting as the primary fuel source during this type of exercise. This is especially imperative over the course of an entire weight training session in which many individual muscles or muscle groups are worked to the point of fatigue (including possible glycogen depletion), which results in an associated prolonged postexercise period of energy-consuming muscle recovery. Because of this, the overall training regimen outcome (e.g., increased strength, power) would likely be affected negatively when carbohydrate ingestion is not optimal.

Another factor to consider regarding ingestion of carbohydrate in the time period surrounding a resistance training bout is its effect on increasing insulin. Carbohydrate ingestion (particularly high-glycemic types) dramatically increases endogenous insulin secretion. The hormone insulin enhances the anabolic stimulus that resistance exercise produces. Specifically, insulin acts as a powerful anabolic hormone in previously exercised muscle in multiple ways, including

- promoting the synthesis of protein,
- decreasing protein breakdown,
- stimulating glucose uptake, and
- stimulating glycogen storage (Biolo et al. 1999; Tipton et al. 2001).

Two of these effects of insulin release—increasing protein synthesis and decreasing protein breakdown—may improve the chronic anabolic adaptations of resistance exercise, particularly if insulin is elevated surrounding the time frame of each resistance exercise bout via carbohydrate consumption. Associated with this is the recommendation to ingest liquid carbohydrate before, during, and after exercise to promote a faster recovery and gains in lean body mass (Haff et al. 2003). Chapter 9 expands on this concept of nutrient timing and the impact that carbohydrate ingestion has on endogenous insulin secretion, as well as the exercise performance improvements observed with such practices.

Athletes can make informed decisions about the use of carbohydrate based on knowledge from multiple perspectives, including the types of carbohydrate that can be ingested; how this ingested carbohydrate is regulated and utilized in the body; and how carbohydrate intake influences aerobic, anaerobic, and strength training. One decision has to do with the choice of food to best restore skeletal muscle glycogen that has been depleted by intense or long-duration exercise.

For example, if a soccer athlete is competing in several matches in a single day (as in tournament play), it is essential that glycogen be restored as soon as possible (within several hours) so that depleted glycogen levels do not induce fatigue for later matches. In this case, it is important that the soccer athlete choose high-glycemic carbohydrate foods, as these have been shown to rapidly restore skeletal muscle glycogen. For an athlete whose primary mode of training is resistance exercise, low-glycemic carbohydrate sources would be recommended for resistance training as part of everyday eating habits while higher-glycemic foods would be recommended for the immediate postexercise period for optimal muscle glycogen repletion and insulin response (Conley and Stone 1996).

The physiological processes of glycogen synthesis, glycogen breakdown, and glycolysis are all ways in which the body deals with ingested carbohydrate. These processes allow for quick ATP production (glycogen breakdown and glycolysis) during intense exercise and allow for the storing of glycogen (glycogen synthesis) in the skeletal muscle and liver for future training and conditioning.

An aerobic endurance athlete, say a long-distance runner, in order to prevent suboptimal carbohydrate stores, should consume approximately 55% to 65% of total caloric intake in the form of carbohydrate (McArdle, Katch, and Katch 2009). While this recommendation provides a general range of carbohydrate ingestion as compared to protein and fat, the absolute amount of recommended carbohydrate (in grams) will vary tremendously depending on the total dietary caloric intake and physical activity level. As a general guide, athletes training or competing on a regular basis should ingest 5 to 7 g of carbohydrate/kg body weight a day and consider increasing this amount to 8 to 10 g/kg body weight per day when the level of training sessions is extreme.

An anaerobic athlete, by comparison, would likely not need more than 5 to 7 g of carbohydrate/kg body weight a day. Even though an anaerobic athlete consistently trains at a high intensity, the relative duration of such intensity is lower than that of an aerobic endurance athlete.

An athlete engaged in a resistance training program will, on a day-to-day basis, require more total energy than a nonactive, healthy counterpart of the same age. By obtaining 55% to 65% of total calories from carbohydrate, a resistance or power training athlete can ensure having near-optimal energy. Athletes on a 3,500 kcal/day diet in which 65% of caloric intake is composed of carbohydrate should aim to consume approximately 570 g of carbohydrate daily (~8 g/kg body weight for a 70-kg [154-pound] individual). In contrast, a nonactive adult consuming 2,500 kcal/day consisting of 55% carbohydrate would require considerably fewer grams of carbohydrate (i.e., 340 g) daily (~5 g/kg body weight per day for a 70 kg [154-pound] individual).

The general carbohydrate prescriptions, based on an athlete's type and extent of energy expenditure, are merely rough guidelines to illustrate the need to be mindful of the percent of carbohydrate per daily caloric intake in an athlete's nutritional program. Specific carbohydrate intake strategies to optimize performance are recommended in chapter 8.

SUMMARY POINTS

- Carbohydrate provides a vital source of energy production during anaerobic and aerobic exercise.

- Reductions of the body's carbohydrate sources during exercise decrease exercise performance and promote fatigue.

- Consumption of adequate carbohydrate on a daily basis (e.g., 55-65% total calories) is critical for optimal athletic performance.

- Dietary carbohydrate is a vital component of exercise preparation, performance, and recovery. Thus, the carbohydrate requirement for athletes is increased due to the repetitive nature of their training.

- During periods of intense physical training, an athlete's daily carbohydrate intake requirement may be as high as 10 g/kg body weight.

- An athlete can take advantage of both high- and lower-glycemic food for optimal performance. Ingesting foods with a high glycemic index during prolonged exercise or immediately after exercise is a vital strategy that athletes are encouraged to use for peak performance and recovery.

- When individuals ingest lower-GI carbohydrate, they can prevent dramatic fluctuations in blood glucose while maintaining a prolonged, lower-level exposure of the previously exercised muscle to blood glucose. Thus it is advantageous for athletes to ingest low-glycemic foods as part of their normal diet between training sessions.

- By planning their carbohydrate feeding schedules, athletes can ensure optimal muscle carbohydrate stores when beginning an exercise bout or training session, carbohydrate provision during exercise, and rapid replenishment of glycogen after exercise and before a subsequent performance.

3

Protein

Richard B. Kreider, PhD, FACSM, FISSN

Proteins are organic compounds composed of a genetically determined sequence of amino acids that serve as the building blocks of protein. Amino acids (figure 3.1) are held together by peptide bonds between the carboxyl and amino groups. For this reason, small sequences of amino acids are called **peptides**. Proteins are found in every cell of the body and are needed to promote growth and to repair damaged cells and tissue, as well as for a variety of metabolic and hormonal activities. For example, some proteins serve as enzymes that catalyze biochemical reactions in the body. Hormones are also proteins that influence metabolic activity in various organs. Other proteins are important in cell signaling processes, while still others influence immunity. Most protein is stored in the form of muscle proteins (e.g., actin and myosin).

➤ peptide—A substance composed of two or more amino acids.

Protein in the Body

Twenty-two amino acids can be used to make proteins; these are listed in the sidebar. This includes eight essential amino acids (nine in infants and children) that must be acquired from the diet because the body cannot

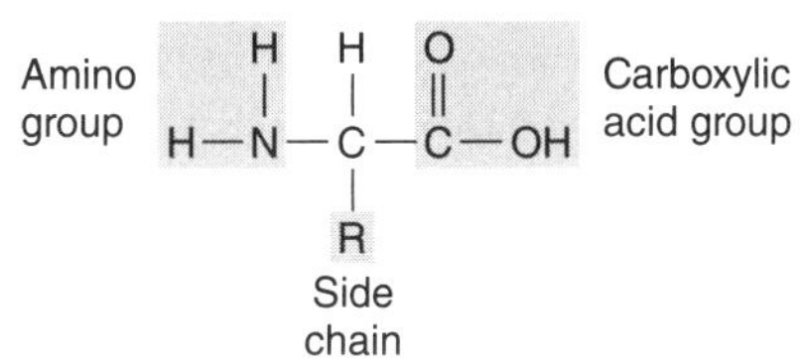

FIGURE 3.1 Structure of an amino acid.

Essential, Conditionally Essential, and Nonessential Amino Acids

Essential Amino Acids

Isoleucine	Methionine	Tryptophan
Leucine	Phenylalanine	Valine
Lysine	Threonine	

Conditionally Essential Amino Acids

Arginine	Histidine	Taurine
Cysteine (cystine)	Proline	Tyrosine
Glutamine		

Nonessential Amino Acids

Alanine	Citruline	Glycine
Asparagine	Glutamic acid	Serine
Aspartic acid		

synthesize them. Protein must be obtained in the diet primarily to provide a source of these essential amino acids (EAAs). Without dietary sources of EAAs, the body must catabolize its own protein stores (e.g., muscle) to provide EAAs to meet essential protein needs. There are also seven conditionally essential amino acids. They are called conditionally essential because the body has difficulty synthesizing them efficiently, so they typically must be obtained from the diet if amounts are to be sufficient. The body can synthesize the remaining amino acids fairly easily, so they are considered nonessential. Dietary protein is classified as *complete* or *incomplete* depending on whether or not it contains adequate amounts of the EAAs. Animal sources of protein contain all EAAs and are therefore considered complete sources of protein, while many plant sources of protein are missing some of the EAAs (i.e., they are incomplete). Protein sources vary in their quality depending on their amino acid profile. Complete protein sources that contain greater amounts of EAAs generally have higher protein quality.

The purpose of protein digestion is to liberate the amino acids from the consumed proteins (Berdanier 2000). During the digestive process, enzymes known as proteases hydrolyze, or break down, whole proteins into their component amino acids, dipeptides, and tripeptides. In contrast to carbohydrate and lipid digestion, which begins in the mouth by way of salivary amylase and lingual lipase, protein digestion does not begin until the food reaches the stomach and is acidified with gastric hydrochloric acid (Berdanier 2000). Once through the stomach, the amino acids are absorbed through the wall of the small intestine; they pass into the blood and then to the liver via the portal vein. The digestion of protein takes several hours, but once the amino acids enter the blood, they are cleared within 5 to 10 minutes (Williams 2002).

A constant interchange of amino acids occurs among the blood, the liver, and the body tissues, with the liver serving as the critical center in amino acid metabolism. The collection of amino acids in these bodily compartments is referred to as the free amino acid pool. The liver is continually synthesizing a balanced amino acid mixture for the diverse protein requirements of the body (Williams 2002). From the liver, the amino acids are secreted into the blood and carried as free amino acids or as plasma proteins (i.e., albumin and immunoglobulins). Metabolic fates of amino acids include the formation of

- structural proteins in the form of skeletal muscle,
- functional proteins such as enzymes, and
- signaling proteins such as hormones.

It is important to note that the various cells of the body use only the amount of amino acids necessary to meet their protein needs. Amino acids in the body's amino acid pool that are used neither for protein synthesis nor to synthesize metabolically important intermediates are deaminated (the amino group [NH_2] is removed), and the carbon skeletons are either oxidized or used for the synthesis of glucose or fatty acids (Berdanier 2000). In the process of deamination, the amino group (NH_2) containing the nitrogen is removed from the amino acid, leaving a carbon substrate known as an alpha-ketoacid. The alpha-ketoacid that is released may have several fates, including (Williams 2002)

- oxidation for the release of energy,
- accepting another amino group and being reconstituted to an amino acid, and
- being channeled into the metabolic pathways of carbohydrate and fat.

The amino group that was formed in the process of deamination must be excreted from the body (Williams 2002). This process occurs in the liver, where the amino group (NH_2) is converted into ammonia (NH_3). Next, the ammonia is converted into urea, which passes into the blood and is eventually eliminated by the kidneys into the urine.

Historically, the adequacy of dietary protein has been assessed using the nitrogen balance technique. **Nitrogen balance** is a laboratory technique by which both consumption and excretion of all nitrogen are meticulously quantified and the net difference calculated. The amount of protein necessary to elicit balance (when intake equals excretion) is thought to be the dietary requirement (Lemon 2001). The type of protein that is ingested in the diet determines the availability of amino acids necessary to repair tissue; promote growth; and synthesize enzymes, hormones, and cells. The Recommended Dietary Allowance (RDA) for protein is 1.0 g/kg per day for children 11 to 14 years of age, 0.8 to 0.9 g/kg per day for adolescents 15 to 18 years of age, and 0.8 g/kg per day for adults (Campbell et al. 2007). However, intense exercise increases protein needs (Campbell et al. 2007). People involved in a general fitness program can generally meet protein needs by ingesting 0.8 to 1.0 g/kg per day. However, individuals who are competitive athletes or who engage in intense training need more protein than this to adequately respond to the stimulus that training provides.

➤ nitrogen balance—The measure of nitrogen output subtracted from nitrogen input.

It is generally recommended that athletes consume 1.5 to 2.0 g/kg body weight of protein to ensure adequate protein intake. Athletes involved in moderate amounts of intense training should consume levels at the lower end of this range (120-140 g/day for an 80-kg [176-pound] athlete), while athletes involved in high-volume intense training should consume levels at the upper end of the range (140-160 g/day for an 80 kg athlete) (Kreider et al. 2009). Later sections of this chapter present more specific recommendations for athletes who perform aerobic and anaerobic training.

Types of Protein

The quality of protein is generally classified in one of two ways. The first method is called the protein efficiency ratio (PER). It is determined via assessment of the weight gain of growing rats fed a particular protein in comparison to a standard protein (egg whites). Types of protein with a higher PER value are considered higher quality. The second method is called the protein digestibility–corrected amino acid score (PDCAAS). This method is recognized internationally as the best method of comparing protein sources for humans. A PDCAAS of 1.0 indicates that the protein exceeds the EAA requirements of the body and is therefore an excellent source of protein. The higher the PDCAAS value, the higher the quality of the protein. Table 3.1 lists the major types of protein found in food and supplements and the quality of the protein as determined by the PER or PDCAAS classification method or both. Gelatin (collagen) protein and wheat protein are relatively poor-quality sources. Meat and fish sources are considered moderately high-quality sources of protein. Soy, egg, milk, whey, and bovine colostrum sources are classified as high-quality protein.

TABLE 3.1 Approximate Quality of Various Forms of Protein in Food and Supplements

Protein	PDCAAS	PER	Comment
Gelatin (collagen)	0.08	–	Inexpensive but poor-quality protein popular as a nutritional supplement in the 1970s and 1980s. Gelatin is still found in some liquid protein supplements.
Wheat	0.43	1.5	Wheat protein has a relatively poor protein quality. However, wheat serves as the starting material for glutamine peptides, which are protein hydrolysates that contain high amounts of glutamine.
Beef, poultry, fish	0.8-0.92	2.0-2.3	Fairly good sources of protein. However, some animal meats contain relatively high amounts of fat, which reduces their utility as a primary means of obtaining protein in the diet.
Soy	1.00	1.8-2.3	Despite lacking the amino acid methionine, soy is an excellent source of protein extracted from soybeans. Soy protein concentrate (70% protein) and isolate (90% protein) are particularly good protein sources for vegetarians. Soy protein also contains isoflavone glucosides, which have several potential health benefits.
Ovalbumin (egg)	1.00	2.8	Protein from egg whites is considered the reference standard for comparing protein quality. Egg protein powders were once considered the best source of protein for supplements; but egg protein is fairly expensive compared to other forms of high-quality protein, and therefore its use in supplements has decreased.
Milk protein	1.00	2.8	Milk protein contains about 80% casein and 20% whey protein. Milk protein is available in concentrated and isolated forms and is about 90% protein. Milk protein is commonly used in supplements due to relatively low cost.
Casein	1.00	2.9	Caseinates are extracted from skim milk and are available as sodium, potassium, and calcium caseinates. The protein quality of casein is high, and it is relatively inexpensive. Amino acid release is generally more delayed than with whey protein.

(continued)

Table 3.1 *(continued)*

Protein	PDCAAS	PER	Comment
Bovine colostrum (BC)	1.00	3.0	One of the two highest-quality sources of protein currently available in protein supplements; may have some added benefit in comparison to other forms of protein due to a high concentration of growth factors, immunoglobulins, and antibacterial compounds. Brands vary in collection methods; the Intact brand uses a low-heat method that keeps the bioactive proteins intact. Although it is higher in cost than most protein supplements, preliminary evidence indicates that BC may promote greater gains in strength and muscle mass during training as compared to whey protein. More research is needed before definitive conclusions can be made.
Whey	1.00	3.0-3.2	One of the two highest-quality sources of protein currently available in protein supplements. Whey protein is digested rapidly, allowing for fast uptake of amino acids. Whey is available as whey protein hydrolysate, ion exchange whey protein isolate, and cross-flow microfiltration whey protein isolate. These have subtle differences in amino acid profile, fat content, lactose content, and ability to preserve glutamine residues. It is unclear whether these small differences would have any impact on training adaptations. Although whey protein is a more expensive form of good protein, it is currently the most poplar protein supplement used by resistance-trained athletes.

Based on Kreider and Kleiner 2000.

Milk

Different types of milk vary primarily in fat content and total calories. However, they also vary slightly in mineral content, vitamin content (particularly fat-soluble vitamins), and amino acid profile. One cup of milk provides about 8 g of protein. Of this protein, approximately 80% is casein and the remainder is whey protein. Milk serves as a fairly good source of essential and conditionally essential amino acids. Therefore, milk has a relatively high protein efficiency ratio of about 2.8 (whey protein is about 3.2). Skim milk also has a very good ratio of carbohydrate to protein (about 1.5 to 1). Consequently, skim milk can serve as a good source of not only protein but also carbohydrate if an individual is not lactose intolerant.

Several studies have indicated that milk before or during exercise (or both before and during) can serve as an effective sport drink (Roy 2008; Watson et al. 2008). Ingesting milk after exercise promotes protein synthesis (Williams 2002; Watson et al. 2008; Bucci and Unlu 2000; Florisa et al. 2003). In addition to promoting protein synthesis, low-fat milk is an effective postexercise rehydration drink (Shirreffs, Watson, and Maughan, 2007). The following sections focus on the two primary types of protein found in milk, whey and casein.

Whey

Whey protein is currently the most popular source of protein used in nutritional supplements, particularly in the sport nutrition market. Whey protein is available as whey protein concentrates, isolates, and hydrolysates. The primary differences among these forms are the method of processing, plus small differences in fat and lactose content, amino acid profiles, and ability to preserve glutamine residues. For example, whey protein concentrates (between 30% and 90% protein) are produced from liquid whey by clarification, ultrafiltration, diafiltration, and drying techniques (Bucci and Unlu 2000). Whey protein isolates ($\geq$90% protein) are typically produced through ion exchange (IE) or cross-flow microfiltration (CFM) techniques. Whey protein hydrolysates (about 90% protein) are typically produced by heating with acid or preferably treatment with proteolytic enzymes followed by purification and filtration.

The different processing methods affect the concentration of whey protein subtypes and peptides (e.g., β-lactoglobulin, α-lactalbumin, immunoglobulins, albumin, lactoferrin, lactoperoxidase, peptides, glycomacropeptides, and proteose-peptose) that reportedly have antioxidant, anticancer, antihypertensive, antihyperlipidemic, antibacterial, antimicromial, and antiviral properties (Florisa et al. 2003; Toba et al. 2001; Badger, Ronis, and Hakkak 2001; FitzGerald and Meisel 2000; Wong et al. 1997; Horton 1995). Some of these proteins and peptides bind to vitamins and minerals and therefore play an important role in nutrient metabolism. Proteins and peptides have also been found to enhance digestion (Pelligrini 2003; Korhonen and Pihlanto 2003). Theoretically, increasing dietary availability of these biologically active proteins and peptides may promote general health. However, it is unclear whether these subtle differences would make one form of whey protein better than the other.

In comparison to other types of protein, whey protein is digested at a faster rate, has better mixing characteristics, and is often perceived as a higher-quality protein. Research has indicated that the rapid increase in blood amino acid levels after ingestion of whey protein stimulates protein synthesis to a greater degree than casein (Tipton et al. 2004; Boirie et al. 1997; Fruhbeck 1998). Theoretically, individuals who consume whey protein frequently throughout the day may optimize protein synthesis (Tipton et al. 2004; Willoughby, Stout, and Wilborn 2007; Tipton et al. 2007; Tang et al. 2007; Andersen et al. 2005; Borsheim, Aarsland, and Wolfe 2004). Whey protein may also offer a number of health benefits in comparison to casein (see next section for discussion of casein), including greater immunoenhancing (Di Pasquale 2000; Gattas et al. 1992) and anticarcinogenic properties (Di Pasquale 2000; Gattas 1990; Puntis et al. 1989). For example, Lands and colleagues (1999) reported that ingesting a supplement containing whey protein (20 g/day) during 12 weeks of training promoted better gains in immune function, performance, and body composition alterations than ingesting casein. These findings have helped position whey protein as a superior source of protein.

Casein

Caseinates are manufactured from skim milk by a processing technique that involves separating the casein from whey (i.e., resolubilizing) and then drying it. Caseinates used in commercial supplements are usually available as sodium caseinates, potassium caseinates, calcium caseinates, and casein hydrolysates. The specific processing method employed affects the amino acid profile slightly as well as the availability of α, β, γ, or κ casein subtypes. The advantage of casein is that it is a relatively inexpensive source of protein. Casein is available in a range of grades that vary depending on quality, taste, and mixing characteristics (Bucci and Unlu 2000). The major disadvantage is that casein tends to clump when mixed in acidic fluid and therefore does not mix well in liquid. It also digests at a slower rate than other forms of protein. Research data have indicated several factors that influence protein synthesis, including the number of calories consumed, the quantity and quality of protein ingested, the insulin response to the meal, and the digestibility of the food (Beaufrere, Dangin, and Boirie 2000).

The time course of amino acid release in the blood is influenced by the digestion rate of food. Protein-containing foods that are digested faster (e.g., whey) generally result in a greater release of amino acids in the blood over a shorter period of time. Protein-containing foods that are digested at a slower rate (e.g., casein) typically promote a smaller but more prolonged increase in amino acids (Di Pasquale 2000). Consequently, casein tends to have a more anticatabolic effect than whey protein (Boirie et al. 1997). Skeletal muscle **catabolism** refers to a process of muscle breakdown. Since protein synthesis (hypertrophy) and protein breakdown (catabolism) are independently regulated mechanisms, any nutrient that acts as an anticatabolic (reduces the breakdown of skeletal muscle) improves recovery from exercise and may accelerate adaptations to the exercise and training stimulus.

➤   catabolism—Tissue breakdown, especially degradation of the protein in the lean body mass.

Egg

Egg protein is typically obtained from chicken egg whites (ovalbumin) or whole eggs through a variety of extraction and drying techniques. Egg whites are recognized as the reference protein that other types of protein are compared to. The PER and PDCAAS of egg protein are similar to that of milk protein and only slightly lower than that of casein, whey, and bovine colostrum. A number of studies have evaluated the effects of egg protein on nitrogen retention and physiological adaptations to training in comparison to other types of protein. Results of these studies generally indicate that egg protein is as effective as milk protein, casein, and whey in promoting nitrogen retention (Gattas et al. 1992; Gattas 1990; Puntis et al. 1989). Nitrogen retention is a key component of the process of nitrogen balance (discussed earlier). Specifically, if nitrogen is retained, then nitrogen balance is said to be positive and is an indication that nitrogen is being used to make lean tissue.

Soy

Soy is a high-quality, complete protein. The PER and PDCAAS of soy protein are similar to that of dietary meat or fish and slightly lower than that of egg, milk, casein, bovine colostrum, and whey protein. Consequently, it has been suggested that soy serves as an excellent source of dietary protein, particularly for vegetarians (Messina 1999).

Research has also indicated several potential health benefits. Soy is a low-fat vegetable source of protein that, when added to the diet, can contribute to lower cholesterol levels, both intrinsically and by displacing foods higher in saturated fat and cholesterol. Hence, consuming a diet high in soy may help reduce cholesterol (Dewell, Hollenbeck, and Bruce 2002; Jenkins et al. 2000; Potter 1995; Takatsuka et al. 2000). Soybeans are also a good dietary source of isoflavone phytoestrogens (e.g., daidzein and genistein). Isoflavones bind to estrogen receptors and have estrogen-like properties (Allred et al. 2001; Kurzer 2002; Messina and Messina 2000; Nicholls et al. 2002; Pino et al. 2000; Tikkanen and Adlercreutz 2000). Because of the high levels of isoflavone phytoestrogens in soy protein, there has been interest in determining whether soy may serve as a nutritional alternative to hormone or ipriflavone therapy (or both) in women.

However, in resistance training studies assessing body composition, comparisons of soy and whey protein showed that soy protein was just as effective as whey protein (Kalman et al. 2007; Brown et al. 2004; Candow et al. 2006). Little if any research exists to document negative outcomes in males ingesting soy protein in terms of training adaptations. In the absence of such studies and given the support from other investigations (Kalman et al. 2007; Brown et al. 2004; Candow et al. 2006; Drăgan et al. 1992), it appears that soy protein supplementation in male athletes is a valid choice.

Bovine Colostrum

Bovine colostrum is the premilk liquid produced from the mammary glands of cows during the first 24 to 48 hours after giving birth (Mero et al. 1997; Baumrucker, Green, and Blum 1994; Tomas et al. 1992). It is primarily available as a supplement, because there are only a few producers (dairy farms) that market raw bovine colostrum. Bovine colostrum has greater nutrient density and higher protein quality than traditional dairy milk. For example, the PER of bovine colostrum is about 3.0, which is higher than the PER of beef, fish, poultry (2.0-2.3), and soy (1.8-2.3) and compares favorably to that of egg (2.8), milk protein (2.8), casein (2.9), and whey protein (3.0 to 3.2). Bovine colostrum has a relatively high concentration of insulin-like growth factor (IGF)-I, growth factors (IGF-II, transforming growth factor [TGF] β), immunoglobulins (IgG, IgA, IgM), and antibacterials (lactoperoxidase, lysozyme, and lactoferrin) not found in other sources of protein (Mero et al. 1997; Baumrucker, Green, and Blum 1994; Tomas et al. 1992). These bioactive compounds may strengthen the immune system and promote growth. For this reason, bovine colostrum has been marketed as a unique source of quality protein, growth factors, and immunoenhancing compounds in numerous food products (e.g., infant formulas, protein supplements).

Gelatin

Gelatin is obtained by boiling of the skin, tendons, and ligaments of animals. Gelatin contains protein, collagen (a primary component of joints, cartilage, and nails), and various amino acids. It is classified as an incomplete protein because it lacks the amino acid tryptophan. Gelatin is commonly used in foods as a stabilizer, as well as by the pharmaceutical industry as an encapsulating agent (Hendler and Rorvik 2001). Because gelatin contains several amino acids (proline, hydroxyproline, and glycine) found in collagen, it is often marketed as a supplement that supports bone and joint health.

Identifying which type of protein is best for nutritional products is difficult. Different types of protein may offer specific advantages over others depending on the population targeted or the outcome desired. For example, soy protein may be the best choice for vegetarians, individuals interested in increasing dietary availability of isoflavones, or people who want to maintain a low-fat diet. Egg protein is generally well accepted among consumers and may be an attractive alternative for lacto-ovo vegetarians. Milk protein is inexpensive and serves as a high-quality source of casein and whey protein for people who are not lactose intolerant. Casein may serve as a good source of protein to minimize protein catabolism during prolonged periods between eating, such as during sleep, or in people maintaining a low-calorie diet. On the other hand, frequent ingestion of whey protein may optimize protein synthesis and immune function. Finally, bovine colostrum appears to be a high-quality protein that may enhance training adaptations, but it is expensive compared to other forms of protein.

Protein and Performance

Adequate protein ingestion is essential for maximizing training-induced adaptations, particularly in strength development. Also, since protein can be metabolized for energy, adequate protein ingestion is of particular concern for athletes in energy-demanding aerobic endurance sports, such as triathlons or marathons. The next sections highlight various aspects of protein intakes for several types of athletes and physical activity preferences—aerobic, anaerobic, and strength training.

Aerobic Exercise

The general understanding is that protein's contribution to prolonged aerobic exercise ranges between 5% and 15% of total energy expenditure, depending on the intensity and duration of the exercise bout (Antonio and Stout 2001; Mero 1999). For this reason, it was once thought that the dietary protein needs for aerobic endurance athletes were no greater than those for an untrained individual. However, research using advanced methods of assessing energy expenditure and protein balance has indicated that protein needs of aerobic endurance athletes are slightly higher than for the general population (e.g., 1.2-1.4 g/kg per day) (Lemon 2001). In a landmark study, Tarnopolsky and colleagues (1988) compared distance runners with sedentary controls relative to two different protein intakes to determine their effects on nitrogen balance. A 10-day period of normal protein intake was followed by a 10-day period of altered protein intake in both groups of male subjects. The nitrogen balance data revealed that the aerobic endurance athletes required 1.67 times more daily protein than sedentary controls. Aerobic endurance athletes excreted more total daily urea than either bodybuilders or controls. The authors concluded that the aerobic endurance athletes required greater daily protein intakes than sedentary individuals to meet the needs of protein catabolism during aerobic exercise.

Using this factor of protein intake, Friedman and Lemon (1989) instructed five well-trained distance runners to consume two different diets for a period of six days each. In one of the six-day intervention periods, the runners consumed the Recommended Dietary Allowance of protein (~0.8 g/kg body weight per day). For the other six days, the runners consumed a protein intake that was 1.7 times higher (~1.5 g/kg body weight per day). During each trial, the runners followed their regular training program (7-10 miles of running daily). Estimates of whole-body nitrogen retention (an indicator of protein synthesis and protein breakdown) were obtained from urinary and sweat nitrogen losses. The differences in protein intake combined with the nitrogen excretion measures showed significant differences in estimated whole-body nitrogen retention between the two protein intakes. Specifically, nitrogen retention remained positive during the high-protein trial but was significantly reduced in the lower-protein trial. The authors stated that the current protein RDA (0.8 g/kg body weight per day) may be inadequate for athletes engaging in chronic high-intensity aerobic endurance exercise. Since approximately 1.5/kg body weight per day resulted in a positive nitrogen retention in this group of athletes, athletes engaged in this mode of training should strive to ingest this amount of protein in their diets.

While it is easy to obtain this amount of protein in the diet, it may be advantageous for aerobic endurance athletes to time protein intake in order to optimize training adaptations (Kerksick et al. 2008). For example, studies have shown that ingesting protein (0.5 g/kg) with carbohydrate (1.5 g/kg) after exercise is more effective in promoting glycogen retention than ingesting carbohydrate alone (Zawadzki, Yaspelkis, and Ivy 1992). Moreover, ingesting creatine (a combination of three amino acids) with carbohydrate reportedly promotes greater glycogen storage than ingesting carbohydrate alone (Green et al. 1996). Also, creatine loading before carbohydrate loading has been reported to promote glycogen supercompensation (Nelson et al. 2001).

Ingestion of EAA and protein with carbohydrate after exercise has also reportedly enhanced protein synthesis (Borsheim et al. 2002; Tipton et al. 1999) and help mediate the immunosuppressive effects of intense exercise (Gleeson, Lancaster, and Bishop 2001). Finally, some evidence suggests that ingestion of branched-chain amino acids with carbohydrate during exercise may help lessen the catabolic effects of exercise (Mero 1999; Coombes and McNaughton 2000; Bigard et al. 1996; Carli et al. 1992; Rowlands et al. 2008). Consequently, for aerobic endurance athletes, it is important to ingest enough protein in the diet to maintain nitrogen balance. There may be some advantage to ingesting a small amount of protein or amino acids before, during, and after exercise in order to help athletes better tolerate training (Kerksick et al. 2008). For more on the timing of nutrient intake, see chapter 9.

Anaerobic Exercise

As previously discussed, for many years the conventional thought was that protein did not contribute significantly to energy metabolism during prolonged exercise. For this reason, the contribution of protein or amino acids to the energy demands of anaerobic exercise was thought to be minimal. Current literature now supports that proteins are degraded and that they contribute to metabolism even during a single bout of high-intensity exercise (Bloomer et al. 2007, 2005) and that training influences the content of enzymes involved in protein metabolism (Howarth et al. 2007). A single bout of resistance exercise also stimulates gene expression related to protein synthesis (Hulmi et al. 2009). Performing a number of sprints or successive bouts of intense exercise promoted protein degradation and oxidation (De Feo et al. 2003). Moreover, performing exercise bouts in glycogen-depleted conditions promoted a greater degradation and utilization of protein as a metabolic fuel (Wagenmakers 1998).

While carbohydrate remains the primary fuel needed for high-intensity exercise, protein can serve as a fuel source during high-intensity, intermittent, and prolonged exercise bouts. For this reason, it is important to ingest carbohydrate along with protein or amino acids (or both) before, during, and after exercise in order to replenish amino acids used during exercise and optimize recovery (Kerksick et al. 2008). In general, athletes participating in anaerobic exercise should consume 1.5 to 2.0 g/kg of protein per day.

Strength Training

Research has established that resistance-trained athletes need to ingest a sufficient amount of protein in the diet to maintain a positive nitrogen balance and **anabolism** (Lemon 2001). Studies also indicate that ingesting protein or amino acids before, during, or after intense exercise (or at more than one of these time points) can influence protein synthesis pathways (Willoughby, Stout, and Wilborn 2007; Esmarck et al. 2001; Tipton and Ferrando 2008; Tipton et al. 2001). Several questions remain:

- Does protein supplementation promote muscle hypertrophy during training?
- Do different types of protein promote greater training adaptations?
- Does nutrient timing influence training responses?

Concerning the first question, a number of studies have shown that supplementing the diet with protein promotes greater training adaptations during resistance training than ingesting an isoenergetic amount of carbohydrate (Andersen et al. 2005; Hulmi et al. 2008; Kalman et al. 2007; Hayes and Cribb 2008; Kerksick et al. 2007, 2006; Kraemer et al. 2006). Moreover, different types of protein (combined with carbohydrate or other ergogenic nutrients like creatine and β-hydroxy–β-methylbutyric acid [HMB]) may have additional benefits (Willoughby, Stout, and Wilborn 2007; Rowlands et al. 2008; Hulmi et al. 2008; Kalman et al. 2007; Solerte et al. 2008; Kendrick et al. 2008; Candow et al. 2008; Cribb, Williams, and Hayes 2007). Consequently, growing evidence indicates that strength athletes should ingest quantities of protein at the upper end of the range of 1.5 to 2.0 g/kg per day, as well as ingest protein or amino acids either before, during, or after exercise (or at more than one of these times) in order to optimize training adaptations (Campbell et al. 2007; Kerksick et al. 2008; Lemon 2001).

➤ anabolism—The building of body cells and substances from nutrients, especially the building of proteins and muscle mass in the body.

Multiple studies have examined the combination of amino acid–carbohydrate supplements in the time frame that encompasses a resistance exercise session, but fewer have addressed supplementation with intact protein (such as whey and casein) after resistance exercise and its effects on nitrogen balance. Tipton and colleagues (2004) studied the ingestion of casein and whey protein and their effects on muscle anabolism after resistance exercise. They concluded that ingestion of whey and casein after resistance exercise resulted in similar increases in muscle protein net balance and net muscle protein synthesis, despite different patterns of blood amino acid responses (a quicker response of plasma amino acids for whey protein and a more sustained response for casein protein). In a similar study, Tipton and coworkers (2007) looked at whether ingestion of whole proteins before exercise would stimulate a superior response compared with after exercise. They reported that net amino acid balance switched from negative to positive after ingestion of the whey protein at both time points. For more specific information on the importance of the timing of protein ingestion and resistance exercise, refer to chapter 9.

Professional Applications

Unlike fat and carbohydrates, protein is not primarily a metabolic fuel that is oxidized during exercise and physical activity. Rather, protein's main function in relation to athletic and exercise performance is to increase muscle mass and functional strength in response to the exercise and training stimulus. This understanding leads to two of the most common questions concerning protein:

- Which types are the best to ingest?
- How much protein should be consumed over the course of a day?

Regarding the best protein type, it is quite clear that animal-based protein (beef, chicken, milk, egg) is superior to plant-based protein. Animal sources of protein contain all EAAs and are therefore considered complete sources of protein, while many sources of plant protein are missing some of the EAAs (i.e., are incomplete). Types of protein vary in their quality depending on their amino acid profile. Complete protein sources that contain greater amounts of EAAs generally have higher-quality protein. Specifically, according to the protein rating system known as the *protein digestibility–corrected amino acid score* (PDCAAS), egg, milk, whey, and bovine colostrum sources of protein are classified as high-quality proteins. Soy protein, a plant protein, also is a high-quality protein according to this ranking system. Lean meats such as chicken breast, roast turkey, and tuna, as well as skim milk, are excellent choices of protein due to their relatively high protein content and low fat content.

Protein supplements are also a good way to obtain high-quality protein. Most commercial protein supplements marketed to athletes contain whey-, casein-, egg-, and soy-based protein. Protein supplements offer high-quality protein and can be prepared relatively easily during traveling. This is the primary benefit of protein supplements—convenience—especially when one considers that whole foods containing protein need to be purchased, prepared or cooked, and then perhaps refrigerated.

Protein intake recommendations has been a popular topic in the sport nutrition field for many years. Ingesting 1.5 to 2 g protein per kilogram body weight is recommended for athletes and physically active individuals. For a 200-pound (91-kg) individual, this equates to approximately 135 to 180 g protein per day. For a 120-pound (54-kg) individual, it equates to approximately 80 to 110 g protein per day. The protein should be ingested with each meal in approximately equal doses. Assuming a 200-pound athlete eats about five times a day, he should ingest about 30 g protein with each meal (20 g protein per meal for the 120-pound athlete). Ingesting high-quality protein regularly throughout the day ensures that the skeletal muscles have the anabolic building blocks (amino acids) to support lean tissue accretion. The concept of when to ingest protein in relation to exercise training and physical activity is referred to as protein timing. This topic is covered in more detail in chapter 9.

SUMMARY POINTS

- Dietary protein is classified as *complete* or *incomplete* depending on whether or not the protein contains adequate amounts of the EAAs.
- Animal sources of protein contain all EAAs and are therefore considered complete sources of protein, while many plant sources of protein are missing some of the EAAs (i.e., are incomplete).
- It is generally recommended that athletes consume 1.5 to 2.0 g/kg body weight of protein to ensure adequate protein intake.
- Milk (whey and casein), egg, soy, and bovine colostrum sources of protein are classified as high-quality protein.
- Adequate protein ingestion is essential for maximizing training-induced adaptations, particularly in strength development.
- Ingesting high-quality protein regularly throughout the day ensures that the skeletal muscles have the anabolic building blocks (amino acids) to support lean tissue accretion.

4

Fat

Lonnie Lowery, PhD, RD, LD

As a "default fuel" source for humans, fat (triacylglycerol) is abundant in the body. A relatively lean athlete with 15% body fat carries approximately 10,000 g of stored triacylglycerol in adipose tissue, providing 90,000 calories (kcal) of energy. This is enough energy to complete multiple marathons and many more resistance exercise sessions. Further, approximately 300 g (2,700 kcal) of triacylglycerol is present in intramuscular lipid droplets.

However, fat is much more than fuel. A complex variety of fats exists, with variations depending on their **fatty acid** makeup and placement on the **glycerol** backbone. These variations can exert pharmaceutical-like effects as they influence biological systems. Many (but not all) of these pharmaceutical-like effects occur because the dietary fats an athlete ingests are incorporated into cell membranes, affecting biochemical processes and the physical nature of the cell. The results can include anti-inflammatory, antidepressive, anticatabolic, and other effects that are of interest to hard-training athletes (Lowery 2004). A large body of literature exists on the various fatty acid types and their physiology, but specific application to athletes is still in the early stages. The section "Dietary Fat and Performance" provides details on the relationship between fats and athletic performance.

➤ fatty acid—A major component of fats that is used by the body for energy and tissue development.

➤ glycerol—A three-carbon substance that serves as the central structural component of triglycerides.

Fat Digestion and Absorption

Of course, in order to take advantage of fat as a fuel source or a "nutra-ceutical," an athlete must digest (break down) and absorb it into the body. Fat digestion begins in the mouth with an enzyme called lingual lipase; the fat is further broken down by gastric and pancreatic lipases. Bile, which is produced in the liver and stored and secreted on demand by the gallbladder, then mixes with and emulsifies the partially digested fat in the proximal small intestine. Then, almost strangely, these broken-up fatty acids and glycerol molecules are recombined in the intestinal cells as they are packaged into chylomicrons and sent into the lymphatic circulation. Ultimately, the absorbed packages of fat enter the blood and have their contents extracted by an enzyme lying in the capillary beds of tissues, lipoprotein lipase. It is only then that the constituent fatty acids can be transported into a fat cell or working muscle cell. Once in muscles, they can enter the mitochondrial "furnace" as a fuel (figure 4.1). During nonfed periods, the scenario changes somewhat. It is mostly at this time that the "free" fatty acids are derived

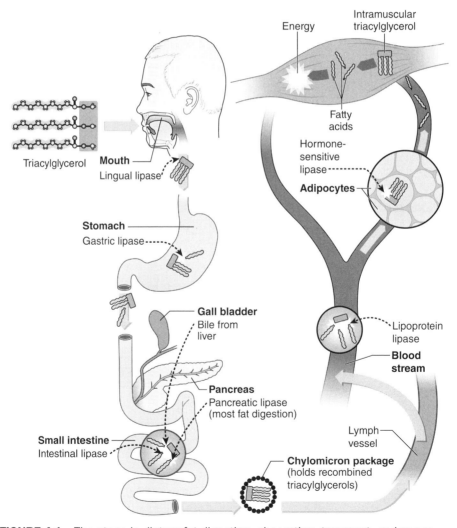

FIGURE 4.1   The steps in dietary fat digestion, absorption, transport, and usage.

from adipose cell storage, under the influence of adrenaline and the enzyme hormone-sensitive lipase. The mobilized free fatty acids can circulate to working muscles escorted by the albumin protein.

Types of Fat

Fat contains only three atoms (carbon, hydrogen, and oxygen), but the ways in which these atoms are bonded to each other and their numbers give fats various classifications and biological functions. The following discussion deals with these differences. An understanding of the differences enables the athlete to choose the proper types of fat in order to optimize health and performance.

Chemical Differences in the Types of Fat

Fats can be categorized into two major types, saturated and unsaturated, but it is important to make distinctions far deeper than this. A look at figure 4.2 will aid in the understanding of these differences. Over the past two decades, nutrition scientists have increasingly appreciated why these many differences affect an athlete's physiology. Indeed, researchers have manipulated different types of fat to enhance exercise performance, impart healthy weight gain, induce body fat loss, and control inflammatory conditions as well as emotional states. So, what are these differences?

- Degrees of saturation: The number of carbon-carbon double bonds.
- Carbon-carbon double-bond position: The placement of the double bonds counted from either end of the fatty acid chain.
- Chain length: The length of the carbon chain that makes up the fatty acids.
- Fatty acid placement. Differences in where the fatty acid chains are attached (or omitted) from the fat molecule's glycerol "backbone." These can be manipulated by food chemists to produce potential ergogenic effects.

Degrees of Saturation

One first notices that fatty acids are the "business end" of a fat (triacylglycerol) molecule. Fatty acid chains have the vast majority of the kilocalories (kcal) and the most pharmaceutical-like effects. It is from their degree of unsaturation (the number of carbon-carbon double bonds) that fatty acids, and thus their parent triacylglycerol molecule, get the designation *saturated*, *monounsaturated*, or *polyunsaturated*. That is, a fatty acid can contain zero, one, or multiple carbon-carbon double bonds, respectively (refer to figure 4.2). The more carbon-carbon double bonds on a fatty acid, the less "saturated" it is with hydrogen atoms.

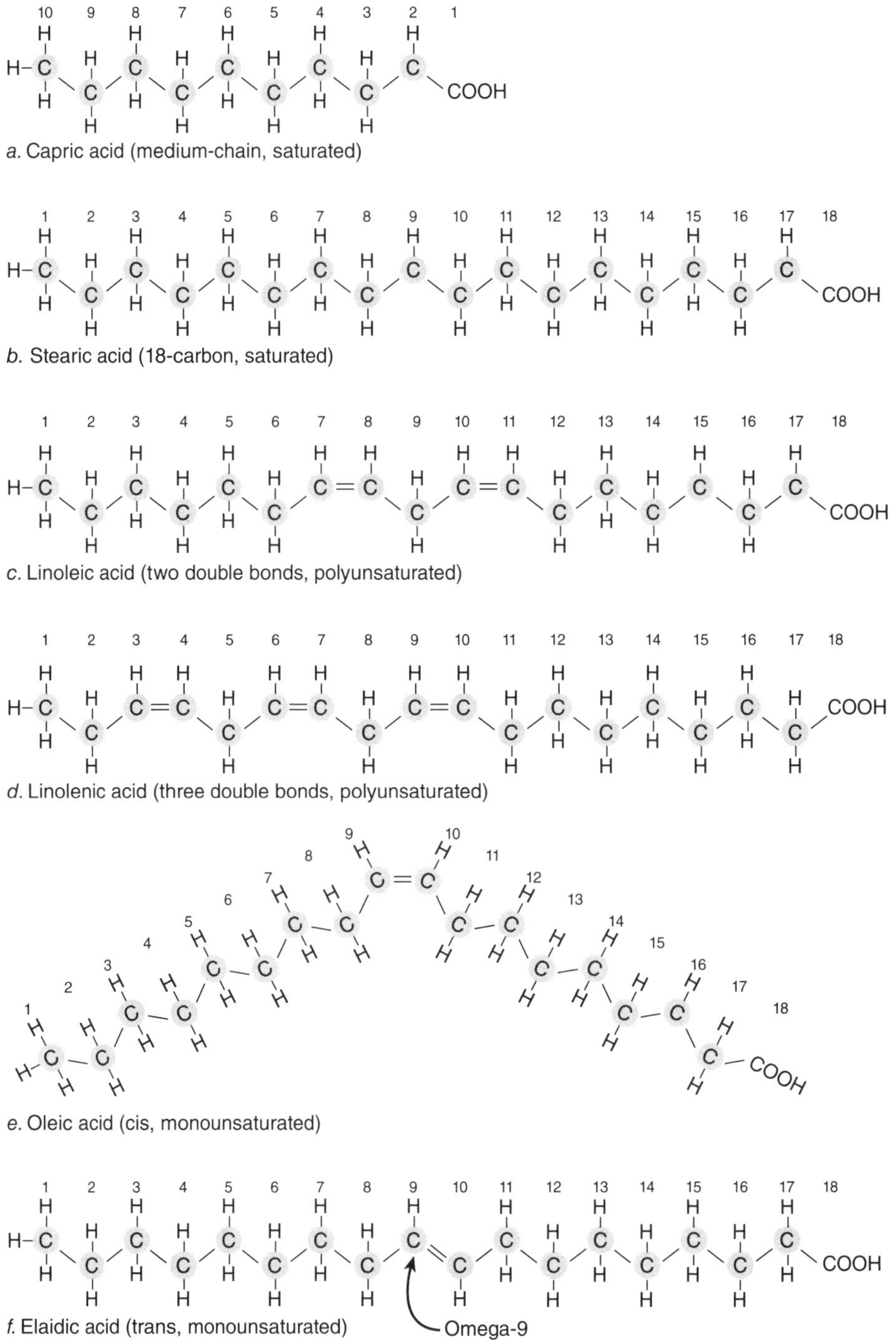

FIGURE 4.2 Six different triacylglycerol molecules show variation in the number of double bonds, placement of double bonds, and chain length. Also, the shape of the molecule varies in cis versus trans fatty acids, as seen in the eladic acid and oleic acid examples.

Saturated fatty acids, the fatty acid chains with zero double bonds (refer to the capric and stearic acid chains in figure 4.2, *a* and *b*), have been condemned for negatively affecting low-density lipoprotein (LDL) cholesterol receptors on the liver and thus increasing serum LDL cholesterol (and therefore heart disease risk). Educational materials since the early 1970s have included this observation, but more recent research suggests that differences exist even among the saturated fatty acids. For example, s*tearic acid*, an 18-carbon fatty acid (figure 4.2*b*), does not appear to be as atherogenic as other saturated fatty acids (Mensink 2005). Further, recent research actually suggests a helpful role for higher serum cholesterol concentrations among strength athletes, as is discussed later in this chapter.

Monounsaturated fatty acids have enjoyed a much more positive reception among dietitians. For example, *oleic acid*, (figure 4.2*e*) which olive oil is so rich in, has been related to enhanced longevity and reduced morbidity. This beneficial effect is apparent from observations that the Mediterranean diet is rich in olive oil and that populations consuming this diet tend to live longer than others. Controlled research indicates that oils rich in this monounsaturated fat improve blood pressure and glucose metabolism compared to diets higher in carbohydrates or polyunsaturates (Park et al. 1997; Rasmussen et al. 1995; Thomsen et al. 1995). Canola oil is also rich in oleic acid, offering a cheaper and slightly more versatile alternative. Tree nuts, peanuts, and nut butters are also excellent sources of oleic acid.

Polyunsaturated fats (i.e., polyunsaturated fatty acids, from which the parent fat molecule gets its designation) have two or more carbon-carbon double bonds. Most notably, these include *linoleic acid* (two double bonds, figure 4.2*c*), which is heavily consumed in Western cultures; *linolenic acid* (three double bonds, figure 4.2*d*), which is underconsumed in Western cultures; and the fish oil fatty acids *eicosapentaenoic acid* (EPA, five double bonds) and *docosahexaenoic acid* (DHA, six double bonds), which are also underconsumed in Western cultures. These latter fatty acids, due to their large number of double bonds, are sometimes called *highly unsaturated fatty acids* (HUFA). A balance of the various polyunsaturates is important, because these fatty acids can have opposing effects in the body. That is, a diet too rich in linoleic acid increases low-grade inflammatory states that have been linked to cardiovascular disease, diabetes, and other chronic diseases prevalent in Western cultures (Boudreau et al. 1991; Calder 2006; Kapoor and Huang 2006; Simopoulos 2002). Also, high-intensity exercise leads to an inflammatory state that can improve or worsen depending on the amounts of linolenic and linoleic acids ingested. Specifically, ingestion of EPA and DHA, which have anti-inflammatory properties, can counteract the low-grade inflammation brought on by high-intensity exercise (for more information on EPA and DHA, see the section "Essential Fatty Acids"). The inclusion of more fish oil–derived fatty acids moderates this effect. Unfortunately, very little information presently exists about whether linoleic acid–based inflammation worsens athletic conditions such as bursitis and tendinitis.

Carbon-Carbon Double-Bond Position

No discussion of polyunsaturated fatty acids (PUFA) would be complete without an explanation of the position of the carbon-carbon double bonds. This is where the categories *omega-3* and *omega-6* become meaningful (monounsaturates are in the *omega-9* category, which tends to get less attention). "Omega" refers to the position of the first carbon-carbon double bond, counting from the methyl end (figure 4.2). This is important in relation to several nutraceutical effects. For example, fish oils contain omega-3 fatty acids and are anti-inflammatory, while most vegetable oils contain predominantly omega-6 fatty acids, which are proinflammatory. Typically two "regular" carbon-carbon single bonds separate the rarer carbon-carbon double bonds on PUFA molecules. These double bonds can also be designated by counting from the "delta" or carboxyl end (the end attaching to a glycerol when a full fat molecule is formed). Thus, linolenic acid, which is underconsumed from sources such as flax meal or walnuts, is fully described by counting from both ends of its chain. It is an omega-3, "delta" 9,12 polyunsaturated fatty acid. A popular supplemental fat is *conjugated linoleic acid* (CLA) found in beef and dairy. It has double bonds closer to each other than is typical; for example, one version of CLA is an omega-7, delta 9,11 fatty acid. The section "Fat Supplements for Athletes" discusses this particular supplemental fat in more detail.

Another positional difference relating to carbon-carbon double bonds does not concern the numerical position on the fatty acid chain. Instead it concerns the localized type of a given double bond. This is the *cis* versus *trans* descriptor. Most "natural" fatty acids exhibit the cis configuration. In these fats, the carbon-carbon double bond is missing hydrogen atoms on the same side of the fatty acid chain. The resulting "hairpin" shape is evident in the oleic acid example in figure 4.2*e*. Conversely, trans-configured fatty acids (or **trans fat**), created by food producers in a process called **hydrogenation**, have the missing hydrogen atoms on the opposite sides of the chain, giving them a straight shape much like the one exhibited by elaidic acid (figure 4.2*f*). Indeed, the deleterious effects of man-made trans fats, such as those in some pastries, crackers, fried chicken, and French fries, are much like those attributed to saturated fats (e.g., cardiovascular disease), both metabolically and physically. For example, a triacylglycerol with three very straight fatty acids attached to its glycerol "backbone" would pack more tightly with its fellows into a cell membrane compared to a triacylglycerol with "bent" fatty acids.

➤ trans fat—Also known as trans fatty acid, typically refers to a type of processed fat that is used in baked goods like doughnuts, breads, crackers, potato chips, cookies, and many other processed food products like margarine and salad dressings.

➤ hydrogenation—A process used in the food industry in which hydrogen gas is bubbled through oil at a high temperature to create trans fatty acids, which increases shelf life or spreadability (or both) of the original oil. Hydrogenated oils also impart certain beneficial "mouth feel" characteristics on finished food products.

Chain Length

On a deeper level than degree of unsaturation, the physical fact of chain length is also important. Fatty acid chains range widely from 4 to 22 carbons in length but are more typically 16 to 22 carbons long. Examples of (rarer) short-chain fatty acids (less than six carbons long) are those made by bacteria in the gut as they act on dietary fiber or those present in cow's butter. Examples of (also rare) medium-chain fatty acids (6-12 carbons long) are capric acid and lauric acid derived from tropical oils that are sold as sport supplements. Long-chain fatty acids (i.e., 16-22 carbons long) are most common and include all of the mono- and polyunsaturated fats previously discussed, including linoleic acid (omega-6, cis type, 18 carbons), linolenic acid (omega-3, cis type, 18 carbons), oleic acid (omega-9, cis type, 18 carbons), elaidic acid (omega-9, trans type, 18 carbons), EPA (omega-3, cis type, 20 carbons), and DHA (omega-3, cis type, 22 carbons). See table 4.1. Fatty acid chains that are classified as medium-chain fatty acids (6-12 carbons long) have been studied in terms of improving aerobic endurance performance. The theoretical rationale of ingesting these medium-chain triglycerides (MCT) is that they may spare muscle glycogen and improve aerobic endurance performance. Unfortunately, the majority of studies investigating this aspect of MCT ingestion have not supported improvements in aerobic endurance performance. However, as noted in the section "Medium-Chain Fatty Acids," there may be other benefits for athletes ingesting these types of fat.

TABLE 4.1 Types of Dietary Fat

Type and examples	Number of carbon atoms: number of c-c double bonds	Dietary sources	Recommended intakes[†]
Saturated fatty acids			
Butyric acid	4:0	Cow's butter	–
Various medium-chain types (e.g., capric and lauric acids)	6-12:0	Tropical oils, dietary and medical supplements	<30 g per serving to prevent intestinal distress
Palmitic acid	16:0	Animal fat, palm oil	Saturated fat <33% of fat intake; <10% of caloric intake
Stearic acid	18:0	Animal fat, cocoa butter	Saturated fat <33% of fat intake; <10% of caloric intake

(continued)

Table 4.1 *(continued)*

Type and examples	Number of carbon atoms: number of c-c double bonds	Dietary sources	Recommended intakes[†]
Monounsaturated fatty acids			
(cis, n-9) Oleic acid	18:1	Olive, canola, peanut oils	>33% of fat intake; ~15% caloric intake
(trans, n-9) Elaidic acid	18:1	Partially hydrogenated oils: some margarines, pastries, crackers, fried chicken, French fries	Minimize
Polyunsaturated fatty acids			
(all cis, n-6) Linoleic acid*	18:2	Most vegetable oils: snack foods, bottled oils including corn, cottonseed, safflower, and so on	Adequate Intake: 17 g daily men, 12 g daily women
(cis + trans, n-7 or n-6) Conjugated linoleic acids**	18:2	Beef and dairy, dietary supplements	3.0-7.5 g research dose; typical intakes <250 mg daily
(all cis, n-3) Linolenic acid*	18:3	Walnuts, flax products, canola oil, and soybean oil (some)	Adequate Intake: 1.6 g daily men, 1.1 g daily women
(all cis) Gamma-linolenic acid	18:3	Primrose, borage and black currant oils, dietary supplements; produced in body from other fatty acids	~500 mg daily research dose
(all cis, n-3) Eicosapentaenoic acid (EPA)	20:5	Salmon, sardines, herring, dietary supplements	160 mg Daily Value (extrapolated); dose–response effects (more = larger effect); limit total EPA + DHA to <3.0 g daily
(all cis, n-3) Docosahexaenoic acid (DHA)	22:6	Salmon, sardines, herring, dietary supplements	160 mg Daily Value (extrapolated); dose–response effects (more = larger effect); limit total EPA + DHA to <3.0 g daily
Uncommon triacylglycerols (2 or 3 fatty acids + glycerol)			
Structured triacylglycerols	–	Research and medical formulas	10 g (oral) research dose
Diacylglycerol	–	Enova oil	14 g per tablespoon serving

[†]Method of recommendations may vary: % of total kilocalories or % of total fat intake, grams or milligrams; recommendations based upon USDA suggestions, Daily Values, Adequate Intakes, intervention and observational studies, and computational estimates by author.

*Essential fatty acid.

**Conjugated linoleic acid is actually multiple fatty acids, commonly cis-9, trans-11 or trans-10, or cis-12 versions.

Fatty Acid Placement

Fatty acid placement is a final difference, and one that can be manipulated; food chemists can specifically arrange or omit fatty acids from the glycerol "backbone" of a triacylglycerol molecule. The result can be what is known as a *structured triacylglycerol* (careful arrangement of different fatty acids on the glycerol molecule) or alternatively a *diacylglycerol* (omitting the middle, or sn-2 fatty acid). These manipulations are perhaps the cutting edge of fat technology for athletes and are discussed in the section "Dietary Fat and Performance" later in the chapter.

Essential Fatty Acids

The potent and varied physiological effects of the many fatty acids are perhaps best exemplified by the fact that humans must consume certain ones to prevent deficiency symptoms. The two nutritionally essential fatty acids are **linoleic acid** (omega-6) and **linolenic acid** (omega-3). Consumption of these fatty acids is necessary because humans lack the enzymes delta-12 and delta-15 desaturase. These cellular enzymes would add carbon-carbon double bonds (points of unsaturation) at the 12 and 15 positions in fatty acid synthesis as the chain is built. Again, note that linolenic acid is an (essential) omega-3 fatty acid with double bonds at the 9, 12, and 15 positions, counting from the delta (carboxyl) end. Without the provision of such double bonds and thus these fatty acids, vertebrates (e.g., humans) exhibit symptoms such as retarded growth, dermatitis, kidney lesions, and even death. This is partly because consumed linoleic acid and linolenic acid are built into longer physiologically important fatty acids that become part of cell membranes and form eicosanoids. Eicosanoids, derived from the essential fatty acids, influence many bodily systems and play key roles in inflammation and immunity.

➤ linoleic acid—One of two essential fatty acids; an 18-carbon fatty acid with two double bonds, also referred to as omega-6 fatty acid. In most Western diets, this fatty acid is overconsumed relative to linolenic acid (omega-3).

➤ linolenic acid—One of two essential fatty acids; an 18-carbon fatty acid with three double bonds, also referred to as omega-3 fatty acid. This fatty acid is underconsumed in most Western diets.

An interesting additional example is the omega-3 fatty acid, docosahexaenoic acid (DHA). As another fatty acid with effects on cell membranes, eicosanoid production (e.g., prostaglandins), and gene interactions, DHA also produces valuable physiological effects (Arterburn, Hall, and Oken 2006). In fact, some have argued for the formal recognition of DHA as an essential fat because these effects are more than merely helpful. Animal, epidemiological, and human intervention studies suggest that DHA improves neurological and visual function in developing infants (Innis 2008; Hoffman et al. 2004; Weisinger, Vingrys, and Sinclair 1996). Docosahexaenoic acid is a major component of cerebral gray matter. Provision of DHA as part of a fish oil supplement improves mood and may benefit psychological depression (Logan 2003; Su et al. 2003).

The benefits of DHA extend beyond the brain and eyes. Supplementation with n-3 fatty acids including DHA lessens the inflammatory component of several chronic diseases, some more than others (Browning 2003; Calder 2006). A fish oil supplement containing 1.1 g EPA and 0.7 g/day DHA has been shown to reduce the cortisol response to stress (Delarue et al. 2003). Supplementing DHA with EPA reduces total serum triacylglycerol concentrations, blood pressure, platelet aggregation, and inflammation and decreases arrhythmic cardiac death (Breslow 2006; Richter 2003). Indeed, research suggests that some of the effects of (essential, omega-3) linolenic acid are more potently exhibited by DHA (Breslow 2006; Calder 2006; Ehringer et al. 1990; Su et al. 1999). For these reasons, DHA is arguably a third essential fatty acid (Muskiet et al. 2004).

Note, though, that more research is necessary to elucidate whether DHA, EPA, or some combination is best for cardiovascular and other benefits (Breslow 2006). This breakdown could be of particular relevance to male athletes, whose higher testosterone concentrations depress tissue levels of DHA (Childs et al. 2008). Regarding dose, Arterburn and colleagues (2006) reported that a large dose (2 g) of DHA daily maximizes plasma concentrations in one month. Table 4.1 shows recommended daily intakes of individual fatty acids. Note also that DHA can be converted in the body to EPA, but the reverse does not occur (Arterburn, Hall, and Oken 2006). Many natural sources and dietary supplements include a mixture of DHA and EPA (mixed omega-3), and some recommend a combined dose of less than 3.0 g daily (Morcos and Camilo 2001).

Discussions of essential fatty acids are, however, insufficient to emphasize the impact of dietary fat on health. In the context of the "balanced diet" concept, it is helpful to realize that Western society does not encourage a balanced intake with regard to dietary fat. According to the Institute of Medicine (IOM), intakes of omega-6 to omega-3 fatty acids should approximate a 7-to-1 ratio (Institute of Medicine 2002). Some researchers and dietitians suggest an even lower ratio. These recommendations, based on physiological, paleonutritional, and other evidence, are very different from the nearly 17-to-1 ratio that Westerners actually consume (Simopoulos 2002). To state this differently, Western populations such as Americans, Britons, and Australians vastly overconsume omega-6 fat while vastly underconsuming omega-3 fat (Simopoulos 2002; Mann et al. 1995; Meyer et al. 2003). Due to the competition of these types of fat with respect to incorporation into cell membranes, prostaglandin production, cytokine concentrations, gene interactions, and other effects, this is a prescription for inflammation, thrombosis, and other physiological aberrations. Also connected to the concept of balance are the well-known health benefits of the Mediterranean diet with its emphasis on olive oil. This rich source of omega-9 fatty acids (oleic acid) is part of the reason the Mediterranean diet is considered healthy (Perez-Jimenez, Lopez-Miranda, and Mata 2002). While considered more "neutral" relative to inflammation, rather than anti-inflammatory in itself, oleic acid can nonetheless alter the ratio of (inflammatory) omega-6 fats to omega-3 fats if it replaces some of the omega-6 fat in the diet.

Scientific research on essential fatty acids and athletic performance is in its infancy. While the health benefits of essential fatty acid ingestion for athletes are clear, performance studies are lacking. However, a recent study examined the effects of omega-3 supplementation on young wrestlers' (approximately 18 years old) pulmonary function during intensive wrestling training. Wrestlers consumed capsules containing 1,000 mg/day of omega-3 (180 mg EPA and 120 mg DHA) while participating in wrestling training three times a week for 12 weeks. At the end of the 12-week study, the authors reported that wrestlers ingesting the omega-3 supplement significantly improved their pulmonary function as compared to a placebo group undergoing the same training and pulmonary testing. With the popularity and attention that essential fatty acids are attaining, more research on essential fatty acids and exercise performance is likely.

Cholesterol

Cholesterol is not classified as a dietary fat but is an important lipid. Although it may hold negative connotations for most Americans, dietary cholesterol is actually a controversial substance. First, interpretations of its deleterious effects differ between the United States and Canada. Canadian authorities deemphasize its impact on actual serum cholesterol concentrations and cardiovascular risk (McDonald 2004) and do not consider the common U.S. recommendation to restrict dietary cholesterol to less than 300 mg per day important enough for inclusion in Canada's dietary guidelines. This is not to say that Canadians view circulating cholesterol as without impact on cardiovascular risk; instead the view is that dietary cholesterol has a relatively minor influence on blood levels of cholesterol and probably cardiovascular disease.

> ➤ cholesterol—A complex fatty substance with many important functions in the body; can be made in the body or supplied through foods of animal origin.

Second, dietary cholesterol may play as yet unrecognized roles in strength athletes. In a sense, dietary cholesterol may actually be emerging as advantageous. Early work by Riechman and colleagues (2007) suggests correlations between dietary cholesterol intake and lean mass and strength gains among older resistance trainers (60-69 years). Although not causal, the relationship with lean mass gain was significant ($R^2 = 0.27$), suggesting that more than a quarter of the variance in observed lean mass gain during resistance training was attributable to dietary cholesterol. Interestingly, this lends some credence to historical, less scientific suggestions from coaches that strength athletes should consume large amounts of whole eggs and beef. More research will be necessary in younger persons. As this cholesterol research is in very early stages, it is not clear how to best reconcile any potential benefits with the controversial potential adverse effects on vascular health.

Dietary Fat and Performance

Certain examples suggest how the effects of fat differ between athletes and sedentary healthy persons or patients in clinical settings. For instance, physical training can favorably change the tissue ratios of fatty acids in the body (Andersson et al. 2000; Helge et al. 2001). This beneficial, nondietary shift toward greater omega-3 content is not seen in nonexercisers. In addition, consumption of the lower-fat diet often pursued by athletes favorably changes tissue ratios of fatty acids (Raatz et al. 2001). This is at least in part due to a lower presence of (and thus less competition from) omega-6 fatty acids. Many athletes do not realize they can reduce (improve) their tissue ratios of omega-6 to omega-3 by simply consuming less overall dietary fat.

Extreme diets can become problematic, however. As one example, the "benefits" of very low-fat, high-fiber diets suggested by some researchers induce changes that athletes may want to avoid. For instance, reduced testosterone concentrations (Dorgan et al. 1996; Hamalainen et al. 1983; Reed et al. 1987) from such intakes may be beneficial to a patient with risk of androgen-dependent prostate cancer but may not be beneficial to an athlete who needs the additional 10% to 15% circulating testosterone. Most athletes are aware that testosterone is advantageous for athletic recovery and muscular growth.

Another popular and sometimes extreme dietary recommendation, decreased kilocalorie intake, may also be problematic for athletes. With the often large kilocalorie expenditures of training or the caloric demands of adding lean mass, it would not be advantageous for athletes to restrict the very energy that drives progress. All things considered, fat content of the diet can range from 20% to 40% of total kilocalories with no effect on strength performance (Van Zant, Conway, and Seale 2002).

Fat as Exercise Fuel

The longer-term effects of dietary fat on an athlete are not the only consideration; it is important to understand more acute issues as well. Regarding dietary fat as fuel during exercise, two major phenomena are the "metabolic crossover effect" (table 4.2) and the "duration effect," or "fat shift" (table 4.3). The former involves a crossover from fat oxidation at rest and at lower intensities toward carbohydrate usage at high intensities. That is, an inverse relationship exists between direct fat "burning" (measured by respiratory exchange ratio) and exercise intensity (measured via heart rate or $\dot{V}O_2max$) (Brooks 1997; Klein, Coyle, and Wolfe 1994; Sidossis et al. 1997). Biochemical control and the immediacy of need for energy are reasons for this crossover. Even highly trained aerobic endurance athletes, with their enhanced capacity to oxidize fat, eventually "cross over" to carbohydrate use, albeit at higher intensities than less aerobically fit persons.

The duration effect, however, involves the opposite relationship. Exercise duration is positively correlated with fat use (Lowery 2004). During prolonged, low-intensity exercise (greater than 30 minutes), the use of carbohydrate to fuel the activity gradually shifts toward an increasing reliance on fat as the fuel. The greater reliance on fat can be demonstrated by measurement of glycerol levels in the blood. Recall that a triglyceride molecule consists of a glycerol molecule and three fatty acids. If fat is going to be used to fuel activity, the triglyceride molecule needs to be broken down (chemists use the term "hydrolysis" to refer to this reaction) into a free glycerol molecule and three free fatty acids. The glycerol and fatty acids are said to be "free" because they are not bound to each other as they were in the triglyceride form. As exercise duration increases, an associated increase of blood glycerol levels occurs (table 4.3), indicating that triglycerides have been broken down and that the fatty acids are being used to fuel the low-intensity exercise.

Two points about exercise for body fat loss are worth reiterating here. First, not all bodily fat is stored in adipose cells. A significant percentage comes from the roughly 300 g of stored intramuscular triacylglycerol. Research

TABLE 4.2 Fat Versus Carbohydrate Oxidation During Fasted Exercise of Different Intensities

Exercise intensity*	RER**	Fuel type	Biochemistry***
Low (<25% $\dot{V}O_2max$)	0.70	Fat	$C_{16}H_{32}O_2 + 23\ O_2 \rightarrow$ 16 CO_2 + 16 H_2O
Moderate (50% $\dot{V}O_2max$)	0.85	Fat + carbohydrate (increasingly carbohydrate)	Mix of palmitate and glucose usage
High (100% $\dot{V}O_2max$)	1.00	Carbohydrate	$C_6H_{12}O_6 + 6\ O_2 \rightarrow$ 6 CO_2 + 6 H_2O

*Low-intensity exercise can be very prolonged (several hours) and moderate-intensity exercise somewhat less (perhaps 1-4 h), while high-intensity exercise is measured in just minutes.

**Respiratory exchange ratio (RER) assessed on a metabolic cart (volume of CO_2 produced / volume of O_2 consumed each minute) is often used interchangeably with respiratory quotient (RQ), which is technically a cellular respiration term. RER measures validate the biochemistry at the far right in the table.

***Note that, as with RER measurements, the CO_2 produced / O_2 consumed for palmitate "burning" = 16 / 23 = 0.70, which rises with intensity toward glucose use where 6 / 6 = 1.00.

TABLE 4.3   Fat Mobilization During Fasted Exercise of Different Durations

Exercise duration	Serum glycerol[†]
Prolonged, >60 min	Higher
Moderate, 30 to 60 min	Moderate
Brief, <30 min	Lower

[†]Serum glycerol concentrations (fat breakdown and mobilization) are high during prolonged fasting (i.e., even at rest) as well as during low- to moderate-intensity prolonged exercise; in general, greater fat mobilization during exercise relates to greater fat oxidation.

has clarified that these muscle lipid droplets are a portion of the oxidized fat seen with use of metabolic cart systems. Second, the crossover and the duration phenomena do not necessarily suggest that body fat reduction is only achieved directly during fasted, low- to moderate-intensity prolonged exercise. Indeed, repeat bouts of high-intensity exercise stimulate mitochondrial biogenesis that would enhance fat usage throughout an athlete's day. Further, high-intensity training reduces glycogen stores that would subsequently be refilled by ingested carbohydrate, a nutrient that may otherwise be converted and stored as body fat (these are key reasons many power athletes are so lean). The choice of exercise intensity and duration, then, is partly determined by the athlete's need for aerobic conditioning versus the need for rest and prevention of (sympathetic type) overtraining.

Fat Loading

To augment and support the adaptations of physical training, athletes have increasingly sought to manipulate dietary fat. This takes the form of both food manipulation and dietary supplement administration. Food manipulations center around the fact that eating more fat—even "fat loading"—can increase muscle concentrations of stored triacylglycerol and increase the activity of "fat-burning" enzymes. Raising the roughly 300 g of stored intramuscular triacylglycerol would appear advantageous regarding simple fuel supply. A look inside a muscle cell reveals lipid droplets immediately adjacent to the mitochondrial furnaces that drive aerobic endurance performance, leading to interest in increasing these readily accessible depots of fuel. This is especially true given that aerobic endurance athletes have an increased capacity to store these fat droplets compared to nonexercisers (van Loon et al. 2004) (interestingly, cellular fat accumulation is part of the mechanism behind diabetes but in athletes is not deleterious). Eating more dietary fat is not intended simply to increase the content of one's intramuscular "gas tank," however. By adapting to a higher-fat diet, an athlete becomes better at using stored fat (Fleming et al. 2003; Zderic et al. 2004). One strategy, then, is to devise a pre-event dietary regimen that allows for one to two weeks of increased lipid storage and (fat oxidative) enzyme enhancement.

Unfortunately, the primary finding of fat loading studies appears to be an increased (rather than decreased) rate of perceived exertion (RPE), with inconsistent or decreased overall performance. Although some studies have suggested a prolonged time to exhaustion after a fat load (which is good), the increased sense of effort coupled with no enhancement of aerobic power (Fleming et al. 2003; Hargreaves, Hawley, and Jeukendrup 2004; Stepto 2002) has led many researchers and coaches to abandon or modify the fat loading strategy. It appears that simply having more intramuscular fat or even enhanced fat oxidation does not equate to better performance in most sports. This has prompted researchers to try fat loading regimens followed by ample pre- and midexercise carbohydrate consumption. Despite showing marked and seemingly favorable changes in fuel metabolism, however, these investigations remain equivocal regarding actual performance (Williams 2005).

Fat Supplements for Athletes

Although they are relatively rare in the Western food supply, specialty fat supplements are of interest due to two biological facts. First, cell membranes will generally incorporate the newly ingested fat, a rather profound phenomenon. For example, in relatively large amounts, EPA and DHA can displace the more inflammatory arachidonic acid (all-cis, n-6, 20:4) in cell membranes, altering the cellular prostaglandin cascade (Boudreau et al. 1991). Using the analogy of a water balloon to depict a cell, this means that the "rubber" of the balloon changes—not simply its contents, as would be true with carbohydrate ingestion. Further, the cell membrane can remain altered for long periods of time. Some studies using fish oils report washout periods of 10 to 18 weeks (Endres et al. 1989; Kremer et al. 1987). Second, cell contents and operations change when uncommon types of fat are provided as fuel. For example, medium-chain triacylglycerol supplements (which are distinguished by the length of the fatty acids rather than their unsaturation) can be more readily absorbed and "burned" (oxidized) in cells, as discussed next.

Fish Oils

Probably the most pervasive type of special lipid supplementation is fish oils. These supply both EPA and DHA at roughly 50% of the total (gel) capsule's contents; EPA is usually predominant. More concentrated products, sometimes called extra-strength fish oils, contain more of the "active ingredients" EPA and DHA and may alter the ratio toward more or less DHA. This is the reason fish oil enthusiasts justifiably look for the total dose of EPA plus DHA in a product rather than simply dosing by total grams of gross fish oil. Fatty foods, on the other hand, provide a sometimes broad mix of fatty acids and tend toward only one predominant type or another.

Typically, claims about sport supplements purported to confer multiple beneficial effects are exaggerated or deliberately misleading, but the myriad effects of consuming EPA–DHA supplements are more evidence based, making them very popular. There are reasons beyond the long washout periods (which could be negative as well as positive). The simple fact that omega-3 fat is underconsumed in most Western cultures creates a state of relative deficiency or imbalance. This relative deficiency is what underlies the various physiological effects noted earlier in the chapter. For example, Archer and colleagues (1998) reported that the U.S. population, particularly in the Midwest, eats too little fatty fish to garner cardioprotective effects. This makes supplementation of interest. Other factors that add to the interest in fish oil supplements include the low level of concern about heavy metal contamination (mercury) in comparison with some seafood (Lowery 2004) and a recommendation from the American Heart Association that supplementation may be necessary in select populations (Breslow 2006). As a general rule, dietitians recognize that correcting a deficiency induces more reliable and potentially broader positive effects than does hypersupplementation of a nutrient that is adequately consumed.

Reviews addressing how EPA and DHA may benefit athletes are rare and include an element of speculation due to a dearth of population-specific research. However, research on healthy persons and those with athletic injuries or issues do exist. A review by Lowery (2004) suggested that the anti-inflammatory and antidepressive (mood elevating) effects of these omega-3 fatty acids may benefit athletes who train hard or who are overtrained. A later study by Simopoulos (2007) also indicated that the anti-inflammatory effects were beneficial for athletes, suggesting 1 to 2 g of daily EPA plus DHA.

Conditions such as tendinitis, bursitis, osteoarthritis, and even overtraining syndrome (e.g., depression) are examples of athlete-specific maladies that may be improved through omega-3 supplementation. The protective effect against cartilage breakdown, for example in arthritic conditions (Curtis et al. 2000), may be beneficial to an athlete's career longevity, as may the bone-protective effects (Fernandes, Lawrence, and Sun 2003), although more sport-specific research is needed. Benefits to exercise-related bronchoconstriction have also been reported (Mickleborough et al. 2003). Further, emerging research may suggest a role for omega-3 fat in reduction of body fat. This has a sound research basis due to the known inflammatory nature of obesity, particularly visceral obesity (e.g., cytokines [Bastard et al. 2006]), and the corrective anti-inflammatory characteristics of fish oils. Such work is in the early stages, however, and has not yet provided the critical mass of evidence needed to call for (body composition related) recommendations. Finally, research on the relation between omega-3 fat and muscle recovery and soreness from exercise is mixed and appears dose and age related (Cannon et al. 1995; Lenn et al. 2002; Phillips et al. 2003).

Conjugated Linoleic Acid

Perhaps the next most popular fatty acid supplement among athletes, which is actually a group of positional **isomers**, is *conjugated linoleic acid* (CLA). Since before the First International Conference on CLA in 2001, however, researchers realized that humans are "hyporesponders" compared to animals such as mice. In a sense this is unfortunate due to the dramatic anticatabolic and body fat–reducing qualities exhibited by CLA in these animals (Pariza, Park, and Cook 2001; Park et al. 1997). A second generation of animal research has since ascribed individual qualities to the cis-9, trans-11 isomer (growth enhancing) versus the trans-10, cis-12 isomer (antilipogenic, lipolytic, or both) (Pariza, Park, and Cook 2001). Any consistent benefits to humans and to athletes in particular have yet to be elucidated, however. Reasons for the relative inefficacy in human studies could include different dosing methods (often 3 g daily in human research versus 0.5% to 1.0% of food weight or total kilocalories in animal studies), study duration, and species differences. The faster metabolic rates and growth curves of rodents compared to humans appear to be confounders.

> ➤ isomers—Compounds that have identical molecular formulas but differ in the nature or sequence of bonding of their atoms.

Human intakes of CLA from foods such as dairy and meats have been reported to be 151 mg daily for women and 212 mg daily for men; almost all of this is the cis-9, trans-11 type (Terpstra 2004). Very limited human research suggests increases in strength or lean body mass, or both, with supplementation (Lowery 1999; Terpstra 2004), while other data suggest a small reduction in body fat (Williams 2005). Strength and body composition protocols in human studies have not been standardized, however, and thus no clear benefits have been substantiated. Since publication of the few positive findings on body composition, concerns have emerged over potentially hampered insulin sensitivity and fatty liver (Ahrén et al. 2009; Wang and Jones 2004) and unimpressive effects regarding body weight and fat reduction in pigs and humans (Wang and Jones 2004). Thus, human studies remain rare compared to animal research, which is continuing. Although one meta-analysis has indicated a modest and variable body fat–reducing effect in humans that approximates 1 kg (2.2 pounds) of loss over 12 weeks (Whigham, Watras, and Schoeller 2007), at the present time CLA isomers do not appear to be as advantageous to humans as other fatty acid supplements.

Medium-Chain Fatty Acids

As mentioned earlier, another important aspect of fatty acid selection in sport nutrition is fatty acid length. Short, medium, and long fatty acids exert different physiological effects. For example, although EPA and DHA are discussed in the "Carbon-Carbon Double-Bond Position" section of this chapter, their length also matters. They are longer than more common fatty acids and thus are distinguished by their chain length and not simply the presence of the omega-3 double bond. About half as long as EPA and DHA are the medium-chain fatty acids capric acid (10 carbons, figure 4.2*a*) and lauric acid (12 carbons), typically derived from coconut oil and palm kernel oil. The relative shortness of the fatty acid chains in medium-chain triglycerides (MCT) makes them behave very differently in the body.

Compared to common 16- and 18-carbon fatty acids, MCT are water soluble enough to be absorbed directly into the blood, without need for the lymphatic vessels as is typical (see figure 4.1). Once in the bloodstream and upon reaching tissues such as liver or skeletal muscle, MCT can also be taken into the mitochondrial furnaces of cells without the usual need for carnitine transferase enzymes. Thus, great interest was generated in the 1980s in testing MCT as an immediate performance fuel. Unfortunately, this research, using approximately 25 to 30 g MCT preexercise and sometimes along with carbohydrate, revealed no benefit regarding improved performance or glycogen sparing during exercise (Horowitz et al. 2000; Vistisen et al. 2003; Zderic et al. 2004). There was then speculation that larger amounts may be needed to offer a benefit, but gastrointestinal distress was already a problem with many subjects. Research has been done with large 71 to 85 g doses of MCT, but symptoms such as cramping and diarrhea were again problematic (Calabrese et al. 1999; Jeukendrup et al. 1998).

Interest in the ergogenic effects of MCT, however logical, may have taken the focus away from other potential benefits to athletes. A good deal of sport nutrition involves weight gain and body recompositioning. This may be an avenue of future interest for MCT. Medium-chain triglycerides are a calorie source that is biochemically less likely to be stored as body fat due to rapid transport to the liver (for beta-oxidation of the fatty acids and ketone formation) and increased thermogenesis compared to long-chain triacylglycerol (Aoyama, Nosaka, and Kasai 2007). Indeed, new research suggests reduced body fat over a period of MCT ingestion (Aoyama, Nosaka, and Kasai 2007; Takeuchi et al. 2008). Researchers have explained that additional fat and calories benefit commonly underfed athletes (Horvath et al. 2000; Lowery 2004; Venkatraman, Feng, and Pendergast 2001; Venkatraman, Leddy, and Pendergast 2000), and MCT or similar nutrients may be an advantageous way to provide them.

Structured Triglycerides

Medium-chain fatty acids are again garnering attention, in part due to the renewed (actually ongoing) research on "structured triglycerides." Structured triglycerides are a special triacylglycerol molecule formed through a chemical process known as esterification. During this process, specifically chosen fatty acids are placed onto a glycerol backbone. Early research suggested body fat–reducing qualities and a lack of intestinal distress surrounding structured triacylglycerols that contain a mix of medium-chain and long-chain fatty acids (Aoyama, Nosaka, and Kasai 2007; Takeuchi et al. 2008). Further, a structured triacylglycerol with a targeted fatty acid at the middle, or sn-2 position, may better deliver that fatty acid into the body. Structured triacylglycerols confer enhanced nitrogen retention and less liver stress than simple physical mixtures of various types of fat in clinical situations (Lindgren et al. 2001; Piper 2008). Nonetheless, barriers, such as technology or cost, have prevented widespread use in sport nutrition.

Apart from structured triglycerides (also known as structured triacylglycerols), the other major adjustment of whole fat molecules is the use of diacylglycerols. These molecules were introduced in Japan in 1999 as cooking oil and have since become available in the United States (Flickinger and Matsuo 2003). In diacylglycerols, the glycerol backbone of the source triacylglycerol has the middle (sn-2) fatty acid removed. These oils are oxidized more readily (rather than stored in the body) when they replace typical oils (Flickinger and Matsuo 2003). The mechanism involves a lack of 2-monoacylglycerol during digestion, which affects absorption and metabolism.

How much fat is recommended in an athlete's diet? Unfortunately, no firm standards exist for optimal lipid intake. The acceptable macronutrient distribution range for fat is 20% to 35% of energy intake (Institute of Medicine 2005). When fat intake is at 30% of total calories, *Dietary Guidelines for Americans* (U.S. Department of Health and Human Services and U.S. Department of Agriculture 2005) recommends that the proportion of energy from fatty acids be 10% saturated, 10% polyunsaturated, and 10% monounsaturated and that sources of essential fatty acids be included. In general, athletes report an average fat intake of 35% of total calories (Hawley et al. 1995). The area in which most athletes need to plan is fat source distribution. A fat intake with an equal balance of saturated, polyunsaturated, and monounsaturated fats is not likely to occur by chance. Saturated fats are abundant in the typical American diet and are found in animal fat such as beef and dark meat in poultry. Monounsaturated fats are found in vegetable oils, such as olive oil and canola oil, and in peanut butter. Polyunsaturated fats are found in nuts, cheese, and fish. Athletes need to make sure that they are selecting a variety of foods to obtain the recommended balance between the types of fat.

While the research is limited, it appears that fat intake can vary as a percentage of total calories and not affect exercise performance. When fat intake was 20% of total calories as compared to 40% of total calories, there was no effect on exercise training or strength exercise performance in moderately trained males (Van Zant, Conway, and Seale 2002). In relation to aerobic exercise, researchers from Switzerland (Vogt et al. 2003) compared the effects of a diet containing 53% fat and a diet containing only 17% fat in 11 male duathletes (a duathlon consists of running and cycling). After subjects ingested the high-fat or low-fat diet for five weeks, there was no difference in the time it took to run a half marathon or in the total work output during a 20-minute all-out time trial on a cycle ergometer.

From these studies it appears that the percentage of total calories derived from fat does not have a large impact on exercise or athletic performance. But while this seems to be the case in most circumstances, athletes need to be careful not to go to extremes—eating too much or too little dietary fat. Consuming too much fat can lead to the overconsumption of total calories, which leads to weight gain in the form of body fat. Because fat tissue does not contribute to movement, it acts as "dead weight" and decreases relative force production. Athletes in sports where greater physical size is beneficial may be more prone to this problem. For example, American football linemen are more likely to consume excess calories and be classified as overweight or obese than other positions (Mathews and Wagner 2008).

On the other hand, if fat intake is too low, performance can be decreased. Athletes that participate in gymnastics, figure skating, and weight class events (e.g., wrestling) are more likely to consume too little dietary fat. Horvath and coworkers assessed the aerobic endurance performance of male and female aerobic endurance athletes after they ingested isocaloric diets with varying fat contents (Horvath et al. 2000). The athletes consumed isocaloric diets consisting of either 16% fat, 31% fat, or 44% fat for four weeks before running at 80% $\dot{V}O_2$max until voluntary exhaustion. The authors reported that the 31% fat diet resulted in a significant improvement in aerobic endurance performance in comparison to the 16% fat diet. There were no differences in aerobic endurance performance between the 31% fat and the 44% fat diet groups, however.

The recommendation is that athletes consume a habitual diet of approximately 30% fat. Of this 30%, 10% should be saturated, 10% polyunsaturated, and 10% monounsaturated. Following these fat intake suggestions avoids the extreme practices of consuming too little or too much dietary fat.

SUMMARY POINTS

- Classification of fat includes degrees of saturation (the number of carbon-carbon double bonds); carbon-carbon double-bond position (the placement of the double bonds counted from either end of the fatty acid chain); chain length (the length of the carbon chain that makes up the fatty acids); and fatty acid placement (differences in where the fatty acid chains are attached or omitted from the fat molecule's glycerol backbone). An understanding of the these differences enables athletes to choose the proper types of fat in order to optimize health and performance.

- Fat is the primary fuel at rest and during low-intensity exercise.

- Fat comes in a wide variety of types, some of which are essential, including linolenic acid from flax and walnuts (omega-3, polyunsaturated), EPA and DHA from fish oil (omega-3, polyunsaturated), and oleic acid from olive and canola oils (omega-9, monounsaturated).

- Fat confers nutraceutical benefits, including helping to maintain sex hormones, potentially enhancing mood, reducing inflammation, and assisting in body fat control.

- It is recommended that athletes consume a habitual diet of approximately 30% fat. Of this 30%, 10% should be saturated, 10% polyunsaturated, and 10% monounsaturated.

- Diets that are too low in fat are associated with reduced testosterone concentrations and exercise performance.

- Consuming too much fat can lead to the overconsumption of total calories, which leads to weight gain in the form of body fat.

- Fat supplements (conjugated linoleic acid, medium-chain fatty acids, and structured triglycerides) have not consistently demonstrated improvements in exercise performance.

5

Fluids

Bob Seebohar, MS, RD, CSCS, CSSD

Water is the most important nutrient for the human body. It composes approximately 60% of an average person's body weight and can fluctuate between 45% and 75% (Dunford and Doyle 2008). The amount of water in a person's body depends on factors such as age, gender, body composition, and overall body size. Water is stored in different locations in the body including fat, bone, muscle, and blood plasma (Dunford and Doyle 2008). Euhydration, the state in which the amount of water is adequate to meet the body's physiological demands, should be the daily goal for any active individual. Hyperhydration, an excess amount of water, and hypohydration (sometimes referred to as dehydration), an insufficient amount of water, are two extremes of fluid intake that can be dangerous.

Total body water is separated into two different compartments in the body: intracellular fluid (ICF), which stores about 65% of the total body water, and extracellular fluid (ECF), which contains the remaining 35% of total body water. Extracellular fluid is further separated into the fluid in the interstitial space between cells; intravascular water within blood vessels; and fluid in other locations, such as cerebrospinal fluid. Despite barriers that separate the compartments, water moves quite easily between the ICF and ECF. The ECF acts as a passageway for water to enter the ICF space (Sawka, Wenger, and Pandolf 1996).

The ICF and ECF are composed of similar substances but in very different concentrations. In the ECF, the major **cation** is sodium and the major **anions** are chloride and bicarbonate. Other substances found in the ECF include potassium and protein. The composition in the ICF is quite different. Potassium is the major cation, and phosphate and protein are the major anions. Sodium is present but in much smaller concentrations. These different compositions between the ECF and ICF are important for the transport of fluid and electrolytes across cell membranes. There is constant pressure for sodium to "leak" into cells and for potassium to "leak" out of cells, and these concentrations are regulated by sodium–potassium pumps on the cell membranes (Sawka, Wenger, and Pandolf 1996). See figure 5.1.

➤ cation—Positively charged ion.

➤ anion—Negatively charged ion.

While there are differences in composition between these two spaces, the total concentration of solutes **(osmolarity)** is the same. If the concentration in either compartment changes, a shift occurs. During heavy sweating, water is lost and plasma volume changes, resulting in a higher concentration of sodium in the plasma. As water moves out of the cells, the cells shrink in volume. The body is very efficient at maintaining homeostasis (equilibrium or balance), and thus the opposite also holds true: If the sodium concentra-

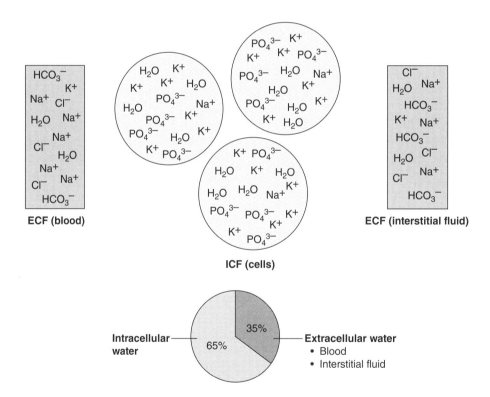

FIGURE 5.1 When the body is in fluid balance, most of the water (H_2O), potassium (K^+), and phosphate (PO_4^{3-}) will be in the intracellular fluid (ICF) and most of the sodium (Na^+), chloride (Cl^-), and bicarbonate (HCO_3^-) will be in the extracellular fluid (ECF). Though the types of compounds in these two spaces are different, the total concentration of solutes (osmolarity) is the same. If the total concentration of solutes changes in either space, the body will move water from one space to the other to maintain balance.

Adapted, by permission, from M. Dunford, 2010, *Fundamentals of sport and exercise nutrition* (Champaign, IL: Human Kinetics), 114. Adapted, by permission, from M. Dunford, 2009, *Exercise nutrition,* version 2.0 (Champaign, IL: Human Kinetics), 33.

tion in the ECF is low, then the osmolarity will be less than in the ICF, and the body will move water into the cells (Sawka, Wenger, and Pandolf 1996).

➤ osmolarity—Concentration of a solution.

When a solution (or beverage) contains a total solute concentration that is equal to the solute concentration of human blood, the solution is considered isotonic. Fluids are absorbed best in the human body when they are isotonic. A **hypotonic beverage** is a solution whose osmolarity is less than that of the body and is emptied from the stomach more quickly; a **hypertonic beverage** is a solution with higher osmolarity than that of the normal body and emptied from the stomach more slowly. For example, many sport drinks are **isotonic beverages**, whereas pure sweetened juice is a hypertonic beverage and therefore is emptied slowly in comparison to a sport drink (Rehrer et al. 1990).

➤ hypotonic beverage—A solution with less osmolarity than that of the body and therefore emptied from the stomach more quickly.

➤ hypertonic beverage—A solution with higher osmolarity than that of the normal body and thus emptied from the stomach more slowly.

➤ isotonic beverage—A beverage with a solute concentration equal to that of blood. Optimal absorption of fluids occurs when the solution is isotonic.

Fluid Balance During Exercise

During exercise, an increase in core body temperature will increase blood flow to the skin and sweat loss in an effort to cool the body. Evaporation is the primary method of heat loss during exercise and can be substantial in warmer environments (Sawka et al. 2007). Individual characteristics such as body weight, genetic predisposition, and state of heat acclimatization influence sweat rate for any activity (Yamamoto et al. 2008). Thus individuals within the same sport, and those in different sports and player positions, have a very large range of sweat and electrolyte losses. Sweat losses profoundly affect total body water (ECF and ICF).

Over a period of 8 to 24 hours, water losses can be fully replaced to establish normal total body water, within 0.2% to 0.5% of body mass if adequate fluid and electrolytes are consumed (Cheuvront et al. 2004). Well-trained athletes can have relatively high total body water values because of their higher lean body mass. Another factor affecting total body water is glycogen. Greater stored glycogen can increase total body water because 3 to 4 g of water is bound to each gram of glycogen stored (Olsson and Saltin 2008). This is an important consideration for some athletes who compete in weight-class or acrobatic sports such as wrestling, weightlifting, boxing, gymnastics, taekwondo, and figure skating. Though keeping glycogen stores "maxed out" is important, eating a high-carbohydrate diet within the days before weigh-in for weight-class sports can alter the weight class an athlete participates in. Athletes in many aesthetic and weight-class sports must eat a diet tailored to their physique and weight needs.

Dehydration

Normal hydration is vital not only for good athletic performance. More importantly, fluid balance is crucial to normal cardiovascular and thermoregulatory functions (Petrie, Stover, and Horswill 2004). Dehydration increases one's risk of developing potentially life-threatening heatstroke. The risk of dehydration and subsequently heat illness is greater in hot, humid environments and at altitude. Athletes exercising at altitudes above 2,300 m (8,200 feet) are likely to experience fluid losses above and beyond those due to exercise (McArdle, Katch, and Katch 2006).

Dehydration greater than 2% of body weight can impair athletic performance (Sawka et al. 2007). The major cause of dehydration in athletes is sweat losses that are not compensated for through fluid intake. Each athlete has a different sweat rate based on environmental conditions, clothing type, equipment worn, metabolic rate, and body surface area. And the onset of sweating is largely determined by an athlete's metabolic rate and core body temperature, which is dependent on exercise intensity and body mass (Godek et al. 2008).

Given the factors that contribute to sweat losses, it becomes obvious that athletes in particular sports and particular positions within those sports are at greater risk for dehydration in comparison to their fellow athletes. American football players, hockey players, and wrestlers all have an increased risk for dehydration based on various factors not related to exercise. The large body surface and protective equipment of American football players put them at an increased risk for dehydration. Within an American football team, linemen have a greater risk for dehydration due to their greater body surface area (Godek et al. 2008). Hockey players, because of their protective equipment, are also at a greater risk (Noonan, Mack, and Stachenfeld 2007). Wrestlers are also at an increased risk because they may engage in harmful weight loss practices, such as dehydration, in an attempt to make a certain weight class (Kiningham and Gorenflo 2001).

Hyponatremia

Exercise-associated hyponatremia, a low concentration of sodium in the blood, is very common in aerobic endurance athletes and was first described in the 1980s. Although the exact mechanism is unclear, factors associated with hyponatremia include

- overconsumption of hypotonic fluids,
- excessive loss of sodium through sweat, and
- extensive sweating with the ingestion of low-sodium fluids.

In general, symptomatic hyponatremia in events lasting less than 4 hours is attributable to drinking too much fluid and taking in little sodium before, during, and sometimes after the event (Laursen et al. 2006). The signs and symptoms of **hyponatremia** include disorientation, confusion, headache, nausea, vomiting, and muscle weakness. If left untreated, this condition can rapidly progress and cause seizures, brain swelling, coma, pulmonary edema, and cardiorespiratory arrest (Montain 2008).

➤ hyponatremia—Dangerously low blood sodium levels. A combination of factors can contribute to hyponatremia; but in athletes, the typical cause is long bouts of exercise combined with consumption of only water.

Women may be at higher risk for developing hyponatremia in longer aerobic endurance events possibly because of a number of psychosocial and biological factors (Swaka et al. 2007). Interestingly, fluid intake recommendations for women have often been based on sweat loss data from men, which are obviously too high for most women and may have led to greater sodium dilution in the body due to smaller total body water stores (Speedy, Noakes, and Schneider 2001).

Athletes who experience hyponatremia may not recognize the early signs and symptoms, which appear when blood sodium concentration reaches 130 mmol/L (Speedy, Noakes, and Schneider 2001). These include bloating, puffiness, nausea, vomiting, and headache (Hew-Butler et al. 2005). As the severity of hyponatremia increases and blood sodium concentration dips below 125 mmol/L, more serious signs and symptoms appear, including altered mental status (e.g., confusion, disorientation, and agitation), seizures, respiratory distress (due to pulmonary edema), and unresponsiveness. At the extreme, hyponatremia can be very dangerous and result in coma and death (Hew-Butler et al. 2005).

It is easy for athletes to become hyponatremic and dehydrated by choosing water alone or food and drink with little to no sodium. For individuals who have a high sweat rate and sweat sodium concentration, commercial sport drinks may not contain enough sodium to help with preventing hyponatremia. In general, the recommendation is to choose a sport drink containing a minimum of 20 mEq sodium (460 mg) per liter of fluid.

There is no concrete recommendation regarding electrolyte intake before exercise, although many athletes consume salty foods and drinks beforehand to prevent hyponatremia. Consuming an adequate amount of salt on a daily basis, especially for salty sweaters, is recommended; and in some cases, the use of salt tablets may be warranted during exercise as long as they are consumed with enough fluid to maintain fluid and electrolyte balance. Active individuals should limit fluid intake to what is needed to minimize dehydration and should consume sodium-rich foods and beverages during exercise longer than 2 hours in order to prevent excessive drinking and limit the risk of developing hyponatremia (Speedy, Noakes, and Schneider 2001).

Measuring Hydration Status

An athlete's hydration status should be assessed during training to ensure adequate hydration both during exercise and at rest. Ideally, the hydration testing method should be sensitive and accurate enough to detect total body water changes of 2% to 3% body weight. Testing hydration status in the field should be practical from a time, cost, and technical standpoint. **Urine specific gravity** (USG) is a quantifiable field test and is the preferred method for assessing hydration status before exercise in athletes. Urine specific gravity devices range from under $100 to $300 and are extremely easy to travel with and use in field settings.

➤   urine specific gravity—A tool used to measure hydration status.

Individuals can assess their own hydration status by examining the quantity of urine they produce, evaluating urine color, and estimating changes in body weight. Using one of these measures of hydration alone is not recommended because each has its own limitations. The color of urine is determined primarily by the amount of urochrome, a breakdown product of hemoglobin (Maughan and Shirreffs 2008). When a large amount of urine is excreted, the urine is dilute and the solutes are less concentrated. This gives the urine a pale color. When a small amount of urine is excreted, the urine is more concentrated. This gives the urine a darker color (Maughan and Shirreffs 2008). The urine color chart shows eight colors on a scale that reflects a linear relationship between the color of urine and its specific gravity and osmolarity (Armstrong et al. 1994). It is important to remember that certain dietary compounds can make urine appear darker, including B-complex vitamins, beta carotene, betacyanins, and some artificial food colors and medications (Maughan and Shirreffs 2008). Athletes should pay particular attention to these factors if they are using urine color frequently to determine hydration status.

When an athlete is hydrated, the urine should be pale in color and plentiful, although athletes should keep in mind that it may appear darker and brighter if they have taken a multivitamin or B complex within an hour or so prior to urinating. In general, urine should be the same color as diluted lemonade. If it is darker and concentrated, the athlete is dehydrated. If urine is orange or brown, it is imperative that the athlete see a physician immediately.

Body weight is another hydration status tool. For well-hydrated individuals who are in energy balance, body weight (measured in the morning after urinating) fluctuations should be plus or minus 1%. Keep in mind that morning body weight changes can be influenced by changes in bowel movements and eating habits. In women, hormonal fluctuations during the menstrual cycle may influence body weight. During the second half of menstruation, body weight increases slightly (Kirchengast and Gartner

2002); and in the days before menstruation, women may have an increase in water retention and body weight gain (Rosenfeld et al. 2008).

Weighing before and after an exercise session can also be useful to help determine if athletes are meeting their fluid needs during training. The easiest approach is for athletes to weigh in the nude before a training session (preferably one at competition intensity) and then immediately after the workout. The difference in weight will provide a good estimate of fluid losses and the amount of fluid that should be ingested subsequently to maintain hydration status; one should keep in mind any potential changes in hydration status based on time point in a female's menstrual cycle. For example, for someone who weighs 170 pounds before a session and 168 pounds afterward, the loss is 2 pounds (32 ounces). Because fluid equaling 150% of the lost weight is needed for rehydration (see p. 79), this athlete should consume 40 to 48 oz (1,120-1,420 ml) of fluid to achieve euhydration. Testing the first urine of the morning for color, assessing USG, and noting changes in body weight should provide enough information to detect any changes in water balance (Sawka et al. 2007).

Hydration and Performance

It is especially important that athletes pay close attention to fluid and electrolyte balance during aerobic endurance exercise because of the increased likelihood of becoming dehydrated, becoming overheated, or experiencing the consequences of altered electrolyte balance. While many think of running and distance cycling as *the* aerobic endurance sports, athletes who play American football, soccer, hockey, and a variety of other sports also have an increased risk for dehydration, heat illness, and low blood sodium levels.

Compared to the attention given to fluid balance in aerobic endurance athletes, significantly less attention has been paid to fluid balance during strength and power exercise. A plausible explanation is that athletes are more likely to become dehydrated during long bouts of aerobic exercise; the short duration of many strength and power events, in addition to readily available fluids, makes dehydration less of a concern.

Aerobic Endurance Exercise

Maintaining fluid and electrolyte balance is crucial for individuals who engage in aerobic endurance exercise. In fact, a fluid loss of a mere 2% of body weight has been shown to reduce exercise performance in both hot and temperate environments (Maughan and Shirreffs 2008). However, in one study of Ironman triathletes, a 3% reduction in body mass during competition had no adverse effects on thermoregulation or body temperature (Institute of Medicine 2005), indicating that some athletes may be better regulators of heat and require different fluid strategies.

Before Exercise

It is important for people to begin exercise euhydrated and with normal electrolyte levels. Good hydration practices during the day, focusing on the consumption of fluids and high water content foods such as fruits and vegetables, should be the main goal. If at least 8 to 12 hours have passed since the last exercise session and fluid consumption is sufficient, the individual should be close to a euhydrated state. On the other hand, for someone who has lost a significant amount of fluid and has not replenished with fluids and electrolytes in the amounts needed to establish euhydration, an aggressive preexercise hydration protocol is in order (Sawka et al. 2007).

At least 4 hours before exercise, athletes should consume approximately 5 to 7 ml fluid per kilogram body weight. They should consume more fluid slowly, approximately 3 to 5 ml/kg body weight, 2 hours before exercise if the individual is not urinating or if the urine is dark (Sawka et al. 2007). Consuming sodium-rich foods at this time can help stimulate thirst and retain fluids. If sodium is consumed in a beverage, the recommended amount is 20 to 50 mEq (460-1,150 mg) per liter (Swaka et al. 2007).

A common practice before an event is for athletes to attempt to hyperhydrate with water. This practice is not advised because it increases the risk of urination during the event and could dilute the sodium levels in the body, thus increasing the risk of hyponatremia (Laursen et al. 2006). For promotion of a euhydrated state before training or competition, fluid palatability is of utmost importance. Palatability or the lack of it will contribute to or detract from preexercise hydration strategies. The fluids should typically be lightly sweetened, should contain sodium, and should be cool in temperature.

During Exercise

The goal of drinking during exercise is to prevent excessive dehydration (greater than 2% of body weight from water loss) and excessive changes in electrolyte balance (Sawka et al. 2007). Although fluid replacement strategies are highly individualized, athletes should aim for 3 to 8 ounces (90 to 240 ml) of a 6% to 8% carbohydrate–electrolyte beverage every 10 to 20 minutes during exercise lasting longer than 60 to 90 minutes. This will assist in hydration and promote better performance during prolonged exercise (Sawka et al. 2007; Jeukendrup, Jentjens, and Moseley 2005).

It is well known that consuming carbohydrate during exercise maintains blood glucose levels and reduces fatigue. A sport drink typically contains the following (Institute of Medicine 2005; Jeukendrup, Jentjens, and Moseley 2005):

- 20 to 50 mEq of sodium (460-1,150 mg) per liter
- 2 to 5 mEq of potassium (78-195 mg) per liter
- About 6% to 8% carbohydrate concentration

Energy bars, gels, and other foods, depending on a person's needs and preferences, can also supply this combination (Institute of Medicine 1994). Consuming beverages with sodium (20-50 mEq/L fluid) or snacks containing sodium will help stimulate thirst and retain water (Ray et al. 1998). In addition to sodium, a sport beverage with protein may also increase fluid retention. In a study examining fluid retention after dehydration (2.5% body weight loss), researchers gave 13 subjects beverages containing carbohydrate plus protein (6% and 1.5%, respectively), carbohydrate only (6% solution), or water at a volume equal to body weight loss over a 3-hour recovery period. Fluid retention was significantly higher for the carbohydrate–protein group than for the carbohydrate group. Both carbohydrate–protein and carbohydrate only were better than water for rehydration. The authors concluded that fluid retention after consumption of a carbohydrate–protein beverage was 15% greater than after consumption of a carbohydrate-only beverage and 40% greater than after consumption of water (Seifert, Harmon, and DeClercq 2006).

After Exercise

After exercise, the goal is to fully replenish any fluid and electrolyte deficit from the exercise bout (Sawka et al. 2007). Athletes must consume 150% of the lost weight to achieve normal hydration within 6 hours after exercise (Maughan and Shirreffs 2008). Therefore, practically speaking, the recommendation is to ingest 20 to 24 ounces (600 to 720 ml) of fluids for every pound of body weight lost during training. Though plain water is effective for rehydration, athletes should consider a sport drink or consume their water with foods that contain electrolytes such as sodium and chloride to replace electrolyte losses (Dunford 2006).

Some research studies have shown that as a whole, alcoholic and caffeinated beverages have diuretic effects; but such effects are transient, and therefore these beverages do contribute to daily hydration recommendations. However, if rapid rehydration is the goal postexercise, it is advisable to avoid alcoholic and caffeinated beverages in the first few hours after activity (Dunford 2006). The fluid chosen in the postexercise period should promote rapid rehydration.

Depending on the amount of time before the next exercise session, consuming sodium-rich foods and beverages with water after competition or a training session should suffice. Sodium is one of the key nutrients athletes should consume in the postexercise period to return to a euhydrated state because it will help retain ingested fluids and stimulate thirst. While sweat sodium losses differ among individuals, which can make individual sodium prescription difficult during this period, a little extra salt added to meals or snacks may be particularly useful for those with high sweat sodium losses (Swaka et al. 2007).

Strength and Power Performance

While a plethora of studies have led to specific recommendations for fluid consumption and measuring hydration status in aerobic endurance athletes, fewer studies have looked at the effects of dehydration on strength and power. Collectively, these studies have yielded mixed results; some indicate that mild dehydration can affect certain aspects of performance, and others suggest that even severe dehydration has no effect. The varying results may be due, in part, to differences in methodology and measures obtained.

In one study, scientists examined the effects of progressive dehydration on strength and power as measured by strength, jump capacity, and neuromuscular function. Twelve recreationally active men completed six bouts of resistance exercise in a progressive state of hypohydration caused by jogging in the heat. No differences were noted in vertical jump height, electromyography data, or isokinetic leg extension at a rate of 120°. However, when subjects lost 1% of their body mass through hypohydration, isometric leg extensions were significantly reduced. At a 2.6% reduction in body mass from hypohydration, isokinetic leg extensions at a rate of 30° were significantly reduced. No dose–response effects were noted in any tested variables except at threshold for isometric and isokinetic strength at 30° (Hayes and Morse 2010). Another study examined the effect of euhydration versus progressive dehydration (2.5% and 5% drop in body mass) on vertical jump height, jump squat, and isometric back squat. No differences were noted between trials in all of these measures. However, hypohydration (at both 2.5% and 5% drops in body mass) significantly decreased resistance exercise performance during sets of a six-set back squat protocol (Judelson et al. 2007b).

In contrast to this study are others that show absolutely no effect of dehydration on strength and muscular endurance. One crossover study measured changes in isometric muscular strength and endurance after a 4% drop in body mass due to dehydration through intermittent sauna exposure in seven men. The authors observed no effect even though this level of dehydration is twice the critical cutoff point most often recommended for athletes competing in aerobic endurance exercise (Greiwe et al. 1998).

While the studies on dehydration and strength and power have provided mixed results, after accounting for methodological differences, researchers reviewing the evidence found that hypohydration appears to decrease strength by approximately 2%, power by approximately 3%, and high-intensity endurance by approximately 10% (Judelson et al. 2007a). In addition to these noted changes in performance, many sports are multifaceted and require muscular endurance, strength, and aerobic endurance, and therefore hypohydration will likely affect performance in these sports. Therefore, dehydration is likely to affect one or more variables contributing to athletic performance. For example, an athlete on a lightweight crew team who dehydrates in order to make weight may be able to participate, but her performance may be subpar at best. In addition, depending on the climate conditions, she may be putting herself at an increased risk of heat illness.

In addition to potentially hampering one's aerobic and muscular endurance and increasing the risk of heat illness, dehydration may increase an athlete's risk of developing rhabdomyolysis, a potentially very serious injury to skeletal muscle that results in leakage of large quantities of intracellular contents to plasma (Beetham 2000; Knochel 1992; Bergeron et al. 2005).

Strength Training

Resistance exercise is associated with unique metabolic demands. However, very little research has evaluated the effect of dehydration on strength training, and there is no clear consensus on whether dehydration decreases muscle performance. In one study investigating the effects of hydration on markers of metabolism, data indicated that inducing a hypohydrated state (up to 4.8%) changed the endocrine and metabolic internal environments before and after the training bout. Specifically, catabolic hormones, cortisol, epinephrine, and norepinephrine increased, which altered the postexercise anabolic response (Judelson et al. 2008). These data suggest that a dehydrated state enhances the stress of a resistance exercise session and may interfere with training adaptations.

Another study addressing the effect of hypohydration on muscle damage, which measured myoglobin and creatine kinase specifically, showed no significant differences in these markers of muscle damage in a euhydrated or a 2.5% or 5.0% hypohydrated state. However, although the finding was not statistically significant, the authors noted that the more dehydrated the participants were, the less total work they performed (Yamamoto et al. 2008).

In summary, while some data indicate that hydration would benefit athletes performing resistance training, it is not yet possible to devise a scientifically based hydration protocol. Therefore, resistance-trained athletes should be encouraged to emphasize good hydration techniques throughout the day in an effort to remain as hydrated as possible before, during, and after training.

Age-Related Fluid Needs

The two population groups that have an increased risk of dehydration and heat illness are children and the elderly. Because these two groups are more likely to experience hydration-related issues and, in the case of elderly persons, alterations in electrolyte balance, it is imperative that sport nutritionists be aware of the issue in these populations and also educate parents and coaches.

Children

Fluid needs for children are more challenging and problematic than for adults because little published research is available on this age group. Several factors contribute to an increased risk of heat illness in children. Children and adolescents generate more heat per unit body mass than adults (Falk, Bar-Or, and MacDougall 1992). Additionally, once a child is dehydrated, his or her core body temperature increases to a greater extent than in an adult (Unnithan and Goulopoulou 2004). Furthermore, voluntary dehydration (not ingesting enough fluid when it is offered during exercise) is very common in children (Bar-Or et al. 1992). Further contributing to the increased risk of heat illness in children is the fact that they have more heat-activated sweat glands per unit skin area (Falk, Bar-Or, and MacDougall 1992) but their sweat rate is lower per sweat gland than in adults (Falk, Bar-Or, and MacDougall 1992; Bar-Or 1980), and they seem to accumulate more heat from the environment (Petrie, Stover, and Horswill 2004). Additionally, the sweating threshold is higher in children than in adults, and more sodium and chloride are lost in sweat (Meyer et al. 1992).

A few studies on children and adolescents have shown that sweat rate per hour ranges from 510 to 1,260 ml, or 17.2 to 42.6 ounces (Ballauff, Kersting, and Manz 1988; Bar-Or 1989; Sawka and Pandolf 1990). Dehydration of 2% of body weight in adults seems to decrease work capacity and decrease performance, whereas a mere 1% dehydration has the same effects in children (Kenney et al. 1990). Therefore, it is very important to provide as much of an individual fluid prescription to active children as possible. General fluid recommendations in the heat include drinking until the child does not feel thirsty plus another 4 ounces and 8 ounces (120 and 240 ml) for children and adolescents, respectively (Unnithan and Goulopoulou 2004). Children should drink 4 to 8 ounces of fluid before activity, 4 ounces every 15 minutes during exercise, and at least 16 ounces (480 ml) after exercise to promote rehydration (Bar-Or et al. 1997). Taste is a critical component in beverages for children. Lightly flavored beverages containing sodium and carbohydrate enhance thirst and effectively reduce or prevent voluntary dehydration in boys. Interestingly, girls may be less prone to voluntary dehydration due to their lower sweat rates (Bar-Or 1996). However, adequate fluid replacement strategies still apply to girls.

Elderly Persons

Fluid and electrolyte imbalances are common in older adults because aging is associated with certain physiological changes in renal adaptation, blood flow responses, sweat rates, thirst sensation, and fluid and electrolyte status that all affect thermoregulation (Rosenbloom and Dunaway 2007). Age-related changes include decreased renal functioning, which can cause kidney water excretion to be higher than in younger adults (Rolls and

Phillips 1990). Additionally, aging leads to structural changes in the blood vessels that decrease blood flow to the skin as a means to dissipate heat. In fact, older adults can have between 25% and 40% less skin blood flow at a given thermic load than younger adults (Kenney et al. 1990). Finally, elderly individuals may have lower sweat rates and may also begin sweating later in an exercise session in comparison to younger adults (Kenney and Fowler 1988). These three changes can predispose older individuals to fluid imbalances, especially when an exercise stimulus is introduced. Additional renal changes due to biological aging include

- a decline in glomerular filtration rate (GFR) (a measure of kidney function indicating the rate at which blood is being filtered by the kidneys),
- reduced urinary concentrating ability (Tarnopolsky 2008),
- less efficient sodium-conserving ability (Reaburn 2000), and
- decreased ability to excrete a large amount of water (Rolls and Phillips 1990).

All of these changes reduce fluid and electrolyte homeostasis, which can predispose people who are elderly to hypovolemia (an abnormal decrease in blood volume) and dehydration (Rosenbloom and Dunaway 2007, Rolls and Phillips 1990).

Elderly persons are also at risk for **hypernatremia**, an increase in plasma sodium concentrations greater than 145 mEq/L. This can result from an excessive loss of water and electrolytes caused by polyuria (excessive urine production), diarrhea, excessive sweating, or inadequate water intake. However, for many elderly individuals, the age-related decrease in thirst may be the primary cause (Epstein and Hollenberg 1976). Although the extent of hypernatremia in the elderly has not been established, it seems that when fluid choices are palatable and no illness is present, elderly persons have no problem maintaining fluid balance during sedentary conditions. Drinking plentiful fluids and eating a reduced-sodium diet can be a dangerous combination for older adults because they may become overhydrated due to a decreased ability to retain sodium and excrete water (Crowe et al. 1987; Kenney and Chiu 2001; Thompson, Burd, and Baylis 1987).

➤ hypernatremia—Elevated blood sodium typically caused by dehydration.

Elderly individuals are less able to regulate the amount of fluid in the body in cases of fluid deprivation or overhydration. And, as already mentioned, urinary concentrating ability decreases (Tarnopolsky 2008; Seckl, Williams, and Lightman 1986; Burrell, Palmer, and Baylis 1992), as well as the ability to excrete a high amount of water (Phillips et al. 1993a). In one study comparing healthy younger and older individuals in a dehydrated state, the older group had a decreased thirst sensation with 24 hours of fluid deprivation, whereas the younger group showed a strong thirst response (Tarnopolsky 2008). The elderly group displayed no increase in mouth dryness, increase in thirst, or unpleasantness of taste in the mouth. Taken together, these data along with other findings, indicate that elderly persons are predisposed to dehydration (Phillips et al. 1993b).

The recommendation is that rehydration periods be longer for older adults, in comparison to younger adults, after they have experienced dehydration (Epstein and Hollenberg 1976). Consumption of fluids should begin early in an exercise session to prevent the onset of dehydration (Campbell and Geik 2004). No published data exist on which to base an exact fluid replacement strategy for elderly people. Fluid replacement guidelines for younger athletes can be used to establish a hydration plan for masters athletes (Rosenbloom and Dunaway 2007).

Professional Applications

Careful monitoring of hydration status and electrolyte balance is crucial not only for athletic performance but also for prevention of heat illness, heatstroke, and hyponatremia. It is therefore essential that sport nutritionists not only help athletes monitor their hydration and electrolyte status but also teach them how to do this for themselves and to be aware of the signs of dehydration, overheating, and hyponatremia.

Athletes can do two easy things to assess their hydration status. First, they should pay attention to the frequency of urination, urine color, and quantity. Urine should be pale yellow and plentiful (though consuming B vitamins in the form of a B complex, multivitamin, or functional food can make urine brighter and darker). Athletes should also get into the habit of weighing themselves before and after each training session. If they lose 2% of their body weight from before to after practice, they need to do a better job hydrating before and during training. For each pound lost, they should consume 20 to 24 ounces (600 to 720 ml) of fluid, preferably in the form of a sport drink or a beverage with added sodium to help maintain blood sodium levels.

Every year, people die from hyponatremia. Though the marathoner who takes a long time to finish (4-5 hours or more) and consumes only water is more likely to suffer from hyponatremia than a basketball player, sport nutritionists should be aware of the potential for hyponatremia in a wide range of athletes. As an example, a 40-something-year-old ultimate Frisbee player, Mike, was playing in a tournament on a Saturday afternoon when he felt dizzy and confused. His teammates did not recognize that there was a problem until he collapsed. After he was rushed to the emergency room he fell into a coma for a few days, and his father was told he had swelling on his brain. Mike had consumed only water during the tournament and neither salted his food nor ate much processed food (which is often higher in sodium), putting him at an increased risk for hyponatremia. Though he recovered fully from the coma, this situation could have been prevented with proper education.

Dehydration can hamper most kinds of athletic performance, from aerobic endurance exercise to sports requiring explosive power movements. Two groups that need to be closely monitored and educated regarding dehydration and heat illness are children and the elderly. The following are some general hydration recommendations for athletes, which should be adapted as necessary to meet the unique needs of the sport and the individual:

- At least 4 hours before exercise, athletes need to drink approximately 5 to 7 ml fluid per kilogram body weight and approximately 3 to 5 ml per kilogram body weight 2 hours beforehand if they are not urinating or if the urine is dark (Sawka et al. 2007).

- The fluid consumed before exercise should contain 20 to 50 mEq (460-1,150 mg) of sodium per liter (Swaka et al. 2007).

- Athletes should consume between 3 and 8 ounces (90 and 240 ml) of a 6% to 8% carbohydrate–electrolyte beverage every 10 to 20 minutes during exercise lasting longer than 60 to 90 minutes (Sawka et al. 2007; Jeukendrup, Jentjens, and Moseley 2005).

- Athletes should choose a sport drink that contains 20 to 50 mEq of sodium (460-1,150 mg) per liter, 2 to 5 mEq of potassium (78-195 mg) per liter, and about 6% to 8% carbohydrate concentration for use during exercise (Institute of Medicine 2005; Jeukendrup, Jentjens, and Moseley 2005).

- For those with high sweat rates and sweat sodium concentrations, commercial sport drinks may not contain enough sodium to assist with preventing hyponatremia. In general, it is recommended that athletes choose a sport drink containing a minimum of 20 mEq of sodium (460 mg) per liter of fluid.

- Athletes should consume 20 to 24 ounces (600 to 720 ml) of fluid for every pound of body weight lost after training. Plain water should be used only after exercise when it is combined with foods that contain sodium (Dunford 2006).

SUMMARY POINTS

- Fluids are of utmost importance to maintaining good health and performance for any individual participating in sport. Many variables affect hydration needs and status; thus proper timing and implementation of different hydration and rehydration strategies throughout the training year are important in order to fine-tune individual fluid prescriptions.

- Normal hydration is essential for athletic performance and normal cardiovascular and thermoregulatory functions. Dehydration greater than 2% of body weight can impair athletic performance. Dehydration also increases the risk of heat illness.

- Athletes may want to consider ingesting a sport drink that contains protein to enhance rehydration during the recovery period after exercise (Seifert, Harmon, and DeClercq 2006).

- There is no conclusive evidence of significant performance decrements in resistance training when it is performed in a hypohydrated state. Resistance-trained athletes should be encouraged to emphasize good hydration techniques throughout the day in an effort to remain as hydrated as possible before and after a training session.

- Factors associated with hyponatremia include overdrinking hypotonic fluids, an excessive loss of sodium through sweat, and extensive sweating with the ingestion of low-sodium fluids. In general, hyponatremia in events lasting less than 4 hours can be attributed to drinking too much fluid and taking in too little sodium before, during, and sometimes after the event (Laursen et al. 2006).

- Athletes should limit fluid intake to only what is needed to minimize dehydration and should consume sodium-rich foods and beverages during exercise longer than 2 hours in order to prevent excessive drinking and hyponatremia (Speedy, Noakes, and Schneider 2001).

- General fluid recommendations for children include drinking until the child does not feel thirsty plus another 4 ounces and 8 ounces (120 and 240 ml) for children and adolescents, respectively (Unnithan and Goulopoulou 2004). Children should drink 4 to 8 ounces of fluid before exercise, 4 ounces every 15 minutes during exercise, and at least 16 ounces (480 ml) after exercise to promote rehydration (Bar-Or et al. 1997).

- No current data provide the basis for an exact fluid replacement strategy for elderly persons; fluid replacement guidelines for younger athletes can be used to establish a hydration plan for masters athletes (Rosenbloom and Dunaway 2007).

6

Vitamins and Minerals

Henry C. Lukaski, PhD, FACSM, FCASN

The growing awareness of the synergy between diet and physical activity stimulates interest in the roles that **micronutrients** (vitamins and minerals) play in the attainment of health and peak physical performance. Evidence of increased activity of micronutrient-dependent and energy-producing metabolic pathways, biochemical adaptations in tissues, and elevated rates of turnover and losses has built interest in the interaction of micronutrient nutrition and physical activity (Rodriguez, DiMarco, and Langley 2009). The food content of vitamins and minerals is small (micrograms [µg] to milligrams [mg]) compared to that of protein, carbohydrate, and fat (up to hundreds of grams [g]). Micronutrients, however, exert potent biological effects as components of proteins. In this capacity, micronutrients enable the complex reactions that are required to utilize the potential energy in macronutrients to fuel the biological processes inherent in physical training and recovery (Lukaski 2004; Volpe 2007).

> ➤ micronutrient—A mineral, vitamin, or other substance that is essential, even in very small quantities, for growth or metabolism.

The Dietary Reference Intakes (DRIs) are recommendations for intake to prevent nutritional inadequacy that could lead to deficiency and impair health and function (Institute of Medicine, Food and Nutrition Board [IOM] 1997, 1998, 2000, 2001, 2005, 2003). The Recommended Dietary Allowance (RDA) is a value that meets the needs of ~98% of healthy people, whereas the Adequate Intake (AI) is the value that is set sufficiently high to prevent inadequacy. An RDA is calculated from data derived from rigorous scientific studies; the AI is derived from less complete research information. Importantly, physical activity was considered a factor in the DRI for only one-third of the nutrients (tables 6.1 and 6.2).

TABLE 6.1   Exercise-Related Functions and Recommended Dietary Allowances (RDAs) of Micronutrients for Individuals (19-50 years)

Nutrient	Function	RDA Males	RDA Females	Physical activity considered	Activity effect on requirement
Vitamins					
Thiamin (B$_1$), mg	Reactions in energy production pathways	1.2	1.1	Yes	Limited evidence[a]
Riboflavin (B$_2$), mg	Electron transfer in oxidative production	1.3	1.1	No	Small effect[b]
Niacin, NE*	Electron transfer in oxidative energy production	16	14	No	–
Pyridoxine (B$_6$), mg	Amino acid and glycogen breakdown	1.3	1.3	Yes	Small effect[c]
Cyanocobalamin (B$_{12}$), µg	Folate recycling and hemoglobin synthesis	2.4	2.4	No	–
Folate, µg DFE*	Cell regeneration and hemoglobin synthesis	400	400	No	–
Ascorbic acid (vitamin C), mg	Antioxidant	90	75	Yes	No demonstrated effect[d]
Retinol (vitamin A), µg RAE*	Antioxidant	900	700	No	–
Tocopherol (vitamin E), mg	Antioxidant	15	15	Yes	–
Minerals					
Iron, mg	Aerobic energy production	8	18	Yes	Increased need[e]
Magnesium, mg	Aerobic energy production	400	310	Yes	Limited effect[f]
Zinc, mg	Energy metabolism and gas exchange	11	8	No	Limited effect[g]
Copper, µg	Iron metabolism, aerobic energy production, and antioxidant	900	900	No	–
Phosphorus, mg	Energy metabolism	700	700	No	–
Selenium, µg	Antioxidant	55	55	No	–

Nutrient	Function	RDA Males	RDA Females	Physical activity considered	Activity effect on requirement
Iodine, µg	Energy metabolism	150	150	No	–
Molybdenum, µg	Unknown	45	45	No	–

*NE = niacin equivalents; DFE = dietary folate equivalents (1 µg folate from food or 0.6 µg folic acid from fortified foods or supplements); RAE = retinol activity equivalents (1 µg retinol = 12 µg beta-carotene) (Institute of Medicine, Food and Nutrition Board 1998).

[a]Limited evidence of increased need with prolonged exercise.

[b]Increased performance with B_2 supplementation of low-status subjects; otherwise inconsistent results.

[c]Based on decreases in B_6 status in athletes and not requirement per se.

[d]Based on physical activity and vitamin C status.

[e]Increase intake for regular heavy, intense exercise (30-70%); beneficial effects in iron-deficient, nonanemic women.

[f]Limited evidence of an effect of magnesium depletion on some measures of performance.

[g]Limited evidence of an effect of low zinc status on some measures of performance.

TABLE 6.2 Exercise-Related Functions and Adequate Intakes (AIs) of Micronutrients for Individuals (19-50 years)

Nutrient	Function	AI Males	AI Females	Physical activity considered	Activity effect on requirement
Vitamins					
Vitamin D, µg	Calcium absorption and utilization	5	5	No	–
Vitamin K, µg	Clotting and bone formation	120	90	No	–
Biotin, µg	Gluconeogenesis	30	30	No	–
Pantothenic acid, mg	Glycogen synthesis	5	5	No	–
Choline, mg	Acetylcholine, creatine, and lecithin formation	550	425	Yes	Possible effects[a]
Minerals					
Calcium, mg	Bone formation	1,000	1,000	Yes	Insufficient evidence
Fluoride, mg	Unknown	4	3	No	–
Chromium, µg	Facilitate insulin	35	25	No	–
Manganese, mg	Antioxidant	2.3	1.8	No	–
Sodium, g	Fluid regulation, nerve conduction, and muscle contraction	1.5	1.5	Yes	–
Potassium, g	Fluid regulation, glucose transport, glycogen storage, and ATP production	4.7	4.7	No	–
Chloride, g	Fluid regulation, nerve conduction, and muscle contraction	2.3	2.3	Yes	–

[a]Strenuous exercise decreased plasma choline concentrations; supplements slightly increased performance.

This chapter provides an overview of the biological roles of vitamins and minerals in support of physiological function during exercise, and it highlights the effects of reduced micronutrient status on measures of physical performance. The chapter also identifies the points at which micronutrients can affect metabolism during physical activity and outlines the effects of reduced intakes of micronutrients on physical activity.

Micronutrient Requirements for Athletes

Micronutrients include vitamins, which are **organic compounds**, and minerals, which are inorganic elements that exist as solids; they cannot be produced by the body and thus must be consumed in food and beverages. Micronutrients form bioactive compounds, generally proteins. They are not direct sources of energy but facilitate energy production and utilization from carbohydrate, fat, and protein; transport oxygen and carbon dioxide; regulate fluid balance; and protect against oxidative damage. As shown in figure 6.1, many of the B vitamins (thiamin, riboflavin, niacin, B_6, and pantothenic acid) and some minerals (iron, magnesium, copper, and zinc) are needed for the metabolism of carbohydrate into energy for muscle work. Iron, copper, B_6, B_{12}, and folate are required for red blood cell (RBC) formation and oxygen (O_2) transport to muscle cells. Zinc is essential for removal of carbon dioxide (CO_2) from working muscle and recycling of lactate to glucose. In the adrenal gland, vitamin C is necessary for the production of epinephrine, which acts to release free fatty acids (FFA) from adipose tissue. Niacin may block the release of FFA during exercise. Vitamins C and E, beta-carotene, and some minerals (zinc, copper, and manganese) neutralize reactive oxygen species (ROS) and prevent free radical damage in muscle and other tissues.

➤ organic compounds—Compounds made mostly of carbon atoms.

Evaluation of micronutrient needs for optimal physical performance requires concurrent assessment of nutrient intake and biochemical measures of nutritional status (Lukaski 2004). Only a limited number of investigations have met these criteria. Sole reliance on self-reported food intake to characterize nutritional status is problematic because of underreporting of food intake (Magkos and Yannakoulia 2003). Assessment of the adequacy of micronutrient intakes relies on the appropriate DRI (RDA or AI) (IOM 2003). Low micronutrient intakes generally result in subclinical deficiencies characterized by decreased biochemical indicators of nutritional status and impaired physiological function. Figure 6.2 presents an overview of how a subclinical deficiency of several minerals (zinc, iron, riboflavin, and magnesium) leads to reductions in exercise performance and markers of performance. Overt or clinical deficiency is rare without excess loss or impaired absorption (IOM 1997, 1998, 2000, 2001).

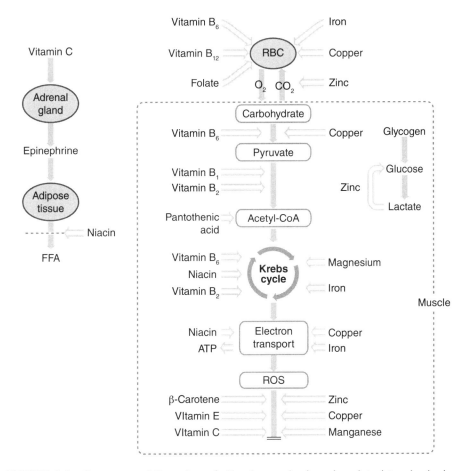

FIGURE 6.1 Summary of the roles of vitamins and minerals related to physical performance.

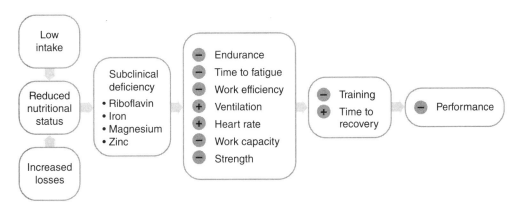

FIGURE 6.2 Outline of the effects of reduced micronutrient nutrition on aspects of physical performance.

Vitamins and Performance

Thirteen vitamins are required for life. They are described as water or fat soluble. Adequate intake of B vitamins (water-soluble vitamins) is important to ensure optimum energy production and the building and repair of muscle tissue (Woolf and Manore 2006). The B-complex vitamins have several major functions directly related to exercise—energy production during exercise and the production of red blood cells, as well as involvement in protein synthesis and in tissue repair and maintenance including the central nervous system. Despite these important roles for vitamins, few studies on vitamin intakes have directly pointed to ergogenic value for athletes. However, some vitamins may help athletes tolerate training to a greater degree by reducing oxidative damage (vitamins E, C), help to maintain a healthy immune system during heavy training (vitamin C), or both. The following sections provide more detail on the specific roles that the vitamins play in an athlete's diet and performance outcomes.

Water-Soluble Vitamins

There are nine **water-soluble** vitamins (eight B vitamins and vitamin C). Their solubility in water limits their storage in the body for extended periods of time. Excessive intake of water-soluble vitamins in supplement form results in excretion of the excess in urine.

➤ water soluble—Capable of being dissolved in water.

Thiamin

Thiamin is the common term for vitamin B_1. The **biologically active** form of B_1 is thiamin pyrophosphate, which acts as a **coenzyme** in the metabolism of carbohydrate and protein to produce energy (IOM 1998). It converts pyruvate to acetyl coenzyme A and α-ketoglutarate to succinyl coenzyme A in the Krebs cycle for oxidative energy production, particularly during exercise (table 6.1). It also participates in the decarboxylation (removal of a CO_2 group) of branched-chain amino acids that contributes to energy production in muscle. Thiamin is widely distributed in foods, including whole grains and enriched cereals and breads, beans, green leafy vegetables, pork, sunflower seeds, and oranges.

➤ biologically active—Referring to a specific substance that has an effect on the metabolic activity of living cells.

➤ coenzyme—Any small molecule that is necessary for the functioning of an enzyme.

The RDA for thiamin is 1.2 and 1.1 mg/day for men and women, respectively, and is also related to energy intake, 0.5 mg/1,000 kcal per day (IOM

1998). According to the research, female gymnasts and wrestlers consume less than RDA levels of vitamin B_1 (Short and Short 1983; Loosli and Benson 1990; Economos, Bortz, and Nelson 1993). Thus, athletes who consume low-energy diets to meet weight standards appear to be at risk for low thiamin status. Evidence of an adverse effect of low thiamin intake is lacking. In a classic study it was reported that neither muscle strength nor running performance was adversely affected in young men fed diets with variable thiamin content (0.23, 0.33, 0.53, and 0.63 mg/1,000 kcal per day) (Keys et al. 1943). Men fed 0.5 and 5 mg thiamin showed no change in aerobic endurance capacity despite impaired biochemical markers of thiamin status (decreased erythrocyte transketolase activity and increased thiamin pyrophosphate activity) (Wood et al. 1980). Other studies failed to show a benefit of supplemental thiamin on muscle strength or exercise performance despite improvements in thiamin nutritional status (Fogelholm et al. 1993; Doyle, Webster, and Erdmann 1997; Webster 1998).

Riboflavin

Riboflavin is the common term for vitamin B_2. Riboflavin functions in the mitochondrial electron transport system as the coenzymes flavin mononucleotide (FMN) and flavin adenine dinucleotide (FAD). These enzymes participate in the transfer of electrons from breakdown of carbohydrate and fat to formation of adenosine triphosphate (ATP). Riboflavin is also necessary for the conversion of vitamin B_6 to its active form (IOM 1998). Food sources of riboflavin include milk and dairy products, eggs, whole grains and cereals, lean meats, broccoli, yogurt, whey protein, and almonds.

The RDA for riboflavin intake is 1.3 and 1.1 mg/day for men and women, respectively, or 0.6 mg/1,000 kcal (IOM 1998). Athletes generally have adequate riboflavin intakes, with the exception of female gymnasts (Short and Short 1983; Loosli and Benson 1990; Economos, Bortz, and Nelson 1993; Beshgetoor and Nichols 2003; Kirchner, Lewis, and O'Connor 1995). Physical training increases riboflavin needs of adults. During training, athletes experience decreased riboflavin status (Fogelholm et al. 1993; Keith and Alt 1991). Metabolic studies of women fed 0.2 compared to 0.6 mg riboflavin daily for 12 weeks, with and without weight loss, showed reduced riboflavin status (decreased erythrocyte glutathione reductase activity) (Belko et al. 1984, 1985). Although gains in peak oxygen uptake after training did not differ with adequate riboflavin intake, the study was not designed to detect performance differences (Belko et al. 1984, 1985). Nineteen percent of adolescent athletes participating in physical training had low riboflavin status at entry; status improved with riboflavin supplementation (2 mg/day, six days a week, for two months), as did physical fitness (Suboticanec et al. 1990). This finding is consistent with a previous observation of improved aerobic endurance performance after supplementation with multiple B vitamins (van der Beek et al. 1994).

Niacin

Niacin is the common term for vitamin B_3. This B vitamin exists as nicotinic acid and nicotinamide, which is metabolized to form nicotinamide adenine nucleotide (NAD) and nicotinamide adenine dinucleotide phosphate (NADP) that serve as coenzymes. The NAD is an electron carrier in the breakdown of carbohydrate, fat, protein, and glycogen to produce ATP; NADP is a hydrogen donor in the pentose phosphate shunt (IOM 1998). High protein content foods are good sources of niacin. Lean meats, fish, poultry, whole-grain products, beans, peanuts, and enriched foods provide ample niacin.

The RDAs for niacin are 14 and 16 mg/day for women and men, respectively (IOM 1998). Although niacin is an essential nutrient for energy metabolism, there is no evidence of any beneficial effect with supplementation at doses exceeding the RDA (Heath 2006). Doses of niacin exceeding 50 mg (compared to the RDA of 14 to 16 mg) administered acutely before exercise blocked fat mobilization and decreased aerobic endurance performance (Pernow and Saltin 1971; Galbo et al. 1976; Murray et al. 1995).

Vitamin B_6

Vitamin B_6 is also commonly referred to as pyridoxine. This term includes all biologically active forms of the vitamin; pyridoxine, pyridoxal, and pyridoxamine are the forms commonly found in foods. Pyridoxal phosphate is a cofactor for enzymes that transform amino acids. It also serves as a cofactor for glycogen phosphorylase that regulates gluconeogenesis and glycogenolysis during exercise (IOM 1998). The highest levels of B_6 are found in high-protein foods (meats, poultry, fish, wheat germ, whole-grain products, and eggs). Other sources are bananas, soybeans, raw carrots, broccoli, spinach, and avocados.

The RDAs for vitamin B_6 are 1.7 and 1.5 mg/day for men and women, respectively (IOM 1998). Approximately one-third of female and 10% of male athletes fail to meet the RDA (Leklem 1990; Manore 2000). Low energy intakes and poor food choices contribute to decreased vitamin B_6 intakes. Surveys of physically active men and women show that 5% to 60% of athletes have decreased B_6 status (Fogelholm et al. 1993; Stacewicz-Sapuntzakis and Borthakur 2006). Aerobic endurance performance did not change in physically active men fed diets containing 2.3 or 22 mg B_6 for nine days (Virk et al. 1999). However, based on increased urinary loss of B_6, data suggest that 1.5 to 2.3 mg of B_6 is needed to maintain adequate B_6 status of adults participating in aerobic endurance training (Fogelholm et al. 1993; Manore 2000).

Folate

Another name for folate is vitamin B_9. This B vitamin acts as a coenzyme for many enzymes facilitating one carbon transfer that is critical for DNA synthesis and amino acid metabolism. It also acts in cell repair and growth, including red blood cell formation (IOM 1998). Dietary sources of folate include green leafy vegetables, fortified cereals, grains, nuts, legumes, liver, and brewer's yeast. Ready-to-eat cereals, bread, and other grain products are good sources of folate.

The RDA for folate is 400 µg of Dietary Folate Equivalents (DFEs) daily. The DFE corresponds to 1 µg of food folate, 0.6 µg of folic acid in fortified foods, or 0.5 µg of folic acid supplement (IOM 1998). Active men have adequate folate intakes, but women tend to consume 130 to 364 µg/day (Woolf and Manore 2006; Keith et al. 1989; Faber and Benade 1991). Among female aerobic endurance athletes, 8% to 33% have low plasma folate concentrations (Matter et al. 1987; Beals and Manore 1998). Plasma folate concentrations were not different between recreational aerobic endurance athletes (median of 8.6 ngl/mL) and gender-matched controls (8.3 ngl/mL) (Herrmann et al. 2005). Folate supplementation of folate-deficient, but not anemic, athletes did not improve physical performance. Female marathoners with low plasma folate (<4.5 ng/ml) supplemented with folate (5 mg/day for 10 weeks) increased hematological parameters but did not improve treadmill performance, cardiorespiratory function, or metabolic response during exercise as compared to placebo-treated, folate-depleted controls (Matter et al. 1987).

Vitamin B_{12}

Vitamin B_{12} is also known as cobalamin. Cobalamin is a general term for the group of cobalt-containing compounds called corrinoids. It functions as a coenzyme for the transfer of methyl groups in the formation of DNA, particularly with folate in the formation of hemoglobin (IOM 1998). Vitamin B_{12} is found only in foods from animal sources such as meats, poultry, fish, eggs, cheese, and milk.

The adult RDA is 2.4 mg/day; the average omnivore diet contains 5 to 15 mg (IOM 1998). Intakes of B_{12} were low in female aerobic endurance athletes (Keith et al. 1989) but adequate in other groups of male and female athletes (Steen et al. 1995; Ziegler, Nelson, and Jonnalagadda 1999). Avoidance of animal-based foods increases the risk for low B_{12} intakes. Evidence of improved performance with B_{12} supplementation is lacking. Early studies clearly established that performance does not improve with B_{12} supplementation. Adolescent males supplemented daily with 50 µg of B_{12} for seven weeks did not improve running performance or work capacity (Montoye et al. 1955). In addition, other supplementation trials with young men undergoing various regimens (injection of 1 mg, three times a week for six weeks [Tin-May-Than et al. 1978] or 0.5 µg/day for six weeks [Read and McGuffin 1983]) failed to show any beneficial effect on strength or aerobic endurance.

Other B Vitamins

Pantothenic acid is a component of coenzyme A that is the major substrate for energy production in the Krebs cycle (table 6.2). It is also involved in gluconeogenesis (IOM 1998). Biotin is a coenzyme involved in amino acid metabolism and a coenzyme for gluconeogenesis (IOM 1998). Pantothenic acid is found in animal and plant products including meats, eggs, legumes, and whole grains. Sources of biotin include egg yolks, liver, legumes, dark green leafy vegetables, nuts, and soybeans.

The RDAs for pantothenic acid and biotin are 5 mg and 30 μg, respectively (IOM 1998). Data on the usual intakes of these B vitamins and biochemical indicators of status are lacking. Supplementation of pantothenic acid (1.8 g/day for seven days) had no beneficial effects on metabolic responses during a 50 km time trial or performance (Webster 1998). Data on the effects of biotin supplementation on performance measures are not available.

Choline functions as a neurotransmitter (acetylcholine) and as a methyl donor in the formation of creatine and a lipid transporter (phosphatidylcholine or lecithin). Although exercise affects plasma choline levels differently (e.g., dependent on intensity and duration), initial evidence suggests that supplemental choline administered regularly during prolonged exercise can improve performance (Deuster and Cooper 2006). More studies are needed to determine if this improvement in performance is consistent and can be repeated.

Vitamin B Complex

Knowledge that B vitamins cumulatively affect energy metabolism has led to research on the effects of supplementation with multiple vitamins on physical performance. Combined restriction of dietary thiamin, riboflavin, and B_6 significantly decreased peak aerobic capacity (~12%), decreased peak power (~10%), and hastened onset of blood lactate accumulation (7%) in trained male cyclists (van der Beek et al. 1994). Although no single B vitamin was identified with any performance impairment, this finding emphasizes the need to view the B vitamins as necessary for optimal performance.

Vitamin C

Vitamin C is also referred to as ascorbic acid. This vitamin has various biological functions that could affect physical performance. Although it does not directly influence enzyme actions, vitamin C is needed to synthesize catecholamines and carnitine, which transports fatty acids into mitochondria for energy production. It reduces inorganic iron for absorption in the intestine and serves as a potent **antioxidant** to regenerate vitamin E from its oxidized by-product (IOM 2000). Food sources of vitamin C include fruits and vegetables (especially citrus fruits and green leafy vegetables), such as broccoli, potatoes, tomatoes, and strawberries.

> antioxidant—A substance that prevents damage caused by free radicals. Free radicals are highly reactive chemicals that often contain oxygen. They are produced when molecules are split to give products that have unpaired electrons. This process is called oxidation.

The RDA for ascorbic acid is 90 and 75 mg for men and women, respectively (IOM 2000). Physiological stressors increase vitamin C needs. Although many athletes consume adequate amounts of vitamin C, 10% to 30% of male collegiate athletes and female aerobic endurance athletes consume less than the RDA (Keith 2006). Up to 15% of athletes have plasma vitamin C concentrations indicative of deficiency (Telford et al. 1992). In a classic study, it was demonstrated that low vitamin C status impairs performance. Adolescents consuming a low vitamin C diet and then supplemented with vitamin C (100 mg/day for four months) improved work capacity by 48% compared to placebo-treated, low vitamin C controls, whose work capacity increased only by 12% (Lemmel 1938). Vitamin C–deficient adults supplemented with vitamin C (500 mg/day for two weeks or RDA levels for eight weeks) significantly increased work efficiency and aerobic power during treadmill exercise (van der Beek et al. 1990; Johnston, Swan, and Corte 1999).

Fat-Soluble Vitamins

Vitamins A, D, E, and K are associated with sources of dietary fat and stored in adipose tissue (IOM 1997, 2000, 2001). These **fat-soluble** vitamins have no direct role in energy production (tables 6.1 and 6.2). Vitamins A and E act as antioxidants in reversing the age-associated decreases in protein synthesis in rodent models (Marzani et al. 2008), and vitamin D status may be related to muscle strength. There is no evidence linking vitamin K to physical performance.

> fat soluble—Capable of being dissolved in fat.

Vitamin A

The physiologically active form of vitamin A is retinol, which can be formed from beta-carotene, a provitamin. Vitamin A protects epithelial cells from damage, plays an important role in vision, and helps maintain immune function (IOM 2001). Its role in exercise is as an antioxidant. Dietary sources of vitamin A include liver, butter, cheese, eggs, and fortified dairy products. Beta-carotene, the precursor of retinol, is found in yellow-orange vegetables and fruits, as well as dark green leafy vegetables.

Different chemical forms of vitamin A (retinol, beta-carotene, and other carotenoids) contribute to meeting the RDA, which is expressed as retinol equivalents (REs). The RDA is 900 RE or 4,500 IU for men, and 700 RE or 3,500 IU for women (IOM 2001). Athletes generally report vitamin A intakes in excess of the RDA. Distance runners (Peters et al. 1986), professional ballet dancers (Cohen et al. 1985), and female (Welch et al. 1987) and male collegiate athletes (Guilland et al. 1989; Niekamp and Baer 1995) have adequate intakes of vitamin A. Some studies that have investigated adolescents and young adults (wrestlers [Steen and McKinney 1986], ballerinas [Benson et al. 1985], and gymnasts [Loosli et al. 1986]) reported that these athletes tend to consume only 30% to 40% of the RDA for vitamin A, which is attributable to avoidance of dietary fat. Conversely, other studies have reported that vitamin A intakes were adequate in adolescent gymnasts and ballet dancers (Soric et al. 2008; Filaire and Lac 2002). Surveys of international athletes show no evidence of low plasma retinol values but do indicate variable ranges (Stacewicz-Sapuntzakis and Borthakur 2006). The effects of vitamin A supplementation on physical performance are not intensively studied. An early study reported no change in running performance of men maintained on a low vitamin A diet for six months followed by a six week repletion phase (Wald, Brougha, and Johnson 1942).

Vitamin E

Vitamin E is sometimes referred to as α-tocopherol, though α-tocopherol is just one of the eight isomers within the vitamin E family. The generic term, vitamin E, refers to naturally occurring compounds termed tocopherols and tocotrienols, of which α-tocopherol is considered the most biologically active. Vitamin E serves as an antioxidant in cell membranes and protects against oxidative stress (IOM 2000). Major sources of dietary vitamin E include vegetables, nuts, whole grains, wheat germ, and peanut butter.

The RDA for vitamin E is 15 mg of α-tocopherol for adults (IOM 2001). Surveys of athletes reveal adequate vitamin E intake (diet and supplements) (Economos, Bortz, and Nelson 1993). However, when only dietary sources were considered, 53% of college athletes (Guilland et al. 1989), 50% of adolescent gymnasts (Loosli et al. 1986), and 38% of ballerinas (Benson et al. 1985) consumed less than 70% of the RDA. Interestingly, the mean intake of vitamin E for athletes was 77% of the RDA as compared to only 60% of the RDA among sedentary controls, which suggests a similar, albeit reduced, vitamin E intake among physically active and sedentary individuals (Guilland et al. 1989).

The effects of supplemental vitamin E on physical performance are inconsistent. Vitamin E supplementation did not affect performance during a 1-mile run, bench step test, 400 m swim test, and motor fitness tests of male adolescents supplemented with 400 mg α-tocopherol daily for six weeks (Sharman, Down, and Sen 1971); work capacity and muscle strength of collegiate male swimmers given 1,200 IU vitamin E for 85 days (Shephard et al. 1974); peak oxygen uptake in ice hockey players given 800 mg daily for 50 days (Watt et al. 1974); aerobic endurance and blood lactate response in competitive swimmers given 600 mg daily for six months (Lawrence et al. 1975); or motor fitness tests, cardiorespiratory function during ergocycle tests, and 400 m swim times in male and female trained swimmers given 400 mg daily for six weeks (Sharman, Down, and Norgan 1976). Thus, supplemental vitamin E does not enhance performance. Similarly, among elite cyclists, supplemental α-tocopherol (400 mg) for five months did not improve performance (Rokitzki et al. 1994). In contrast, α-tocopherol (400 mg for 10 weeks)-supplemented men at altitude had lower levels of lactate during exercise compared to the placebo group (Simon-Schnass and Pabst 1988). One potential benefit of supplemental vitamin E, alone or in combination with vitamin C, is decreased production of oxidative stress. Performance effects of these combined antioxidants are inconclusive (Gaeini, Rahnama, and Hamedinia 2006; Aguilo et al. 2007; Ciocoiu, Badescu, and Paduraru 2007).

Vitamin D

Vitamin D is sometimes referred to as cholecalciferol. Although the central role of vitamin D is calcium absorption and bone metabolism (IOM 1997), epidemiological data suggest a role for vitamin D in muscle strength. Vitamin D deficiency has been associated with musculoskeletal pain and neuromuscular dysfunction (Plotnikoff and Quigley 2003; Hoogendijk et al. 2008). Food sources of vitamin D are fortified dairy products, eggs, tuna, salmon, herring, oysters, shrimp, and mackerel. Further, vitamin D synthesis is promoted through sun exposure on skin.

The adequate intake of vitamin D is 5 µg (200 IU) for adults (IOM 1997). Knowledge that vitamin D receptors exist in skeletal muscle raises interest in the interaction of this nutrient and physical performance (Pfeifer, Begerow, and Minne 2002). In a review of athletic performance and vitamin D, the authors indicate that physical and athletic performance is seasonal; it peaks when vitamin D levels peak, declines as they decline, and reaches its nadir when vitamin D levels are at their lowest (Cannell et al. 2009). Consistent with this, athletes who practice and compete indoors while avoiding sun exposure are at risk for decreased vitamin D levels at any time of the year (Cannell et al. 2009, 2008; Holick 2007). Older adults with low serum 25-hydroxy vitamin D concentrations (<40 nmol/L) have decreased lower body strength (Pfeifer, Begerow, and Minne 2002; Bischoff-Ferrari et al. 2004). Whether low vitamin D status predicts impaired strength remains to be determined in younger adults, adolescents, and children. Likewise, associations between supplemental vitamin D and strength gains need to be investigated.

Minerals and Performance

Minerals are inorganic elements that exist as solids (IOM 1997, 2001, 2005). Sodium, potassium, chloride, calcium, phosphorus, magnesium, and sulfur are designated as macrominerals because the recommended intakes exceed 100 mg/day and the body contains more than 5 g. Hormones control the levels of many of the macrominerals in the body. Iron, copper, chromium, selenium, and zinc are termed trace elements because recommended intakes are less than 100 mg/day. Precise mechanisms for absorption and excretion regulate the trace element content of cells. Fluoride, boron, iodine, manganese, and molybdenum are ultratrace elements with intakes less than 5 mg/day (tables 6.1 and 6.2, pp. 88-89).

In contrast to the situation with vitamins, there are burgeoning data on the adverse effects of low intakes of some minerals on measures of physical performance. Research on the interactions among performance, intake, and status of copper, phosphorus, selenium, iodine, molybdenum, potassium, and chloride is lacking. Therefore, this section focuses on iron, magnesium, zinc, and chromium and emphasizes findings since the publication of the DRIs for minerals.

Macrominerals

Minerals fall into two categories: macrominerals and trace minerals. The total mineral content of the body is approximately 4 percent of body weight. Macrominerals are present in the body in larger amounts than trace minerals and include calcium, phosphorus, magnesium, sodium, chloride, and potassium.

Sodium, Potassium, and Chloride

These minerals exist as electrolytes principally in body fluids (IOM 2005). Sodium is an extracellular cation that maintains body fluid and acid–base balance, as well as nerve function. Potassium is predominantly an intracellular cation and regulates water balance, impulse transmission from nerves to muscle, energy utilization in muscle cells, and production of ATP. Chloride is largely an extracellular anion that participates in fluid balance and nerve impulse transmission. Sodium is distributed widely in foods along with chloride. Potassium is found in fruits and vegetables, dairy products, meat, and fish.

Sodium, chloride, and potassium modulate fluid exchange within the body's fluid compartments, allowing a well-regulated exchange of nutrients and waste products between the cell and its external fluid environment. Individualized recommended sodium intakes may depend on sweat rate and sodium losses during exercise. For example, Division I collegiate football players differed in their sodium losses during a "two-a-day" training camp. Specifically, football players with a history of heat cramps lost about two times more sodium in their sweat when compared to football players without a history of heat cramps (Stofan et al. 2005). For most individuals without a history of heat cramps, attainment of the recommended intake of sodium (1.5 g/day) is adequate to maintain sodium balance.

Calcium and Phosphorus

These minerals have key roles in the formation of bone, with more than 90% contained in bone (IOM 1997). Calcium is needed for nerve conduction and muscle contraction, as well as the synthesis and breakdown of glycogen. Phosphorus is present in every cell as a component of DNA, ATP, phosphocreatine, and 2,3 diphosphoglycerate (2,3 DPG) that regulates the release of oxygen to muscles during exercise. Dietary sources of calcium and phosphorus are milk, dairy products, broccoli, kale, turnip greens, nuts, and legumes.

The adequate intake for calcium for adults is 1,000 mg per day. The adult RDA for phosphorus is 700 mg for both men and women. Clinical studies utilizing athletes and calcium supplementation are rare; when conducted, they supply the research participants with an amount of calcium or phosphorus well above the adequate intake or recommended dietary intake for these minerals.

One such study provided 35 mg calcium per kilogram body weight per day for a four-week period in conjunction with 90 minutes of aerobic endurance training per day, five days per week. The investigators assessed the total and free testosterone production in response to the calcium supplementation before and after an intense training routine. At the end of the four-week exercise training and calcium supplementation intervention, there were no significant differences in either total or free testosterone in athletes ingesting the calcium supplement as compared to athletes assigned to an exercise-only group. Scientific data on phosphorus supplementation are more prevalent, but most of the published studies do not support improvements in aerobic endurance exercise performance (Bredle et al. 1988; Kreider et al. 1990).

Magnesium

Bone contains almost 60% of the magnesium in the body. Only a small percentage of magnesium, which exists as a component of more than 300 enzymes, is in soft tissue (IOM 1997). Magnesium regulates many physiological processes, including energy metabolism as a component of adenosine triphosphatase (ATPase) and 2,3 DPG, and gluconeogenesis. Food sources of magnesium include fruits, vegetables, nuts, seafood, and whole-grain and dairy products. Some bottled waters and hard water are practical sources of magnesium.

The RDA for men and women is 400 and 310 mg/day, respectively (IOM 1997). Dietary surveys of athletes reveal that magnesium intakes equal or exceed the RDA for males but not female athletes, who consume 60% to 65% of the RDA (Nielsen and Lukaski 2006). Regardless of gender, athletes participating in sports that have weight classifications, or in which the competition includes an aesthetic component, tended to consume inadequate amounts of dietary magnesium (<55% of the RDA) (Hickson, Schrader, and Trischler 1986). However, magnesium intakes of athletes assessed as they ate in a training center environment exceeded the RDA (Fogelholm et al. 1992).

Loss of magnesium from the body increases after heavy exercise. Intense anaerobic exercise caused 21% more urinary magnesium losses on the day of exercise, as compared to control or nonexercise conditions; values returned to nonexercise levels on the day after the exercise (Deuster et al. 1987). The amount of urinary magnesium was related to the degree of exercise-induced anaerobiosis, indexed by postexercise oxygen consumption and plasma lactate concentration (Deuster et al. 1987). Thus, magnesium needs increase when glycolytic metabolism is dominant.

Magnesium supplementation of competitive athletes can improve cellular function. Among competitive female athletes with plasma magnesium concentrations at the low end of the range of normal values, serum total creatine kinase decreased after training in the women supplemented daily with magnesium (360 mg/day for three weeks) compared to the athletes receiving placebo (Golf, Bohmer, and Nowacki 1993). Serum lactate concentration and oxygen uptake during an exhaustive rowing performance test decreased in elite female rowers with initial low serum magnesium and supplemented with magnesium (360 mg/day) for four weeks, as compared to the rowers receiving placebo (Golf, Bohmer, and Nowacki 1993). In response to a seven-week strength training program, leg strength increased more in young men consuming supplemental magnesium (250 mg) in addition to the magnesium included in the diet (totaling 8 mg/kg body weight) compared to placebo (Brilla and Haley 1992).

Alterations in dietary magnesium affect magnesium nutrition and performance (Lukaski and Nielsen 2002). Women given a controlled low compared to adequate magnesium intake (180 vs. 320 mg) had negative retention (intake – losses) and decreased indicators of magnesium status (red blood cell and muscle magnesium concentrations). During submaximal exercise, heart rate increased (10 beats per minute) and work efficiency decreased (10%) with the low-magnesium intake.

Trace Elements

By definition, trace elements are chemical components that naturally occur in soil, plants, and animals in minute concentrations. Though required in much smaller quantities than macrominerals, trace elements, also known as trace minerals, are necessary for optimal health and performance.

Iron

This metallic element is critical in the formation of compounds needed for oxygen transport and utilization. Hemoglobin, the principal iron-containing compound, transports oxygen to cells. Cellular iron compounds include myoglobin, the cytochromes, and some enzymes in the Krebs cycle (aconitase, NADH dehydrogenase, and succinate dehydrogenase). Almost 30% of iron is stored in tissues, with 70% involved in oxygen metabolism (IOM 2001). Food sources of iron include heme protein (hemoglobin and myoglobin) found in animal flesh foods. Nonheme iron sources include dried fruits, vegetables, legumes, whole-grain products, and fortified cereals. Heme iron is better absorbed and used than nonheme iron (10-35% vs. 2-10%) (IOM 2001). Heme iron absorption is not significantly affected by dietary components (Monsen 1988), whereas nonheme iron absorption is affected (IOM 2001; Hallberg, Hulten, and Gramatkovski 1997). Meat protein and vitamin C both increase the absorption of nonheme iron (IOM 2001; Siegenberg et al. 1991); and tannins (found in tea, wine, and some foods), calcium, polyphenols, and phytates (found in whole grains) decrease the absorption of nonheme iron (IOM 2001; Siegenberg et al. 1991; Cook et al. 1997; Hallberg et al. 1991; South and Mille 1998).

The RDA for iron is 8 and 18 mg/day for men and women, respectively (IOM 2001). Male athletes generally consume adequate amounts of iron, but female athletes participating in aerobic endurance sports or activities requiring low body weight (e.g., ballerinas and gymnasts) tend to consume less than the RDA for iron (Haymes 2006). Iron intakes of female athletes consuming supplements exceed the RDA (Deuster et al. 1986). Low intake of iron is the principal cause of iron deficiency in women.

Iron deficiency occurs in stages. Early tissue iron depletion, characterized by low serum ferritin (<12 µg/L) and increased total iron-binding capacity (>400 µg/dl), is prevalent in 15% to 20% of women and 20% to 37% of female athletes and in 20% to 25% of girls and 25% to 47% of young female athletes. While the <12 µg/L for serum ferritin is accepted as the clinical cutoff, in female athletes the cutoffs for iron depletion range between 20 and 35 µg/L (at least in the practical setting). Low serum ferritin signals increased iron absorption. Next, the iron content of red blood cells decreases; the number of transferrin receptors on cells increases, and then the number of these receptors increases in serum. Elevated soluble serum transferrin receptor (sTfR) concentrations (>8.5 mg/L) indicate a functional iron deficiency. The final stage of iron deficiency is preceded by stage 2 iron deficiency without anemia, or IDNA. The final stage of iron deficiency is **anemia** with decreased hemoglobin (<130 g/L for men and <120 g/L for women). The prevalence of anemia is 5% in women, 5% to 12% in female athletes, and 6% for girls regardless of athletic participation (IOM 2001).

> ➤ anemia—A decrease in the number of red blood cells, which reduces the amount of oxygen transported to the tissues.

It is well established that anemia reduces peak oxygen uptake, reduces work capacity and aerobic endurance, and raises plasma lactate; these impairments are corrected with iron supplementation (Gardner et al. 1977; Edgerton et al. 1981). Controversy, however, exists regarding the effects of

IDNA on performance and metabolism (Haas and Brownlie 2001). Although supplementation trials of female athletes with IDNA showed increased serum ferritin and decreased lactate during exercise without improvements in performance (Matter et al. 1987; Schoene et al. 1983; Lukaski, Hall, and Siders 1991), other studies of adolescent female athletes and women with IDNA showed improved aerobic endurance performance or peak oxygen uptake (Rowland et al. 1988). One factor that could explain the inconsistency in findings is the confounding effect of inflammation that reduces circulating ferritin levels (McClung et al. 2006). To clarify this issue, it is necessary to discriminate between the effects of inflammation and iron intake on markers of iron status.

Accumulating evidence supports beneficial effects of iron supplementation on performance of individuals with IDNA. During aerobic training, women with IDNA who were supplemented with iron (8 mg/day for six weeks) significantly decreased sTfR and increased ferritin without any change in hemoglobin. Although both groups improved cycling times, the iron-supplemented women improved 15 km cycle time trial and decreased plasma lactate more than the placebo-treated women (Hinton et al. 2000). Also, women with IDNA (sTfR >8.5 mg/L) supplemented with iron (8 mg/day for 10 weeks) and trained on cycle ergometers significantly reduced time to complete a simulated 15 km trial by exercising at a significantly higher work rate and using a lower percentage of aerobic capacity than women treated with placebo (Brownlie et al. 2004). Similarly, iron supplementation (10 mg/day for six weeks) compared to placebo reduced muscle fatigue during knee extensor exercise in women with IDNA (Brutsaert et al. 2003). The DRI panel summarized research findings showing that regular aerobic endurance training raised iron losses up to 3 mg/day (IOM 2001). Thus, individuals who regularly engage in aerobic endurance training should increase iron intakes 30% to 70% to accommodate the increased iron loss.

Copper

Copper functions as a metalloenzyme needed for nonheme iron uptake and hemoglobin formation (ceruloplasmin), for energy production in the mitochondria (cytochrome c oxidase), and as an antioxidant (superoxide dismutase) (IOM 2001). Despite these possible opportunities to influence performance, clear evidence of impaired performance with inadequate copper intake is lacking. Copper is widely distributed in foods, with appreciable amounts in nuts, beans, whole-grain products, shellfish, and organs. The RDA for copper is 900 µg/day for adult males and females.

Zinc

Zinc is found in all tissues of the body as a component of more than 100 metalloenzymes. Zinc-containing enzymes regulate some aspects of energy metabolism, including oxygen–carbon dioxide transport (carbonic anhydrase) and lactic acid metabolism (lactate dehydrogenase), as well as controlling breakdown and synthesis of macronutrients, growth and development, immune function, and wound healing (IOM 2001). Seafood, meats, lima beans, black-eyed peas, white beans, whole-grain products, and fortified cereals are sources of zinc. Diets high in protein provide substantial amounts of zinc. Zinc availability is reduced from diets high in fiber and phytic acid.

Physically active adults generally consume the RDA for zinc (11 and 8 mg/day for men and women, respectively) (Lukaski 2006). Female athletes in aerobic endurance sports and gymnastics have marginal intakes partially due to food restriction (Short and Short 1983). Zinc status is an indicator of performance. Serum zinc levels were low, compared to the range of normal values, in 25% of male distance runners and were inversely correlated with training distances (Dressendorfer and Sockolov 1980). Surveys of aerobic endurance athletes and runners revealed that the prevalence of low serum zinc was 20% to 25% compared to 13% for gender-matched controls (Singh, Deuster, and Moser 1990; Lukaski et al. 1990).

Accumulating evidence indicates that low zinc status affects physical performance. Zinc enhances in vitro muscle contraction (Isaacson and Sandow 1963; Richardson and Drake 1979). Zinc supplementation, compared to placebo, in middle-aged women increased muscle strength and endurance (Krotkiewski et al. 1982). Because these muscle functions rely on recruitment of fast-twitch glycolytic muscle fibers, zinc supplementation may enhance the activity of lactate dehydrogenase, a zinc-dependent enzyme. Male subjects fed diets with low, compared to adequate, zinc content (1 vs. 12 mg/day) had decreased serum zinc and zinc retention, as well as decreased upper and lower body muscle strength (Van Loan et al. 1999). Serum zinc concentrations of adolescent gymnasts were decreased compared to values in nonathletic age- and gender-matched controls; half of the athletes were characterized as subclinically zinc deficient. Serum zinc was positively correlated with adductor muscle strength in the gymnasts (Brun et al. 1995). Elite male soccer players with low, compared to normal, serum zinc concentrations had decreased peak power output and increased blood lactate during cycle ergometer tests (Khaled et al. 1997). Men fed whole-food diets moderately low in zinc (3-4 mg/day) had increased ventilation rates with decreased oxygen uptake and decreased carbon dioxide output and respiratory exchange ratio during prolonged submaximal cycle ergometer exercise (Lukaski 2005). The low-zinc diet resulted in decreased zinc status (serum zinc and zinc retention). The activity of carbonic anhydrase (a zinc-dependent enzyme) in red blood cells decreased with the low-zinc diet.

Selenium

Selenium exists as selenoproteins that exert biological actions including protection against oxidative damage to cells (glutathione peroxidase). Selenium acts with vitamin E as an antioxidant (IOM 2000). Evidence supporting a role for selenium in performance is lacking. Selenium is linked with protein content of the diet. Foods high in selenium include seafood, meats, whole-grain products, liver, wheat bran, and some vegetables (broccoli and cauliflower). The RDA for selenium is 55 µg/day for adult males and females.

Chromium

Emerging evidence suggests that chromium facilitates the action of insulin in cells of individuals with insulin resistance. Its role in promoting physical performance is controversial (Short and Short 1983). Whole grains, cheese, beans, mushrooms, oysters, wine, apples, pork, chicken, and brewer's yeast are sources of chromium.

Chromium is provisionally essential; adequate intakes are 35 and 25 µg/day for men and women, respectively (IOM 2001). Assessment of dietary chromium and chromium nutritional status is problematic (Lukaski 1999), which limits evaluation of its importance in physical activity. Because of the putative role of chromium in regulating glucose metabolism and potentially anabolism (Evans 1989), numerous studies have been conducted to determine the effect of supplemental trivalent chromium, generally as chromium picolinate, on strength gain and body composition change. Consistent results showing a beneficial effect of supplemental chromium on strength gain, muscle accretion, or glycogen synthesis after exercise in healthy men and women are lacking (Vincent 2003; Volek et al. 2006; Lukaski 2007).

Other Minerals

Boron, vanadium, cobalt, fluoride, iodine, manganese, and molybdenum have reported biological functions that theoretically would negatively affect performance when consumed in suboptimal amounts (IOM 1997, 2001). However, there is no published research that presents evidence that restricted intakes of these minerals actually has negative effects on physical performance. Further, vanadium and manganese play roles in carbohydrate and lipid metabolism in animals, but dietary deficiencies in humans are rare.

Professional Applications

Vitamins and minerals function in the human body as metabolic regulators, influencing a number of physiological processes important to exercise or sport performance. For example, many of the B-complex vitamins are involved in processing carbohydrate and fats for energy production, an important consideration during exercise of varying intensities (Williams 2004). Several B vitamins are also essential to help form hemoglobin in red blood cells, which is a major determinant of oxygen delivery to the muscles during aerobic endurance exercise. Additionally, vitamins C and E function as antioxidants, important for preventing oxidative damage to cellular structure and function during exercise training and theoretically optimizing preparation for competition (Williams 2004).

Minerals are important to athletes because they are involved in muscle contraction, normal heart rhythm, nerve impulse conduction, oxygen transport, oxidative phosphorylation, enzyme activation, immune functions, antioxidant activity, bone health, and acid–base balance of the blood (Williams 2005; Speich, Pineau, and Ballereau 2001). Because many of these processes are accelerated during exercise, adequate amounts of minerals are necessary for optimal functioning. Athletes should obtain adequate amounts of all minerals in their diet because a mineral deficiency may impair optimal health, and health impairment may adversely affect sport performance (Williams 2005).

Because vitamins and minerals cannot be produced by the body, but rather must be consumed in the diet, it is essential that athletes and physically active people consume a balanced diet. A balanced diet is one that contains adequate amounts of all the necessary nutrients required for healthy growth and activity. To help ensure a balanced diet, athletes should regularly ingest the following types of foods:

- Lean meats (poultry, fish, low-fat pork, low-fat beef, etc.)
- Fruits (apples, bananas, grapes, oranges, pineapple, blueberries, etc.)
- Vegetables (broccoli, spinach, green beans, carrots, etc.)

This is not a comprehensive list of foods that athletes should ingest on a daily basis, but rather of the types of food choices they should make frequently and consistently. For an athlete or physically active individual who does not consistently eat these types of foods as part of the diet, it is prudent to take a multivitamin to prevent deficiencies. This recommendation has been advanced by the American Medical Association (Fletcher and Fairfield 2002). Athletes that consistently restrict food intake are at greater risk for nutrient deficiencies. Athletes that participate in gymnastics, ballet, cheerleading, and wrestling are typically the types of athletes that restrict food intake and would benefit from a multivitamin supplement.

Some athletes and coaches believe that ingesting a vitamin and mineral supplement will confer athletic advantages, but scientific investigations have not supported this theory. For example, several studies have provided multivitamin–mineral supplements over prolonged periods and shown no significant effects on either laboratory or sport-specific tests of physical performance (Williams 2004; Singh, Moses, and Deuster 1992; Weight, Myburgh, and Noakes 1998). In a long-term study, Telford and colleagues (1992) evaluated the effect of seven to eight months of vitamin–mineral supplementation (100 to 5,000 times the RDA) on exercise performance of nationally ranked athletes in training at the Australian Institute of Sport. They reported no significant effect of the supplementation protocol on any measure of physical performance when compared to results for athletes whose vitamin and mineral RDAs were met by normal dietary intake (Williams 2004; Telford et al. 1992).

In summary, vitamin and mineral supplements will not improve performance when dietary intake of these nutrients is adequate. However, if a vitamin or mineral deficiency is present (as is the case more commonly in weight control sports), a vitamin and mineral supplement could improve performance by eliminating the deficiency.

SUMMARY POINTS

- Vitamins and minerals cannot be produced by the body and thus must be consumed in foods and beverages.

- The content of vitamins and minerals in food is small (micrograms to milligrams) compared to that of protein, carbohydrate, and fat (up to hundreds of grams).

- Vitamins and minerals are not direct sources of energy but facilitate energy production and utilization from carbohydrate, fat, and protein; transport oxygen and carbon dioxide; regulate fluid balance; and protect against oxidative damage.

- Subclinical deficiencies of some vitamins and minerals occur in physically active individuals.

- Vitamins are characterized into two main groups: water soluble and fat soluble. The water-soluble vitamins include the B vitamins and vitamin C. The fat-soluble vitamins are vitamins A, D, E, and K.

- Minerals are classified as either major minerals or trace minerals. Major minerals are those needed by the body in amounts greater than 100 mg/day. Trace minerals are those required in daily quantities of less than 100 mg.

- Vitamin supplements are not necessary for an athlete on a balanced diet, but health professionals may recommend them to athletes if their diet is not balanced, if they are on a very low-calorie diet, or for other special dietary needs.

7

Strength and Power Supplements

Colin Wilborn, PhD, ATC, CSCS, FISSN
Bill I. Campbell, PhD, CSCS, FISSN

Different sports place unique metabolic requirements on bioenergetic systems, and these differences alter the nutritional requirements among athletes involved in various types of strength and power sports. Particularly important to the strength and power athlete are

- increasing lean muscle mass that translates into functional sport-specific strength,
- increasing power and speed over short distances, and
- increasing explosiveness.

These goals typically drive strength–power athletes to seek various options in their training methodologies to maximize the training stimulus. In addition to intense training, a proper nutrition program is also responsible for maximizing the performance of a strength–power athlete. More specifically, precise nutritional supplementation can provide the impetus for maximizing lean muscle mass, power, speed, and explosiveness. Therefore, any nutritional program (including sport supplements) that enhances lean muscle mass, power, speed, and explosiveness, when combined with a proper training program, should translate into improvements in exercise and sport performance.

To stay on the cutting edge of nutritional supplementation, it is important to identify supplements that have been shown to be effective and safe when ingested appropriately. Many experts in the field have identified and separated the leading sport supplements into categories, ranging from those that are safe to those that have harmful side effects or those whose effectiveness has not been demonstrated in the literature. A comprehensive analysis of the sport supplements that may benefit the strength and power athlete must be based on three simple questions:

- Is the sport supplement legal and safe?
- Is there any scientific evidence that the sport supplement may affect health or exercise performance?
- Is there a sound scientific rationale?

Claims of enhanced exercise performance have been advanced for hundreds of sport supplements. Rather than addressing each and every sport supplement with claimed **ergogenic** potential, this chapter will cover the most popular sport supplements that have been demonstrated to be safe, effective, and legal relative to increasing lean muscle mass, strength, and power. These are creatine, HMB, protein, and beta-alanine. Table 7.1 summarizes other popular sport supplements not discussed in the chapter.

➤ ergogenic—Having the ability to enhance work output, particularly as it relates to athletic performance.

TABLE 7.1 Summary of Popular Sport Supplements

Nutrient	Theoretical ergogenic value	Summary of research findings and recommendations
Arginine	Arginine is an amino acid that has numerous functions in the body. It is used to make compounds in the body such as nitric oxide, creatine, glutamate, and proline and can be converted to glucose and glycogen if needed. In large doses, arginine also stimulates release of the hormones growth hormone and prolactin. Arginine has been purported to be advantageous for strength athletes.	The research on arginine shows conflicting results. However, there is some evidence that arginine supplementation can increase strength, muscle mass, and growth hormone levels (Campbell et al. 2006; Elam et al. 1989; Besset et al. 1982). At this point there is not enough evidence to strongly support its use.
Aromatase inhibitors	Aromatase, an enzyme involved in the production of estrogen, acts by catalyzing the conversion of testosterone to estradiol. Aromatase inhibitors have been used medically to inhibit the conversion of testosterone to estrogen; one use is for estrogen suppression in breast cancer patients. Theoretically, if the conversion of testosterone to estrogen is inhibited, endogenous testosterone levels would subsequently increase.	While aromatase inhibitors are relatively new as a nutrition supplement, research suggests that they can increase endogenous levels of testosterone (Willoughby et al. 2007; Rohle et al. 2007).

Nutrient	Theoretical ergogenic value	Summary of research findings and recommendations
Glutamine	Glutamine is the most abundant amino acid in the body, representing about 60% of the amino acid pool in muscles. It is considered a "conditionally essential amino acid" because it can be manufactured in the body; but under extreme physical stress, the demand for glutamine exceeds the body's ability to make it. Glutamine serves a variety of functions in the body including cell growth, immune function, and recovery from stress.	Research has shown that glutamine contributes to the prevention of muscle breakdown, increase in growth hormone, protein synthesis, and improved immune system function (Candow et al. 2001; Castell and Newsholme 1997; Welbourne 1995). However, most of the research has not been done on strength-trained athletes, and it does not appear at this time that it increases strength and power in these athletes.
Antioxidants	Oxidative stress is the steady-state level of oxidative damage in a cell, tissue, or organ, caused by free radicals or the reactive oxygen species (ROS). Reactive oxygen species, such as free radicals and peroxides, represent a class of molecules derived from the metabolism of oxygen that is increased during exercise. Antioxidants block the process of oxidation by neutralizing free radicals.	Research has determined that antioxidants are effective at reducing free radicals. However, their effect on the strength and power athlete has yet to be determined.
Caffeine	Caffeine is one of the most widely used stimulants in the world. It acts as a stimulant on the central nervous system, which causes heart rate and blood pressure to increase. Caffeine ingestion may cause an improvement in time to exhaustion and work output during aerobic exercise.	Caffeine has been shown to have a positive effect on both exercise and energy expenditure (Clarkson 1993; Armstrong 2002; Costill et al. 1978; Graham and Spriet 1991). Whether it benefits the strength athlete is currently unknown. Further research is needed to enable conclusive recommendations.
Prohormones	Prohormones or hormone precursors are naturally derived precursors to the synthesis of testosterone. The rationale for supplementing with prohormones is to aim to increase the body's ability to synthesize testosterone, which could lead to increases in lean mass, strength, and bone density and improvements in body composition.	Despite the rampant claims associated with taking prohormones, research does not support these claims, and it is thought that prohormones have no benefit on strength and body composition (Brown et al. 1999; Joyner 2000; Rasmussen et al. 2000). Several reports have shown that supplementing prohormones can significantly elevate estrogen (Brown et al. 2000; King et al. 1999), which can have negative effects on body composition and strength.

It is important to note that some argue against the use of sport supplements. Individuals who hold to this position cite ethical considerations relating to unfair advantage during competition. Inherent in this viewpoint is the belief that athletes who would normally refrain from using sport supplements feel pressured to use them just to stay abreast of their competitors (Hoffman and Stout 2008). The intent of this chapter is not to address these concerns but instead to focus on those few sport supplements with demonstrated safety and effectiveness.

Creatine

The sport supplement creatine has been the gold standard to which other nutritional supplements are compared (Greenwood, Kalman, and Antonio 2008) because it improves performance, increases lean body mass, and has an excellent safety profile when consumed in recommended dosages (Greenwood, Kalman, and Antonio 2008). Creatine is one of the most widely researched sport nutrition supplements on the market. Among several methods of ingestion, the most common is to mix creatine as a powder into a drink. Creatine is also commonly ingested in the form of a capsule.

Chemically, creatine is derived from the amino acids glycine, arginine, and methionine; it is obtained from the ingestion of meat or fish and is also synthesized in the kidney, liver, and pancreas (Balsom, Soderlund, and Ekblom 1994; Heymsfield et al. 1983). When creatine enters the muscle cell, it accepts a high-energy phosphate and forms phosphocreatine. Phosphocreatine is the storage form of high-energy phosphate, which is used by the skeletal muscle cell to rapidly regenerate adenosine triphosphate (ATP) during bouts of maximal muscular contraction (Hirvonen et al. 1987). The conversion of ATP into adenosine diphosphate (ADP) and a phosphate group generates the energy needed by the muscles during short-term, high-intensity exercise. The energy for all-out maximal-effort exercise lasting up to approximately 6 seconds (typical duration of activity for a strength and power athlete) is primarily derived from limited stores of ATP in the muscle. Phosphocreatine availability in the muscles is vitally important in energy production since ATP cannot be stored in excessive amounts within the muscle and is rapidly depleted during bouts of exhaustive or high-intensity exercise.

Oral creatine monohydrate supplementation has been reported to increase muscle creatine and phosphocreatine content by 15% to 40%, enhance the cellular bioenergetics of the **phosphagen system**, improve the shuttling of high-energy phosphates between the mitochondria and cytosol via the creatine phosphate shuttle, and enhance the activity of various metabolic pathways (Kreider 2003a). Relative to dosage, the majority of published studies on creatine supplementation divided the typical dosage pattern into two phases: a loading phase and a maintenance phase. A typical loading phase comprises 20 g of creatine (or 0.3 g/kg body weight) in divided doses four times a day for two to seven days; this is followed by a maintenance dose of 2 to 5 g daily (or 0.03 g/kg body weight) for several weeks to months at a time.

> ➤ phosphagen system—The quickest and most powerful source of energy for muscle movement.

Scientific studies indicate that creatine supplementation is an effective and safe nutritional strategy to promote gains in strength and muscle mass during resistance training—both important attributes for the strength and power athlete (Greenwood et al. 2000; Kreider 2003a, 2003b; Stout et al. 2000; Volek et al. 1997). Specific to lean body mass, creatine supplementation has been shown to be effective in several cohorts, including males, females, and the elderly (Branch 2003; Brose, Parise, and Tarnopolsky 2003; Chrusch et al. 2001; Kreider et al. 1998; van Loon et al. 2003). Short-term creatine supplementation increases total body mass by approximately 0.8 to 1.7 kg (~1.8 to 3.7 pounds). Longer-term creatine supplementation (e.g., six to eight weeks) in conjunction with resistance training increased lean body mass by approximately 2.8 to 3.2 kg (~7 pounds) (Greenwood, Kalman, and Antonio 2008; Earnest et al. 1995; Kreider et al. 1996; Stout, Eckerson, and Noonan 1999).

Unequivocally, one of the most visible effects of creatine supplementation is an increase in body mass. However, for the strength and power athlete, an increase in body mass will impart benefit only if the weight gain is in the form of lean tissue. Fortunately, several scientific investigations have demonstrated that gains in body mass are partially attributable to actual increases in the cellular protein content of muscle tissue (Volek et al. 1999; Willoughby and Rosene 2001). For more information on the changes in skeletal muscle protein content and overall changes in body composition in response to creatine supplementation, refer to chapter 10.

Creatine can also be advantageous to strength athletes given its ability to promote strength gains during training. Studies indicate that creatine supplementation during training can increase gains in 1-repetition maximum (1RM) strength and power. Peeters, Lantz, and Mayhew (1999) investigated the effect of creatine monohydrate and creatine phosphate supplementation on strength, body composition, and blood pressure over a six-week period. Strength tests performed were the 1RM bench press, 1RM leg press, and maximal repetitions on the seated preacher bar curl with a fixed amount of weight. Subjects were matched for strength and placed into one of three groups—a placebo, creatine monohydrate, or creatine phosphate group. All subjects performed a standardized strength training regimen and ingested a loading dosage of 20 g/day for the first three days of the study, followed by a maintenance dose of 10 g/day for the remainder of the six-week supplementation period. Significant differences were noted between the placebo group and the two creatine groups for changes in lean body mass, body weight, and 1RM bench press. Eckerson and colleagues (2004) also studied the effects of two and five days of creatine loading on anaerobic working capacity using the critical power test. Ten physically active women randomly received two treatments separated by a five-week washout period: (a) 18 g dextrose as placebo or (b) 5 g creatine plus 18 g dextrose taken four times a day for five days. Ingesting the placebo resulted in no significant changes in anaerobic working capacity; however, creatine ingestion significantly increased anaerobic working capacity by 22.1% after five days of loading.

Elsewhere, Kreider and colleagues (1998) conducted a study in which 25 National Collegiate Athletic Association Division IA football players supplemented their diet for 28 days with creatine or a placebo during resistance and agility training. Before and after the supplementation protocol, the football players performed a maximal-repetition test on the isotonic bench press, squat, and power clean and also performed a high-intensity cycle ergometer sprint test. The creatine group showed significantly greater gains in bench press lifting volume; the sum of bench press, squat, and power clean lifting volume; and total work performed during the first five 6-second cycle ergometer sprints. Ingestion of creatine promoted greater gains in fat-free mass, isotonic lifting volume, and sprint performance during intense resistance and agility training.

The studies reviewed here are only a few among dozens that have shown an increase in strength, power, and high-intensity performance. Combined, these three studies indicate that creatine supplementation can increase maximal strength, high-intensity exercise performance, and lifting volume. The International Society of Sports Nutrition (Buford et al. 2007) stated in its comprehensive review on creatine supplementation and position stand:

- Short-term adaptations include increased cycling power; total work performed on the bench press and jump squat; and improved sport performance in sprinting, swimming, and soccer (Volek et al. 1997; Mero et al. 2004; Wiroth et al. 2001; Tarnopolsky and MacLennan 2000; Skare, Skadberg, and Wisnes 2001; Mujika et al. 2000; Ostojic 2004; Theodorou et al. 1999; Preen et al. 2001).

- Long-term adaptations when creatine monohydrate supplementation is combined with training include increased muscle creatine and PCr [phosphocreatine] content, lean body mass, strength, sprint performance, power, rate of force development, and muscle diameter (Kreider et al. 1998; Volek et al. 1999; Vandenberghe et al. 1997).

- In long-term studies, subjects taking creatine monohydrate typically gain about twice as much body mass, fat-free mass, or both (i.e., an extra 2 to 4 pounds of muscle mass during 4 to 12 weeks of training) as subjects taking a placebo (Stone et al. 1999; Noonan et al. 1998; Kirksey et al. 1999; Jones, Atter, and Georg 1999).

- The only clinically significant side effect reported in the research literature is weight gain (Kreider, Leutholtz, and Greenwood 2004; Kreider et al. 2003); however, many anecdotal claims of side effects, including dehydration, cramping, kidney and liver damage, musculoskeletal injury, gastrointestinal distress, and anterior (leg) compartment syndrome, still appear in the media and popular literature. While athletes who are taking creatine monohydrate may experience these symptoms, the scientific literature suggests that these athletes have no greater, and a possibly lower, risk of these symptoms than those not supplementing with creatine monohydrate (Greenwood et al. 2003; Kreider et al. 2003).

The position stand also included the statement, "The tremendous numbers of investigations conducted with positive results from creatine monohydrate supplementation lead us to conclude that it is the most effective nutritional supplement available today for increasing high-intensity exercise capacity and building lean mass."

HMB

β-Hydroxy-β-methylbuteric acid, or HMB, is a **metabolite** of the essential amino acid leucine. HMB has been shown to play a role in the regulation of protein breakdown in the body. HMB helps inhibit proteolysis, which is the natural process of breaking down muscle that occurs especially after high-intensity activity. HMB is typically available as a powder that is mixed with water, as well as in capsule form. It appears that HMB supplementation has a protective effect on muscle and may help the body get a head start on the recovery process by minimizing the amount of protein degradation after intense exercise. The theoretical rationale behind HMB supplementation is that it could slow the breakdown of protein in the body, thus increasing muscle mass and strength (Greenwood, Kalman, and Antonio 2008). Many of the early scientific investigations on HMB were conducted in animal models, with results such as the following:

- Enhanced growth rates in pigs (Nissen et al. 1994)
- Increased muscle mass and decreased body fat in steers (Van Koevering et al. 1994)
- Improvement in several markers of immune function in chickens (Peterson et al. 1999a, 1999b)

On the basis of these early findings, subsequent researchers on HMB supplementation during training in humans set out to determine its effects on inhibiting protein degradation and increasing muscular strength and muscle mass. Nissen and coworkers (1996) conducted the first research study to highlight HMB's anticatabolic potential. Untrained subjects ingested one of three levels of HMB (0, 1.5, or 3.0 g/day) and two protein levels (117 or 175 g/day) and resistance trained three days per week for three weeks. Among other markers of muscle damage, protein breakdown was assessed through measurement of urinary 3-methyl-histidine. After the first week of the resistance training protocol, urinary 3-methyl-histidine increased by 94% in the control group and by 85% and 50% in the individuals ingesting 1.5 and 3 g of HMB per day, respectively. During the second week, urinary 3-methyl-histidine levels were still elevated by 27% in the control group but were 4% and 15% below basal levels for the groups taking 1.5 and 3 g HMB per day. Interestingly, urinary 3-methyl-histidine measures at the end of the third week of resistance training were not significantly different between the groups (Nissen et al. 1996). Other studies demonstrating an **anticatabolic** effect or suppression of muscle damage have supported these findings (Knitter et al. 2000; van Someren, Edwards, and Howatson 2005).

> metabolite—Any substance produced by, or taking part in, a metabolic reaction.

> anticatabolic—Describing a substance that reduces muscle breakdown and prevents catabolism.

Van Someren and colleagues (2005) instructed their male subjects to ingest 3 g of HMB in addition to 0.3 g **alpha-ketoisocaproic acid** daily for 14 days before performing a single bout of eccentric-dominant resistance exercise. This supplemental intervention including HMB resulted in a significant reduction of plasma markers of muscle damage. Gallagher and associates (2000a) evaluated the effects of HMB supplementation (0.38 and 0.76 mg/kg per day) during eight weeks of resistance training in previously untrained men. The researchers reported that HMB supplementation promoted significantly less muscle creatine kinase excretion and greater gains in muscle mass (in the 0.38 mg/kg per day group only) than in subjects taking a placebo. Collectively, these findings support contentions that HMB supplementation may lessen catabolism, leading to greater gains in strength and muscle mass.

> alpha-ketoisocaproic acid—An intermediate in the metabolism of leucine.

HMB supplementation may suppress protein breakdown and markers of muscle damage, but does this anticatabolic effect lead to gains in lean body mass? The scientific literature on this topic is equivocal. In a second arm of the study by Nissen and colleagues (1996), male participants ingested 3 g of HMB or a placebo for seven weeks in conjunction with resistance training six days per week. Fat-free mass increased in the HMB-supplemented group at various times throughout the investigative period but not at the end of the study (the seventh week). Vukovich and coworkers (2001) reported that HMB supplementation (3 g/day for eight weeks during resistance training) significantly increased muscle mass, reduced fat mass, and promoted greater gains in upper and lower extremity 1RM strength in a group of elderly men and women initiating training.

Not all studies have shown that HMB ingestion results in an accretion of lean body mass (Kreider et al. 1999; Slater et al. 2001; O'Conner and Crowe 2003; Hoffman et al. 2004). In studies not showing this effect, subjects received approximately the same amount of HMB as in the studies demonstrating increases in lean body mass.

One of the greatest concerns with the literature on the effectiveness of HMB supplementation in strength athletes is that many of the studies have not used trained populations (Nissen et al. 1996; Van Someren et al. 2003, 2005; Gallagher et al. 2000a). In addition, some studies used elderly populations (Falkoll et al. 2004). It is unwise to extrapolate research findings in an untrained population to a trained population given the variance in training adaptations among these groups. To further convolute the data, many of the studies using trained populations were not effective at enhancing training adaptations (Hoffman et al. 2004; Kreider et al. 1999; O'Conner et al. 2003).

Taking these observations into account, Hoffman and colleagues (2004) stated that if HMB supplementation has any ergogenic benefit in attenuating muscle damage, it is likely to be most effective in untrained individuals, who have the greatest potential for muscle damage during exercise. In relation to safety, no side effects have been reported in human studies using as much as 6 g/day (Gallagher et al. 2000a, 2000b). In conclusion, it appears that HMB may be beneficial (relative to increasing lean body mass) for an individual beginning a strength training program, but not for athletes who are already resistance trained.

Protein and Amino Acids

For years, many have believed that excess protein intake is necessary for optimal muscle growth in response to strength training (Greenwood, Kalman, and Antonio 2008). Skeletal muscle hypertrophy occurs only when muscle protein synthesis exceeds muscle protein breakdown. The body is in a continuous state of protein turnover as old proteins are destroyed or degraded and new proteins are synthesized. When synthesis of contractile proteins is occurring at a faster rate than degradation, the net result is a positive protein balance (i.e., myofibrillar hypertrophy). At rest, in the absence of an exercise stimulus and nutrient intake, net protein balance is negative (Biolo et al. 1995; Phillips et al. 1997, 1999; Wagenmakers 1999).

One must remember that resistance exercise is essential for creating the stimulus needed in order for skeletal muscle hypertrophy to occur. However, when resistance exercise is performed in the absence of nutritional and supplemental nitrogen, net protein balance still does not increase to the point of becoming anabolic. Specific nutrients and supplements (nitrogen-containing compounds) are needed in conjunction with the resistance training in order for net protein balance to become positive.

On the basis of this knowledge, it is clear that protein or the building blocks of proteins, amino acids, need to be available to ensure attainment of a positive balance. Amino acids are made available from the amino acid pool. The amino acid pool is a mixture of amino acids available in the cell that is derived from dietary sources or the degradation of protein. Amino acids enter this pool in three ways:

- During digestion of protein in the diet
- When body protein decomposes
- When carbon sources and amino groups ($-NH_2$) synthesize the non-essential amino acids

The amino acid pool exists to provide individual amino acids for protein synthesis and oxidation, and it is replenished only by protein breakdown or amino acids entering the body from the diet. Thus, the free amino acid pool provides the link between dietary protein and body protein in that both dietary protein and body protein feed into the free amino acid pool.

Protein Intake

One of the most controversial debates that has pervaded the science of sport nutrition surrounds protein intake. The main controversy has centered on the safety and effectiveness of protein intake above the current Recommended Dietary Allowance (RDA). Currently, the RDA for protein in healthy adults is 0.8 g/kg body weight per day. This recommendation accounts for individual differences in protein metabolism, variations in the biological value of protein, and nitrogen losses in the urine and feces. When determining the amount of protein that must be ingested to increase lean body mass, one needs to consider many factors, such as the following:

- Protein quality
- Energy intake
- Carbohydrate intake
- Amount and intensity of the resistance training program
- Timing of the protein intake

While 0.8 g of protein per kilogram body weight per day may be sufficient to meet the needs of nearly all non-resistance-trained individuals, it is likely not sufficient to provide substrate for lean tissue accretion or for the repair of exercise-induced muscle damage (Tarnopolsky 2004). In fact, many clinical investigations indicate that individuals who engage in physical activity or exercise require higher levels of protein intake than 0.8 g/kg body weight daily, regardless of the mode of exercise (e.g., aerobic endurance, resistance) (Forslund et al. 1999; Friedman and Lemon 1989; Lamont, Patel, and Kalhan 1990; Meredith et al. 1989; Phillips et al. 1993) or training state (i.e., recreational, moderately or well trained) (Greenwood, Kalman, and Antonio 2008; Lemon 1991; Lemon et al. 1992; Tarnopolsky et al. 1992).

So, the question remains: How much protein is required for individuals who engage in resistance training and want to increase lean body mass? As stated in chapter 3, a general recommendation relative to protein ingestion is 1.5 to 2.0 g/kg per day (Lemon 1998; Campbell et al. 2007). More specifically, individuals engaging in strength or power exercise should ingest levels at the upper end of this range.

At the cellular level, studies have found that with dietary protein or amino acid supplementation, muscle protein synthesis rate is increased. Biolo and colleagues (1997) evaluated the interactions between resistance training and amino acid supplementation and the corresponding effects on protein kinetics. Six untrained men served as subjects in this study. Each participant was infused with a mixed (phenylalanine, leucine, lysine, alanine, glutamine) amino acid solution. Baseline and postresistance training (five sets of 10 leg presses; four sets of eight Nautilus squats, leg curls, and leg extensions) samples were taken. The results revealed increased protein synthesis and no change in protein degradation.

Although researchers have concluded that postexercise amino acid supplementation has a positive effect on protein synthesis, amino acid infusion is not a practical means of obtaining amino acids. Hence, Tipton and colleagues (1999) investigated the effects of orally administered amino acids; subjects received 40 g mixed amino acids (essential + nonessential), 40 g essential amino acids only, or 40 g of a carbohydrate placebo. They also sought to determine whether there would be a difference in the anabolic effect of amino acid supplementation if they used a mixed amino acid source or essential amino acids alone. The findings indicated that postexercise amino acid supplementation elicits a positive protein balance as compared to the negative balance seen with resistance training alone. The authors also concluded that supplementation with the essential amino acids alone is equivalent to a mixed amino acid supplement.

Elsewhere, Esmark and colleagues (2001) investigated the timing of protein intake after exercise on muscle hypertrophy and strength. This study used a milk and soy protein supplement (10 g protein from skim milk and soybean), 7 g carbohydrate, and 3.3 g of lipid instead of an amino acid mixture. Although the investigators did not calculate protein synthesis, they did measure hypertrophy. The results indicated that skeletal muscle hypertrophy significantly increased after resistance training when subjects took a protein supplement.

Ingesting between 1.5 and 2.0 g/kg per day of protein is not the only parameter to consider, however, because it is important to note that not all protein sources are the same. Not all protein sources contain the same amounts of amino acids. Protein is classified as *complete* or *incomplete* depending on whether or not it contains adequate amounts of the essential amino acids. Complete protein sources that contain greater amounts of essential amino acids generally have higher protein quality. Complete proteins are typically found in sources such as beef, chicken, pork, milk, and cheese, whereas incomplete proteins are typically found in nuts, beans, grains, and seeds.

Common Types of Protein in Sport Supplements

Three of the most common types of protein found in protein supplements are whey, casein, and egg protein. Each of these types of protein is a complete protein, and all are classified as high quality (for an in-depth discussion of the classification of the quality of various proteins, refer to chapter 3) and are administered as a powder. Whey protein, derived from milk protein, is currently the most popular source of protein used in nutritional supplements. Of the three common types of protein found in protein supplements, whey protein appears to have been investigated most thoroughly relative to protein synthesis and lean tissue accretion. Cribb and colleagues (2006) investigated the differential effects of whey versus casein protein on strength and body composition. Subjects ingested either whey or casein (1.5 g/kg body weight per day) for 10 weeks while following a structured resistance training program; the whey protein group experienced significantly greater gains in strength and lean body mass than the casein group.

Casein, also a milk protein, is often characterized as a slower-acting protein (Boirie et al. 1997; Dangin et al. 2001). In comparison to whey protein, casein takes longer to digest and absorb. The reason is most likely that casein takes more time to leave the stomach (Boirie et al. 1997). Although casein stimulates protein synthesis, it does this to a much lesser extent than whey protein (Boirie et al. 1997). Unlike whey, casein helps decrease protein breakdown (Demling and DeSanti 2000) and therefore has anticatabolic properties.

Given the findings that whey protein stimulates protein synthesis and casein helps decrease muscle breakdown, some supplement manufacturers include both whey and casein in their formulations. An investigation by Kerksick and colleagues (2006) illustrated the effectiveness of the combination. Subjects performed a split body resistance training program four days a week for 10 weeks. They received 48 g of carbohydrate, 40 g of whey + 8 g of casein, or 40 g of whey + 5 g of glutamine + 3 g of branched-chain amino acids. After 10 weeks, the group that received both whey and casein had the largest increase in lean muscle mass. Willoughby and colleagues (2007) investigated the effect of a combination whey and casein protein on strength, muscle mass, and markers of anabolism. Their findings agree with those of Kerksick and associates in that the whey and casein combination elicited a superior response in strength and muscle mass compared to placebo. It appears that a combination protein mixture is adequate to stimulate protein synthesis and promote positive training adaptations (Willoughby et al. 2007; Tipton et al. 2004; Kerksick et al. 2006).

Egg protein is also a high-quality protein and has the advantage of being miscible (it mixes easily in solution) (Driskell and Wolinsky 2000). However, egg protein supplements generally do not taste very good and are typically more expensive than other protein supplements. For these reasons, along with the availability of other high-quality protein sources such as whey and casein, egg protein is not as popular a supplement as whey and casein.

In a review, Rennie and colleagues (2004) concluded that there is no doubt that increasing amino acid concentration by intravenous infusion, meal feeding, or ingestion of free amino acids increases muscle protein synthesis. They also concluded that in the postexercise period, increased availability of amino acids enhances muscle protein synthesis. Whey, casein, and egg protein are all high quality and are commonly found in protein supplements marketed to strength-trained athletes.

Beta-Alanine

Within the past few years, beta-alanine has appeared on the sport nutrition market. Beta-alanine is typically administered as capsules or as a powder that is mixed with a liquid (usually water). While several clinical trials have shown increases in markers of aerobic endurance performance, body composition, and strength with beta-alanine, others have demonstrated no ergogenic benefits. This section discusses beta-alanine as a sport supplement, beginning with its parent compound carnosine.

Carnosine is a dipeptide composed of the amino acids histidine and beta-alanine. Carnosine occurs naturally in the brain, cardiac muscle, kidney, and stomach, as well as in relatively large amounts in skeletal muscles (primarily Type II muscle fibers). These Type II muscle fibers are the fast-twitch muscle fibers used in explosive movements like those in weight training and sprinting. Interestingly, athletes whose performance demands extensive anaerobic output have higher concentrations of carnosine.

Carnosine contributes to the buffering of hydrogen ions, thus attenuating (slowing down) a drop in pH associated with anaerobic metabolism. Carnosine is very effective at buffering the hydrogen ions responsible for producing the ill effects of lactic acid. Carnosine is believed to be one of the primary muscle buffering substances available in skeletal muscle. In theory, if carnosine could attenuate the drop in pH noted with high-intensity exercise, one could possibly exercise at high intensities for a longer duration. Relative to ingestion, however, carnosine is rapidly degraded into beta-alanine and histidine as soon as it enters the blood through the activity of the enzyme carnosinase. Thus there is no advantage to ingesting carnosine. However, independent ingestion of beta-alanine and histidine allows these two compounds to be transported into the skeletal muscle and to be resynthesized into carnosine. It appears that beta-alanine is the amino acid that most influences intramuscular carnosine levels because it is the rate-limiting substrate in this chemical reaction (Dunnett and Harris 1999). In fact, studies have demonstrated that 28 days of beta-alanine supplementation at a dosage of 4 to 6 g/day resulted in an increase of intramuscular levels of carnosine by approximately 60% (Harris et al. 2005; Zoeller et al. 2007).

Researchers have begun extensive research in the area of beta-alanine supplementation for strength athletes. Stout and colleagues (2006) examined the effects of beta-alanine supplementation on **physical working capacity at fatigue threshold (PWCFT)** in untrained young men. The participants ingested 6.4 g of beta-alanine for six days followed by 3.2 g for three weeks. The results revealed a significantly greater increase in PWCFT in the beta-alanine as compared to the placebo group. Stout and colleagues (2008) then investigated the effects of 90 days of beta-alanine supplementation (2.4 g/day) on the PWCFT in elderly men and women. They found significant increases in PWCFT (28.6%) from pre- to postsupplementation for the beta-alanine treatment group but no change with the placebo treatment. In a study using collegiate American football players, Hoffman and colleagues (2008a) found that subjects supplementing with beta-alanine (4.5 g) increased training volume significantly over 30 days compared to subjects taking a placebo. Elsewhere, Hoffman and associates (2008b) investigated the effect of 30 days of beta-alanine supplementation (4.8 g/day) on resistance exercise performance and endocrine changes in resistance-trained men. The beta-alanine group experienced a significant 22% increase in total number of repetitions as compared to the placebo group at the end of the four-week intervention. There were no significant differences between groups in hormonal responses.

> ➤   physical working capacity at fatigue threshold (PWCFT)—This parameter, often obtained using a cycle ergometer test, can identify the power output at the neuromuscular fatigue threshold.

Several studies have investigated the effects of supplementing creatine and beta-alanine together (Stout et al. 2006; Zoeller et al. 2007; Hoffman et al. 2006). The proposed benefit would increase work capacity and increase time to fatigue. Hoffman and colleagues (2006) studied the effects of creatine (10.5 g/day) plus beta-alanine (3.2 g/day) on strength, power, body composition, and endocrine changes as collegiate American football players underwent a 10-week resistance training program. Results demonstrated that creatine plus beta-alanine was effective at enhancing strength performance. Creatine plus beta-alanine supplementation also appeared to have a greater effect on lean tissue accruement and body fat composition than creatine alone. However, Stout and colleagues (2006) found that creatine did not appear to have an additive effect over beta-alanine alone.

While many studies have highlighted the positive results of beta-alanine supplementation, several other investigations have shown no improvements. In the study of collegiate American football players already mentioned, Hoffman and colleagues (2008a) examined the effects of 30 days of beta-alanine supplementation (4.5 g/day) on anaerobic performance measures. Supplementation began three weeks before preseason football training camp and continued for an additional nine days during camp. Results showed a trend toward lower fatigue rates during 60 seconds of maximal exercise; however, three weeks of beta-alanine supplementation did not result in significant improvements in fatigue rates during high-intensity anaerobic exercise. Elsewhere, Kendrick and colleagues (2008) assessed whole-body muscular strength and changes in body composition after 10 weeks of beta-alanine supplementation at a dosage of 6.4 g/day. Participants included 26 healthy male Vietnamese physical education students who were not currently involved in any resistance training program. The authors reported no significant differences between the beta-alanine group and a placebo group in whole-body strength and body composition measures after 10 weeks of supplementation.

Beta-alanine supplementation is relatively new and is a potentially useful ergogenic aid. It is important to realize that there have been only a few well-designed clinical investigations on this compound, and the published results to date have been equivocal. One of the potential limitations in the existing literature is the inconsistencies in dosing regimens. While much of the research has been positive, the dosing regimens have varied from 3 to 6 g/day. This problem is confounded by the fact that the higher doses were less effective in some cases. In relation to side effects and dosage, research from Harris and colleagues (2006) has revealed that relatively high single doses of beta-alanine are responsible for unpleasant symptoms of paresthesia (tingling sensation in the skin) that may last up to an hour. This sensation can be eliminated if the maximum single dose is 10 mg/kg of body weight, which corresponds to an average of 800 mg of beta-alanine in a single dose (Harris et al. 2006).

Professional Applications

Athletes whose performance requires high levels of strength and power spend considerable time training to improve these performance characteristics. A proper nutrition program is also responsible for maximizing the performance of a strength–power athlete. In addition to optimal training techniques and sound nutritional principles, certain sport supplements have been shown to enhance muscular strength and power. The four sport supplements that may benefit the strength–power athlete are protein, creatine, HMB, and beta-alanine.

Protein can be ingested from whole food sources, but modern technology has enabled manufacturers to isolate some of the highest-quality sources of protein (i.e., whey and casein). In addition, supplemental protein is often more convenient for athletes who travel and ingest protein several times throughout the day. Protein supplements make ingesting the recommended 1.5 to 2.0 g/kg per day a manageable task for many athletes who are busy with training and competitive schedules.

The other three sport supplements discussed in this chapter, creatine, HMB, and beta-alanine, have different levels of scientific support and reported benefits in relation to athletic and exercise performance. It has been scientifically demonstrated that creatine monohydrate can improve performance and increase lean body mass in resistance-trained athletes. This finding is very important: Even if an athlete has been resistance training for several years, when creatine monohydrate is introduced at recommended doses (20 g/day for approximately one week followed by a maintenance dose of 2 to 5 g daily), resistance training performance will likely improve. For strength–power athletes, this means that they can ingest creatine at any time during the training year—in the off-season (to increase muscle mass) and during the season (to maintain muscle mass).

In contrast, HMB supplements (typically dosed at 3 g/day) have not consistently demonstrated effectiveness relative to strength improvements and increases in lean body mass in resistance-trained individuals. However, in untrained athletes (athletes beginning a resistance training program) or in athletes who are significantly increasing their training volume, HMB supplementation may inhibit protein degradation and increase strength and lean body mass. It appears that HMB supplementation is more effective when the potential for muscle damage during exercise is greatest, as is the case for an athlete beginning a resistance training program or during periods of a competitive season in which training volume and intensity are both elevated.

In some scenarios, creatine and HMB supplementation can potentially be cycled to maximize strength and performance. For instance, American football involves three distinct periods over the year—the off-season, preseason, and the competitive season. During the off-season, sport-specific skill acquisition training decreases, and emphasis is on maximizing strength and lean muscle mass. During this period, ingesting a creatine supplement in addition to the athlete's training program would likely result in muscular strength and lean body mass gains above those that would be elicited by the training program. After the off-season at the end of the summer, the American football player enters into the preseason. The preseason is associated with an enormous amount of training and conditioning. It is not uncommon for football players to have practices multiple times per day (which include conditioning drills) and still be expected to resistance train. During this time in which training volume drastically increases (and the potential for muscle damage increases), HMB supplementation may be a wise choice to limit the amount of muscle damage incurred. After the preseason, the American football season begins; this typically lasts about three or four months and involves daily practices and one competitive game per week. In order to maintain the strength, muscle mass, and power improvements attained during the off-season, the athlete may want to supplement with creatine again, as the volume of resistance training decreases due to the practice and game schedule.

The last of the supplements discussed in this chapter, beta-alanine (typically dosed at 3-6 g/day), does not improve maximal strength but has been shown to improve short-term high-intensity exercise. More specifically, beta-alanine has the demonstrated ability to delay fatigue during high-intensity exercise. This can be advantageous for athletes such as sprinters (800 m), short-distance swimmers, and any athlete engaged in high-intensity conditioning aimed at optimizing metabolic adaptations, regardless of the sport.

SUMMARY POINTS

- While there is no replacement for a balanced diet, sport supplements can help maximize training adaptations, leading to increased strength, power, and lean muscle mass.

- Creatine has been shown to increase strength, muscle mass, and sprint performance; and no other supplement is supported by the same level of positive research.

- Protein and amino acids are required for protein synthesis to remain in a positive nitrogen balance.

- Several clinical investigations have shown that HMB acts as an anti-catabolic supplement.

- While relatively new, beta-alanine appears to be generating scientific support for its ability to improve certain aspects of high-intensity exercise performance.

- A final consideration with these sport supplements is the fact that each has been found to be safe when ingested at the recommended dosages.

Aerobic Endurance Supplements

Bob Seebohar, MS, RD, CSCS, CSSD

Before thinking about taking any ergogenic aid, athletes should consider the safety, legality, and efficacy of the supplement. Nutrition supplements are substances meant to be added to one's normal or typical eating program. These supplements are plentiful and come in a number of forms, including drinks, pills, powders, drinks, gels, chews, and bars. Some aerobic endurance supplements are efficacious, and others are not backed by any research. This chapter discusses supplements that have been shown to enhance aerobic endurance performance, or minimize muscle soreness and inflammation resulting from strenuous, prolonged exercise, or both.

Sport Drinks as Ergogenic Aids

Research on sport drinks originated in the 1960s when a then-assistant University of Florida (UF) football coach, who was also a former UF and National Football League player, asked a UF kidney specialist why the football players lost a significant amount of weight during practice but didn't urinate much. The answer was simple, but the question sparked the development of a new category in the drink market. The players lost so much fluid through sweat that they didn't have the need to urinate. The scientists found that after practice, the players they tested had low total blood volume, low blood sugar, and alterations in their electrolyte balance. The scientists then went to work developing a drink to replace fluid, sodium, and sugar. Over the next few years, the drink formula was tweaked and was made available on the sidelines of all UF football games and practices. This drink, which at the time propelled UF to power over teams in the second half of the game, eventually became known as Gatorade. Since the development of Gatorade, many research studies have examined various sport drink formulations and their ergogenic potential. Research indicates that consuming fluids, electrolytes, and carbohydrate benefits athletes in events lasting longer than 1 hour—making sport drinks potential ergogenic aids for athletes.

The main purpose of a sport beverage is to help maintain body water, carbohydrate stores, and electrolyte balance. A drastic decrease in body water or alteration in electrolyte balance could lead to serious medical conditions such as heat exhaustion, heatstroke, or hyponatremia. In fact, just a 1% decrease in body weight from fluid losses can stress the cardiovascular system by increasing heart rate and decreasing the ability to transfer heat from the body to the environment (Sawka et al. 2007). In addition, a 2% loss in body fluid may impair aerobic endurance performance (Paik et al. 2009; Barr 1999). On a practical level, research shows that many athletes can lose 2% to 6% of their body weight in fluids during exercise in the heat (Sawka et al. 2007). Therefore, the effect of fluid replacement on preventing aerobic endurance performance decrements may be greater in exercise lasting longer than 1 hour and in extreme environmental conditions such as the heat.

Maintaining Carbohydrate Stores

Aside from helping enhance hydration, sport drinks help athletes fuel their performance with carbohydrate. Initially during prolonged strenuous aerobic endurance exercise, the main storage form of carbohydrate in the body, muscle glycogen, provides the majority of the carbohydrate needed to fuel activity. However, muscle glycogen stores are limited, and as they become depleted their contribution to fueling performance also declines (Coggan and Coyle 1991). In fact, the trained athlete typically has only enough muscle glycogen to fuel a few hours of exercise at most (Acheson et al. 1988). Therefore, blood **glucose**, maintained by carbohydrate from a sport drink, gel, beans, and so on, becomes an important factor for providing the necessary energy to maintain activity (Coggan and Coyle 1991). In addition to provoking potential performance decrements, low levels of muscle glycogen are associated with protein degradation, reduced muscle glycogenolysis, and impaired excitation–contraction coupling (the process that enables a muscle cell to contract) (Hargreaves 2004).

> ➤ glucose—A monosaccharide, $C_6H_{12}O_6$, that is the major source of energy for all body cells.

Sport drinks increase levels of blood glucose, improve carbohydrate oxidation, and may help reduce fatigue during aerobic endurance training (Sawka et al. 2007). Improved carbohydrate oxidation (metabolism) reduces the reliance on limited internal carbohydrate stores (Dulloo et al.

1989). Therefore, the more carbohydrate a person can oxidize, the more she can rely on supplemental carbohydrate consumption through sport drinks, energy gels, and bars while sparing muscle glycogen.

The important components of a sport drink that can influence fluid consumption before, during, and after exercise are the type of carbohydrate and electrolytes, color, temperature, palatability, odor, taste, and texture (Sawka et al. 2007). People should consider all of these factors when choosing a sport drink. Athletes' needs vary tremendously; the choice of a sport drink should be as individualized as possible, and time should be taken to determine the proper match for an athlete's physiological needs and taste.

Carbohydrate added to a sport drink may facilitate rehydration and improve the intestinal uptake of water and sodium (Shirreffs, Armstrong, and Cheuvront 2004; Seifert, Harmon, and DeClercq 2006). A carbohydrate concentration between 6% and 8% is considered ideal for providing the needed fuel for performance without unduly slowing the gastric emptying rate (Bernadot 2006; Maughan and Murray 2001). Gastric emptying refers to how quickly fluids leave the stomach. A delay in gastric emptying indicates a delay in the absorption of the contents of the drink, and stomach upset may occur (Maughan and Murray 2001). Beverages up to 2.5% carbohydrate will leave the stomach as rapidly as water. As the carbohydrate content increases, the gastric emptying rate slows; and even a carbohydrate concentration of 6% has a gastric emptying rate significantly slower than that of water, though obviously faster than that of more concentrated drinks (Maughan and Murray 2001).

In addition to total carbohydrate, the type of carbohydrate can have a major impact on performance and carbohydrate oxidation rates. Research indicates that during exercise, consuming a drink containing more than one kind of sugar may be preferential to consuming a beverage with just one type of sugar. In one study examining carbohydrate oxidation rates, eight well-trained cyclists cycled on three separate occasions for 150 minutes each time. Glucose and **fructose** were fed at a rate of 108 g/hour (2-4 g/minute), which led to 50% higher carbohydrate oxidation rates in comparison to the ingestion of only glucose at the same rate (Currell and Jeukendrup 2008). A previous study by the same authors showed that a mixture of glucose + sucrose + fructose resulted in high peak carbohydrate oxidation rates (Jentjens, Achten, and Jeukendrup 2004). Each sugar has its own intestinal transport mechanism; therefore the researchers concluded that once the glucose-only transporter becomes saturated, carbohydrate oxidation cannot increase if glucose is the only carbohydrate ingested.

➤ fructose—A monosaccharide found in many foods.

This research is applicable to the aerobic endurance athlete because it proves that the body is able to absorb more total carbohydrate when a combination of various sugars is used versus a single type of sugar (Currell and Jeukendrup 2008; Jentjens, Achten, and Jeukendrup 2004). Using a combination of sugars will lead to an enhanced carbohydrate oxidation rate; as already mentioned, this could preserve internal stores of carbohydrate. It is also worth noting that fructose is more slowly absorbed than either sucrose or glucose. Therefore it is advisable to avoid ingesting high amounts of fructose, because accumulation in the gastrointestinal tract may lead to intestinal discomfort during exercise (Murray et al. 1989; Fujisawa, Riby, and Kretchmer 1991).

Electrolyte Replacement

The five main electrolytes are sodium, chloride, potassium, calcium, and magnesium. Sodium is the most important because it is lost to the greatest extent during exercise yet is vital for maintaining hydration and plasma volume (Rehrer 2001). When sodium levels are low, fluid loss through urine may increase, leading to a negative fluid balance (Sawka et al. 2007). Typical sweat sodium usually ranges from 10 to 70 mEq/L, and chloride ranges from 5 to 60 mEq/L, although these levels can vary tremendously and are increased by sweat rate and decreased with training adaptations and heat acclimation. Note that a large amount of sodium is typically found in individuals with high sweat rates, so these people may need to be especially cognizant of their sodium consumption.

Sodium deficiency becomes a much greater issue with longer-duration exercise and when fluid low in sodium is consumed (Rehrer 2001). Potassium sweat loss ranges are only 3 to 15 mEq/L, followed by calcium at 0.3 to 2 mEq/L and magnesium at 0.2 to 1.5 mEq/L (Brouns 1991). Potassium deficiency is rare with fluid loss from exercise (Rehrer 2001). In fact, 8 to 29 times more sodium is lost compared to potassium (Otukonyong and Oyebola 1994; Maughan et al. 1991; Morgan, Patterson, and Nimmo 2004).

Sport drinks should contain about 176 to 552 mg sodium per fluid liter (Shirreffs et al. 2007); and if potassium is present, it should be in significantly smaller amounts since it is not excreted in great amounts in sweat. In ultra-aerobic endurance exercise, an even greater concentration of sodium may be beneficial, 552 to 920 mg per fluid liter (Rehrer 2001). It is important to note that in order to remain in positive fluid balance, people need to consume more sodium than they lose through sweat (Shirreffs and Maughan 1998). Aerobic endurance athletes seldom consume enough fluids to replace sweat losses. According to one research study, athletes consumed less than 0.5 L/hour of fluid while their sweat rates ranged from 1.0 to 1.5 L/hour (Noakes 1993). Thus, sodium becomes of utmost importance and can help reduce cardiovascular strain when ingested with fluid. Additionally, when combined with water, sodium can assist in decreasing fluid deficits seen during exercise (Sanders, Noakes, and Dennis 1999).

The American College of Sports Medicine recommends consuming 0.5 to 0.7 g of sodium per liter of fluid per hour; other researchers recommend a higher range, 1.7 to 2.9 g per liter of fluid per hour (Maughan 1991). Regardless of the quantities suggested by research, it is important for the health professional to help athletes determine sweat sodium losses during training of different durations and intensities and in varying environmental conditions. Electrolyte needs vary among athletes and can exceed 3 g/hour (Murray and Kenney 2008). Regular sodium intake is important for improving cardiovascular functioning and performance in that it replaces lost sodium, continues the thirst response, and enhances voluntary drinking (Baker, Munce, and Kenney 2005).

Amino Acids and Protein for Aerobic Endurance Athletes

Some researchers believe that protein requirements for aerobic endurance athletes are higher than for non-aerobic endurance-trained individuals (Jeukendrup and Gleeson 2004; Lamont, McCullough, and Kalhan 1999) because branched-chain amino acids (BCAAs) are oxidized in greater amounts during exercise than at rest. However, just as some research supports this theory, there is also evidence that training does not have this effect on leucine (Wolfe et al. 1984) or BCAAs (Lamont, McCullough, and Kalhan 1999). Additionally, some scientists believe that exercise increases protein efficiency, which makes additional protein in the diet unnecessary (Butterfield and Calloway 1984). In contrast, other investigations (utilizing the nitrogen balance technique) have found that athletes require more daily protein than the average 0.8 g/kg body weight recommended for nonexercising individuals (Lemon and Proctor 1991). Therefore, aerobic endurance athletes should consume 1.2 to 1.4 g of protein per kilogram body weight (Lemon 1998).

Interestingly, protein exhibits a high satiety response; and in athletes seeking weight loss or weight maintenance, intakes up to 2.0 g/kg body weight could prove useful in curbing hunger (Halton and Hu 2004; Latner and Schwartz 1999). However, a daily protein intake over 2 g/kg body weight per day did not elicit any performance advantage for aerobic endurance athletes (Tipton and Wolfe 2004). What is certain is that individuals who participate in aerobic endurance exercise must consume enough protein to help build and repair their body based on the physical demands of their training. If training volume and intensity fluctuate throughout a year with different aerobic endurance and resistance exercise goals, it makes sense to readjust the diet and protein intake accordingly (Dunford 2006). Research in aerobic endurance athletes has examined the effect of both BCAAs and different types of protein on performance and recovery from exercise.

Branched-Chain Amino Acids

Amino acids are the building blocks of protein and can serve as an energy source for skeletal muscle (Ohtani, Sugita, and Maryuma 2006). Protein synthesis can also occur at rest even when essential amino acids are consumed in relatively small amounts, for example 15 g (Paddon-Jones et al. 2004). Branched-chain amino acids are becoming more popular in aerobic endurance exercise due to their potential performance benefits. The BCAAs include leucine, isoleucine, and valine. They can be oxidized by the skeletal muscle to provide the muscles with energy, can enhance postexercise muscle protein synthesis, and can reduce exercise-induced muscle damage (Koopman et al. 2004). The average BCAA content of food proteins is roughly 15% of the total amino acid content (Gleeson 2005); therefore individuals regularly consuming good-quality protein-rich foods are probably consuming adequate amounts of BCAAs to support daily body protein needs.

During aerobic endurance exercise, the BCAA pool, in particular, is maintained through muscle protein breakdown, which makes it even more important that the body remain in protein balance. In longer-duration aerobic endurance exercise, the oxidation of BCAAs in skeletal muscle usually exceeds their supply from protein. This causes a decline of BCAAs in the blood and may facilitate the progression of "central fatigue." According to the central fatigue hypothesis, central fatigue occurs when tryptophan crosses the blood–brain barrier and increases the amount of serotonin forming in the brain (Ohtani, Sugita, and Maryuma 2006). The hypothesis predicts that during exercise, free fatty acids (FFAs) are mobilized from fat tissue and transported to the muscles to be used as energy. Because the rate of FFAs being mobilized is greater than their uptake in the muscles, the concentration of FFAs in the blood increases. Free fatty acids and the amino acid tryptophan compete for the same binding sites on **albumin**. Because FFAs are present in high amounts in the blood, they bind to albumin first, thus preventing tryptophan from binding and leading to an increase in free tryptophan concentration in the blood. This increases the free tryptophan–to–BCAA ratio in the blood, resulting in an increased free tryptophan transport across the blood–brain barrier. Once free tryptophan is inside the brain, it is converted to serotonin, which plays a role in mood and the onset of sleep (Banister et al. 1983). Thus, an end result of more serotonin production in the brain may be central fatigue, forcing individuals to either stop exercise or reduce the intensity.

> ➤ albumin—A water-soluble protein found in many animal tissues.

Although several studies show a drop in BCAA concentration in the blood and although BCAAs may help with mental performance during or after exhaustive exercise, supplementation may have little impact on actual aerobic endurance performance. A few studies have examined changes in amino acid concentration after exhaustive exercise. Researchers in one study examined these changes in 22 subjects participating in a marathon and eight subjects participating in a 1.5-hour army training program. Both groups experienced a significant decline in their plasma concentration of BCAAs. No change was noted in the concentration of total tryptophan in either group, though the marathon subjects showed a significant increase in free tryptophan leading to a decrease in the free tryptophan/BCAA ratio (Blomstrand, Celsing, and Newsholme 1988). Other studies also show a decrease in BCAA concentration and increase in free or total tryptophan after exhaustive exercise (Blomstrand et al. 1997; Struder et al. 1997). In a double-blind examination of the direct effect of BCAAs on tryptophan, 10 aerobic endurance-trained males cycled at 70% to 75% maximal power output while ingesting drinks that contained 6% sucrose (control) or 6% sucrose + one of the following: 3 g tryptophan, 6 g BCAAs, or 18 g BCAAs. Tryptophan ingestion resulted in a 7- to 20-fold increase in brain tryptophan levels, whereas BCAA supplementation resulted in an 8% to 12% decrease in brain tryptophan levels at exhaustion. No differences were noted in exercise time to exhaustion, indicating that the changes in amino acid concentrations did not affect aerobic endurance exercise performance (Van Hall et al. 1995).

In addition to studying changes in amino acid concentration, it makes sense to examine whether there is a subsequent change in cognitive performance. In a study examining the central fatigue hypothesis and changes in cognition, subjects received either a mixture of BCAAs in carbohydrate or a placebo drink. The investigators measured cognitive performance before and after a 30 km cross country race. Subjects given BCAAs showed an improvement from before to after the run in certain parts of a color–word test; the placebo group showed no change. The BCAA-supplemented group also maintained their performance in shape rotation and figure identification tasks, whereas the placebo group showed a significant decline in performance in both tests after the run. The authors noted that BCAA supplementation had a greater effect on performance in more complex tasks (Hassmen et al. 1994). In another study of cognitive functioning after exhaustive exercise, participants ran a 42.2 km cross country race during which they were supplemented with either BCAAs or placebo. The BCAA supplementation improved running performance in the slower runners only. What is more interesting is that the BCAAs positively affected mental performance. The BCAA-supplemented group showed significant improvement in the Stroop color and word test postexercise compared to preexercise (Blomstrand et al. 1991).

Branched-chain amino acid supplementation can also influence recovery from exercise. Feeding BCAAs before aerobic exercise increases the concentration of human growth hormone and helps prevent a decrease in testosterone, which results in a more anabolic environment (Carli et al. 1992). Prolonged exercise will reduce the body's amino acid pool; thus it is important to maintain higher levels, specifically BCAA levels, to suppress cell signaling cascades that promote muscle protein breakdown (Tipton and Wolfe 1998). Creating an anabolic environment through BCAA use may assist in faster recovery from exercise. Branched-chain amino acids also have a positive effect on lessening the degree of muscle damage. In one study, untrained men performed three 90-minute cycling bouts at 55% intensity and consumed a 200-calorie beverage consisting of carbohydrate, BCAA, or placebo before and at 60 minutes during exercise. The BCAA-supplemented beverage trial lessened the amount of muscle damage resulting from the exercise session compared to the placebo trial at 4, 24, and 48 hours after exercise and the carbohydrate trial at 24 hours after exercise (Greer et al. 2007).

Protein and Recovery

Studies examining the effect of protein + carbohydrate on glycogen resynthesis are equivocal; some indicate that protein + carbohydrate is more effective (though some of these studies also provided more total calories), and others show no difference. In one small study, six male cyclists received an **isocaloric** liquid carbohydrate–protein supplement (0.8 g/kg carbohydrate, 0.4 g/kg protein), a carbohydrate-only supplement (1.2 g/kg carbohydrate), or placebo immediately, 1 hour, and 2 hours after a 60-minute cycling time trial. Six hours after the initial trial, the cycling protocol was repeated. Though cycling performance in the subsequent time trial was not different between groups, muscle glycogen resynthesis was significantly greater in the carbohydrate + protein group versus the carbohydrate-only or placebo group during the 6 hours of recovery (Berardi et al. 2006). Another study in nine male subjects yielded similar results, though it is unclear whether the enhanced glycogen resynthesis was due to the addition of protein to carbohydrate or to the greater overall calories in this supplement. In this particular trial, subjects cycled for 2 hours on three separate occasions to deplete muscle glycogen. Immediately and 2 hours postexercise, they ingested 112 g carbohydrate, 40.7 g protein, or 112 g carbohydrate + 40.7 g protein. The rate of muscle glycogen storage during the carbohydrate + protein trial was significantly faster than during the carbohydrate-only trial. Both were significantly faster than the protein-only trial (Zawadzki, Yaspelkis, and Ivy 1992).

➤ isocaloric—Having similar caloric values.

Though these results seem promising, a few studies indicate that the addition of protein to carbohydrate may not further augment muscle glycogen synthesis. In a small study, five subjects received either 1.67 g/kg body weight sucrose or water or 1.67 g/kg body weight sucrose + 0.5 g/kg body weight whey protein hydrolysate immediately after intense cycling and every 15 minutes for 4 hours during the recovery period. There were no significant differences in glycogen resynthesis rates between the carbohydrate-only and carbohydrate + protein groups (Van Hall, Shirreffs, and Calbet 2000). One potential weakness of this study was that it did not use a crossover design as in the other studies (Berardi et al. 2006; Zawadzki, Yaspelkis, and Ivy 1992). A crossover design uses the same subjects for all treatments, which allows the researchers to make more definitive statements about the effectiveness of a given nutrient intervention.

Another investigation in six men yielded similar results. In this crossover study, the men performed two bouts of running on the same day (with a 4-hour recovery period in between) and repeated this protocol 14 days later. At 30-minute intervals during the recovery period, the subjects consumed either carbohydrate only (0.8 g/kg body weight) or carbohydrate (0.8 g/kg body weight) + whey protein isolate (0.3 g/kg body weight). Muscle glycogen resynthesis was not different between groups. However, during the second run, whole-body carbohydrate oxidation (utilization of carbohydrate) was significantly greater in the carbohydrate + protein treatment group, indicating a potential benefit of this combination (Betts et al. 2008).

Though the effect of protein added to carbohydrate on muscle glycogen resynthesis is unclear, the addition of protein to a carbohydrate beverage may increase net protein balance, which in turn may help prevent muscle soreness and damage and thereby promote recovery. In a crossover study examining this, eight aerobic endurance-trained athletes ingested carbohydrate (0.7 g/kg body weight per hour) every 30 minutes during 6 hours of aerobic endurance exercise, and protein + carbohydrate (0.7 g carbohydrate/kg body weight per hour + 0.25 g protein/kg body weight per hour) every 30 minutes during a subsequent 6-hour exercise bout. Whole-body protein balance during exercise with carbohydrate only was negative, whereas the ingestion of carbohydrate + protein resulted in either positive balance or less negative balance (depending on the tracer used to examine whole-body protein balance) (Koopman et al. 2004).

Including protein or BCAAs in the postexercise nutrition plan may enhance muscle recovery and decrease the effect of muscular damage sometimes seen after heavy aerobic endurance exercise. Researchers observed significant reductions in creatine kinase, a blood marker of muscle damage, when cross country runners consumed a beverage with vitamins C and E and 0.365 g of whey protein per kilogram body weight versus a carbohydrate-only beverage (Luden, Saunders, and Todd 2007). Another study showed that feeding 12 g of BCAAs for 14 days before aerobic endurance exercise as well as immediately afterward reduced creatine kinase levels (Coombes and McNaughton 2000).

Though these studies highlight positive results from the addition of protein or BCAAs postexercise, other researchers have found no benefit to adding protein to the postworkout nutrition plan as evidenced by no changes in the level of markers of muscle damage. In one study showing no performance benefit to adding protein to a 4-hour recovery feeding, subjects cycled, recovered, and then cycled the next day. This crossover design study used a small sample and used the subjects as their own controls; subjects received a protein-enriched recovery feeding in the first part of the experiment, followed by a two-week washout period and an isocaloric recovery feeding in the second phase (Rowlands et al. 2007). Additionally, in a study looking at the addition of protein to a carbohydrate drink postexercise in an eccentric exercise model that induced muscular injury, protein did not have a significant effect on returning creatine kinase levels to normal after 30 minutes of downhill running (Green et al. 2008).

Combined, these studies indicate that protein or BCAA may or may not benefit aerobic endurance athletes when consumed postexercise. However, it makes sense for aerobic endurance athletes to eat 1.2 to 1.4 g protein per kilogram body weight daily to ensure an adequate pool of amino acids that the body can rely on during times of need to reduce the catabolic effects of prolonged aerobic endurance exercise (Lemon 1998).

Glutamine

Glutamine rounds out the list of most important single amino acids for aerobic endurance athletes. Glutamine is found in the highest concentration in the free amino acid pool. More of it is present in slow-twitch muscle (Turinsky and Long 1990), which suggests a greater need for this amino acid during aerobic endurance exercise. Plasma glutamine usually follows a pattern of increasing during exercise and decreasing afterward. Intense, long-duration aerobic endurance exercise suppresses the immune system especially if athletes are overtrained (Castell 2003). Because glutamine is an important fuel for the immune system, maintaining an adequate level is extremely important for aerobic endurance athletes. Plasma glutamine concentrations are lower after prolonged, exhaustive exercise; and including glutamine in supplemental form after exercise helped reduce the incidence of infections and illnesses, which quite often plague aerobic endurance athletes after intense training or competition (Bassit et al. 2000).

High Molecular Weight Carbohydrates

Fatigue can be influenced by muscle glycogen stores because adenosine triphosphate (ATP, the energy used in cells) cannot be generated at the rate needed during exercise. Higher muscle and liver glycogen concentrations before exercise can be beneficial to aerobic endurance exercisers. Additionally, the rapid resynthesis of muscle glycogen is important for individuals who participate in many training sessions per day or in longer-duration submaximal exercise sessions. The latter is common for most aerobic endurance athletes, irrespective of the competition distance. Aerobic training is a staple in almost every aerobic endurance athlete's plan, and maintaining consistent carbohydrate stores is of utmost importance.

Blood glucose concentrations are influenced by the movement of ingested glucose from the stomach to the intestine and finally into the blood. This becomes important because the osmolality of a solution influences the gastric emptying rate from the stomach (Vist and Maughan 1994). Carbohydrate sources with high osmolality may delay glucose transportation by slowing gastric emptying (Aulin, Soderlund, and Hultman 2000). A steady supply of glucose without much delay of delivery to the blood and the working muscles and brain is ideal for maintaining physical and cognitive functioning. Additionally, restoring a high amount of glycogen after aerobic endurance exercise is important for subsequent training sessions. Because muscle glycogen resynthesis is highest during the first 2 hours after exercise (Kiens et al. 1990), the type of carbohydrate consumed in the postworkout window becomes even more important in the recovery from the training stimulus.

Patented High Molecular Weight Carbohydrates

Many high molecular weight (HMW) carbohydrates are marketed as substances that can help replenish glycogen stores rapidly. However, this is a misconception. It is not necessarily the size that matters but instead the biology of the carbohydrate. One patented highly branched HMW glucose polymer solution increased the rate of gastric emptying (Leiper et al. 2000), postexercise muscle glycogen resynthesis (Aulin, Soderlund, and Hultman 2000), and subsequent work output. In three separate visits, eight men cycled to exhaustion at 73% maximum oxygen uptake (cycling between 88 and 91 minutes). Immediately postexercise, subjects consumed either 1 L sugar-free flavored water (control), 100 g low molecular weight glucose polymer (maltodextrin), or 100 g of the patented very high molecular weight glucose polymer. They then rested in a bed for a 2-hour recovery period, after which they performed a 15-minute time trial on a cycle ergometer. In comparison to maltodextrin (a common ingredient in sport drinks and supplements), the patented very high molecular weight carbohydrate resulted in faster and greater increases in blood glucose, serum insulin, and work output on the subsequent time trial, presumably due to increased glycogen storage.

Waxy Maize

Waxy maize products are marketed as carbohydrate that can enhance glycogen resynthesis to a greater extent than other types of carbohydrate. However, the published studies on waxy maize show no ergogenic benefit when compared to other types of carbohydrate commonly used in sport nutrition products. Waxy maize produces a blunted blood glucose and insulin response in comparison to maltodextrin (Roberts et al. 2009) and decreased glycogen resynthesis in comparison to an equivalent intake of glucose (Jozsi et al. 1996).

In one study on waxy maize and performance, 10 college-aged men competed in four protocols in which they ingested 1 g/kg body weight of glucose, waxy starch, resistant starch, or artificially flavored placebo 30 minutes before a bout of cycling (90 minutes of a constant load at 66% $\dot{V}O_2$max followed by a 30-minute experimental protocol). Mean carbohydrate oxidation rates were higher during the glucose, waxy starch, and resistance starch trials compared to placebo; and subjects who ingested waxy maize or glucose performed more work (Roberts et al. 2009). Other studies indicate that waxy maize starch is no more beneficial than glucose or maltodextrin for glycogen resynthesis or subsequent time-trial performance after glycogen-depleting exercise (Jozsi et al. 1996) and that glucose may be superior to waxy maize starch for increasing glucose and insulin response (Goodpaster et al. 1996). For a breakdown on waxy maize starch studies, refer to table 8.1.

Caffeine

Caffeine is a multifaceted supplement used in athletics and is one of the most popular among aerobic endurance exercisers. Caffeine has many

TABLE 8.1   Summary of the Research on Waxy Maize

Authors	Participants	Supplement and dosage	Time given	Type of exercise	Study findings
Roberts et al. 2009	10 male cyclists	1 g/kg body weight: • WMS • Maltodextrin	Before and after exercise	Cycling 150 min at 70% $\dot{V}O_2$peak	• WMS compared to maltodextrin led to a blunted spike in blood glucose postingestion. • Significantly lower insulin increase with WMS compared to maltodextrin. • Greater fat breakdown and oxidation during exercise and recovery with WMS compared to maltodextrin.
Goodpaster et al. 1996	10 college-aged male competitive cyclists	1 g/kg body weight: • WS • RS: 70% amylose and 30% amylopectin • GL • Placebo	30 min before exercise	120 min cycling (30 min self-paced and 90 min constant load)	• GL elicited a greater increase in glucose and insulin compared to WMS, RS, and placebo. • Subjects completed more work after ingesting GL or WS compared to placebo.

Authors	Participants	Supplement and dosage	Time given	Type of exercise	Study findings
Jozsi et al. 1996	8 male cyclists	Mixed meal (3,000 calories) with 15% as: • Glucose • Maltodextrin • WS (100% amylopectin) • RS (100% amylose)	12 h after glycogen-depleting exercise	30 min cycling time trial 24 h after glycogen-depleting exercise (12 h after supplemental food intake)	• No differences in time trial performance between groups. • Glycogen concentration increased significantly less in RS (+90 ± 12.8 mmol/kg d.w.) versus GL (+197.7 ± mmol/kg d.w.), maltodextrin (+136.7 ± 24.5 mmol/kg d.w.), and WS (+171.8 ± 37.1 mmol/kg d.w.).
Johannsen and Sharp 2007	7 aerobic endurance–trained men	1 g/kg body weight: • Dextrose • Modified cornstarch • Unmodified cornstarch	30 min before exercise	2 h of cycling	• Only modified cornstarch raised carbohydrate oxidation throughout exercise. • Exogenous carbohydrate oxidation was higher with dextrose compared to modified cornstarch and unmodified cornstarch until 90 min exercise.

Abbreviations: WMS = waxy maize starch; WS = waxy starch (100% amylopectin); RS = resistant starch; GL = glucose; d.w. = dry weight.

potential sport applications. Studies show that doses of 4 mg/kg caffeine can increase mental alertness and improve logical reasoning, free recall, and recognition memory tasks (Smith et al. 1994). In addition, caffeine can help increase time to exhaustion in aerobic endurance exercise bouts (Bell and McLellan 2003; Doherty and Smith 2004), decrease ratings of perceived exertion during submaximal aerobic endurance exercise (Demura, Yamada, and Terasawa 2007), and improve physical performance during periods of sleep deprivation (McLellan, Bell, and Kamimori 2004). Caffeine also has the potential to decrease muscle soreness and augment glycogen resynthesis (Pederson et al. 2008).

Despite the many uses of caffeine, research is equivocal regarding caffeine and improved sport performance. However, this may be attributable to study design factors such as the caffeine dose, the form of caffeine (pill, coffee, or with carbohydrate sources), normal dietary use of caffeine, timing and pattern of caffeine intake before exercise, and the environment in which the exercise testing takes place (Graham 2001).

Caffeine is a stimulant that acts on the central nervous system by crossing the blood–brain barrier and binding to adenosine receptors causing a decrease in adenosine bound to these receptors and a subsequent increase in circulating dopamine activity (Fredholm et al. 1999). According to one theory, this affects the perception of effort and neural activation of muscular contractions. This is the most popular of the main theories aimed at explaining the ergogenic effect of caffeine and also has the most value in terms of scientific support and field validation with exercisers. Another theory surrounding the benefits of caffeine involves a muscle performance effect on enzymes that control the breakdown of glycogen. Most of the support for this theory has come not from in vivo (within the body) but from in vitro (outside the body) research; so it is difficult to draw any formal conclusions related to the theory. Finally, caffeine can acutely increase **lipolysis** and **thermogenesis** (Dulloo et al. 1989) and potentially increase both over a period of time. Also, it may exert a glycogen-sparing effect (Graham 2001). Caffeine is thought to enhance the enzymes that break down fat or increase the levels of **epinephrine**, which can mobilize stored fat (Graham and Spriet 1996). However, research examining this theory is not conclusive (Graham 2001). The current consensus lends more support to the effect on the central nervous system and the reduced perception of effort. Support also comes from athletes undergoing training sessions and competitions encompassing various modes of activity. Caffeine is rapidly absorbed and can reach a maximum level in the plasma within 1 hour. Because it is broken down slowly (half-life of 4-6 hours), concentration can usually be maintained for 3 to 4 hours (Graham 2001).

➤ lipolysis—The breakdown of fat stored in fat cells.

➤ thermogenesis—Heat production in organisms. An increase in thermogenesis will increase calories burned (at least temporarily).

➤ epinephrine—A catecholamine released by the adrenal glands as part of a person's fight-or-flight response. Epinephrine release results in an increase in heart rate, blood vessel contraction, and dilation of air passages.

Ergogenic benefits of caffeine have been shown with doses ranging from 3 to 9 mg/kg body weight (about 1.5-3.5 cups of automatic drip coffee in a 70-kg [154-pound] person) (Hoffman et al. 2007). The performance effects are usually evident when caffeine is consumed within 60 minutes before exercise but are also noticeable when it is consumed during prolonged exercise (Yeo et al. 2005).

Researchers have also looked at the effect of caffeine on carbohydrate absorption and the effects of consuming caffeine combined with a carbohydrate source. Caffeine increases carbohydrate absorption in the intestine. This has been observed with small amounts (1.4 mg/kg body weight) (Van Nieuwenhoven, Brummer, and Brouns 2000) and larger amounts (5 mg/kg body weight); carbohydrate oxidation rates increase by 26% during the last 30 minutes of a 2-hour exercise bout (Yeo et al. 2005). Taken together, these data indicate that caffeine could have a positive impact on carbohydrate use in the body with faster delivery to the working muscles. Additional research has confirmed the improvement of work capacity (15-23%) and lower ratings of perceived exertion when caffeine is consumed with a carbohydrate beverage (Cureton et al. 2007). Caffeine has been thought to act as a diuretic, but the addition of caffeine to a sport drink does not affect fluid delivery or produce any adverse fluid balance or thermoregulation issues during moderate- to high-intensity exercise (Millard-Stafford et al. 2007).

While it is considered a drug, caffeine appears to be safe when used properly; and for most aerobic endurance sports, an ergogenic benefit is seen in doses ranging from 3 to 9 mg/kg body weight taken about 1 hour before exercise. Caffeine is permitted for use by the International Olympic Committee and is on the National Collegiate Athletic Association (NCAA) restricted list (urine concentrations of caffeine must not exceed 15 μm/ml) (U.S. Anti-Doping Agency 2010; National Collegiate Athletic Association 2009).

Sodium Bicarbonate and Citrate

The use of sodium bicarbonate is not new, and its popularity seems to ebb and flow in aerobic endurance sports. Sodium bicarbonate is used as a buffer. A decrease in pH, a more acidic environment, is associated with fatigue; this can have negative performance implications such as increased ratings of perceived exertion and reduced force production (Hawley and Reilly 1997). Supplements that provide a more pH-friendly, alkaline base have been used for years and can delay the onset of fatigue by buffering acidic levels during higher-intensity exercise. The use of these buffering agents proves more beneficial in higher-intensity, short-duration exercise that entails larger muscle involvement and faster motor unit recruitment. In equally high intense but longer-duration exercise, results on the efficacy of these products have been conflicting and have not provided absolute proof of their performance enhancement abilities (Requena et al. 2005).

Sodium bicarbonate has been the most frequently used buffering agent, but sodium citrate is a better option due to its lower incidence and risk of gastrointestinal distress. Better implementation protocols using sodium bicarbonate have also helped resolve some of the gastrointestinal discomfort issues associated with this supplement.

Because the results of research studies have not been consistent, some athletes are turning to newer ergogenic aids such as beta-alanine (discussed in more detail in chapter 7). Current evidence indicates that sodium bicarbonate, citrate, or both can be useful in sports using different energy systems but may be most beneficial to performance of shorter, higher-intensity bouts. These must be used with caution due to the potential for gastrointestinal upset.

Advising athletes on supplements must be done with great care and with full knowledge of their health status, medications, and other supplement usage. When making recommendations for aerobic endurance athletes, practitioners must always keep in mind three important nutrition factors: hydration, electrolyte balance, and carbohydrate intake.

Aerobic endurance events can be won or lost by a matter of minutes, making ergogenic aids popular tools among athletes. The ergogenic aids discussed in this chapter are those for which research has shown benefits to aerobic endurance performance. Table 8.2 summarizes these supplements, their potential ergogenic effects, and potential drawbacks to their use.

TABLE 8.2 Popular Aerobic Endurance Supplements

Sport supplement	Proposed function	Performance benefits	Potential drawbacks
Branched-chain amino acids (BCAAs)	Reduced muscle damage; enhanced recovery from exercise; decrease in central fatigue	BCAAs can improve measures of cognitive performance after long, exhaustive bouts of exercise. They can also enhance recovery from exercise by creating a more anabolic protein balance environment postexercise and decreasing markers of muscle damage. BCAAs may show the greatest potential benefit when consumed during long, exhaustive exercise in a variety of aerobic endurance athletes.	None documented with normal use in healthy adults.
Caffeine	Increased time to exhaustion in aerobic endurance performance; enhanced mental alertness; decreased muscle soreness; enhanced glycogen resynthesis	Caffeine can decrease feelings of fatigue, increase time to exhaustion, and may decrease muscle soreness (especially after eccentric exercise such as downhill running); it may enhance glycogen resynthesis. Anhydrous caffeine (pills vs. in a liquid such as coffee) may have the most pronounced ergogenic effect. Any athlete may benefit from caffeine in one or more ways.	Pregnant women should limit consumption to 300 mg/day due to potentially adverse affects in the fetus; caffeine may adversely affect those with anxiety disorders, cardiac disorders, glaucoma, and hypertension. Anecdotally, some individuals claim that they have an increase in anxiety or increase in cardiac rhythm abnormalities with even small amounts of caffeine.

Sport supplement	Proposed function	Performance benefits	Potential drawbacks
Electrolyte replacement (sodium tablets)	Prevention of hyponatremia	All aerobic endurance athletes engaging in long, exhaustive bouts of exercise can benefit from consuming electrolytes, primarily sodium. Electrolytes prevent hyponatremia, increase thirst, and therefore encourage drinking; they can increase overall hydration, preventing dangerous drops in total body water.	Sodium use is contraindicated in those with hypertension and people with kidney disease. Healthy athletes without hypertension should have no problem with sodium.
Glutamine	Reduced incidence of infections and illness; promotion of recovery by preventing muscle soreness	It remains unclear exactly who glutamine can benefit. Athletes more likely to become ill or those prone to infections (as well as those who tax their bodies by running "ultras," Ironman races, etc.) may want to try glutamine.	None documented with normal use in healthy adults.
Highly branched high molecular weight glucose polymer (patented)	Increased glycogen resynthesis compared to maltodextrin	Fast gastric emptying compared to a combination of maltodextrin + sugars; it quickly replaces muscle glycogen. Best for athletes who train hard more than once per day.	None documented with normal use in healthy adults. Diabetics need to closely monitor their carbohydrate intake and insulin dosing schedule.
Protein	May enhance glycogen resynthesis postexercise when combined with carbohydrates	Every athlete can benefit from taking protein postworkout (taking during a workout may cause stomach upset). Research shows that postworkout protein can decrease protein breakdown and may speed up recovery.	None documented with normal use in healthy adults.
Sodium bicarbonate and citrate	Decrease in pH, which may attenuate fatigue	Though in some instances, sodium bicarbonate and sodium citrate have been found to effectively buffer muscle fatigue, these supplements are not the best option as they may cause gastrointestinal distress.	These supplements, especially sodium bicarbonate, may cause gastrointestinal distress.
Sport beverages	Hydration; sodium can help prevent hyponatremia; enhanced performance; maintenance of blood glucose; reduced fatigue during long bouts of exercise	Sport drinks are one of the best ergogenic aids for aerobic endurance athletes. They have three research-validated purposes: preventing hyponatremia, maintaining total body water, and reducing fatigue during long bouts of exercise.	High intake of fructose may cause gastrointestinal upset during exercise.

*All supplements should be tested during training before being used during competition.

Sport drinks are one of the most widely used ergogenic aids among aerobic endurance athletes. Why choose a sport drink instead of plain water? As first discovered on the football field at the University of Florida in the 1960s, water only may not suffice. Sport drinks can help maintain body water, carbohydrate stores, and electrolyte balance. And athletes are more likely to consume a greater quantity of a drink that they perceive as tasting good in comparison to water. Athletes engaging in strenuous exercise, especially in the heat, can lose 2% to 6% of their body weight in fluid. Not only will they overheat when they lose this much fluid; they are more likely to experience a significant drop in performance as well. Sport drinks have proven time and time again to be effective in blunting this potential drop in performance.

Ideally, an athlete who consumes a sport drink should opt for a 6% to 8% carbohydrate solution and consume 3 to 8 ounces every 10 to 20 minutes during aerobic endurance exercise lasting longer than 60 to 90 minutes. Athletes who choose not to consume a sport drink but instead opt for water will need to consume carbohydrate both during and immediately after training and competition. In addition, they should consume a source of electrolytes, especially sodium. While an athlete who walks or jogs a marathon may be able to get away with consuming a variety of real foods during competition with little stomach upset, most competitive athletes opt for the convenience and ease of digestibility of various sport nutrition products, including gels and "gummies."

Aerobic endurance athletes should aim for 30 to 60 g of carbohydrate per hour while exercising, although those consuming multiple types of carbohydrate can consume 90 g of carbohydrate per hour. And athletes should consume approximately 0.8 to 1.2 g carbohydrate per kilogram body weight postexercise, depending on the intensity and duration of the exercise and the amount of carbohydrate consumed during exercise. In addition, athletes will benefit from ingesting some protein, approximately 0.3 to 0.4 g/kg body weight, with their carbohydrate postexercise to facilitate muscle repair.

Ideally, athletes will consume their postworkout snack within 30 minutes. Waiting will decrease glycogen resynthesis, and subsequent bouts of exercise (especially if the rest period is <24 hours) may be compromised. Even trained athletes have enough stored carbohydrate, in the form of glycogen, to fuel them for only a few hours. In addition to potential performance decrements, low levels of muscle glycogen are also associated with protein degradation, which could result in the breakdown of muscle tissue especially if the athlete is not consuming enough total protein and calories.

Excellent examples of postworkout snacks that meet the criteria for a 150-pound (68-kg) athlete are 20 ounces (600 ml) of low-fat chocolate milk or a blended shake made with 1 cup of sliced strawberries, 1 cup grapes, 1 banana, and 1 scoop of protein powder in water. Athletes can use a variety of combinations to refuel themselves, including cereal with skim milk, salted crackers with low-fat cheese, or combinations of sport supplement products and food (a sport drink followed by nonfat yogurt with fruit on the bottom, for instance).

Athletes who opt for water should also consider their electrolyte needs. Every athlete loses a different amount of the electrolytes (sodium is the electrolyte lost in the greatest quantity). The sport nutrition professional should help athletes determine approximate sweat sodium needs for different durations of training and in different environments. Unless otherwise told by their physician, aerobic endurance athletes should not follow the general recommendations to the public—1,500 to 2,000 mg sodium per day. Instead, they should consume about 500 to 700 mg sodium per liter of fluid during exercise. However, from a practical standpoint, some athletes need quite a bit more than this and will still cramp and lose too much fluid even if they consume the upper limit of this range. Again, the sport nutrition professional can work with athletes to find a range that better suits their needs. After exercise, athletes should consume at least 500 mg sodium for every pound of water weight they lose.

Aside from fluid, electrolytes, and carbohydrate, athletes looking to get an edge on their competition may look toward a variety of other ergogenic aids to help them perform better and enhance recovery. Branched-chain amino acids may help decrease central fatigue so that the aerobic endurance athlete can perform well on mental tasks immediately after exercising (this is helpful for a college athlete who has to study for a test after a long run). Branched-chain amino acids may also help mitigate muscle soreness and inflammation, thereby speeding up recovery from long bouts of exercise. Studies have used anywhere from 6 to 12 g of BCAAs for this purpose, though it is unclear exactly how much should be given and whether BCAAs should be dosed based on per kilogram body weight, on the intensity and duration of exercise, or both.

While BCAAs may help mitigate soreness and inflammation postexercise, some athletes looking to buffer muscular fatigue during exercise have tried sodium bicarbonate and citrate. Even though these two supplements may work, they are not recommended ergogenic aids because of the potential for gastrointestinal upset. No ergogenic aid should come at a price that could impair performance. A better option is beta-alanine, which is discussed in detail in chapter 7.

Some aerobic endurance athletes use glutamine to help boost immunity. Plasma glutamine concentrations are lower after prolonged, exhaustive exercise; and including glutamine in supplemental form after exercise helps reduce the incidence of infections and illnesses, which frequently plague aerobic endurance athletes after intense training or competition. Some studies indicate that glutamine shows promise, though the proper dosage is unclear. Glutamine will not likely affect performance in any way, but staying healthy is vital for maintaining one's training load.

One of the best ergogenic aids for aerobic endurance athletes is caffeine. In doses of 3 to 9 mg/kg body weight (about 1.5-3.5 cups of automatic drip coffee in a 70-kg [154-pound] person) consumed either before exercise (typically 60 minutes) or during prolonged exercise, caffeine is ergogenic. It can decrease feelings of perceived exertion, improve work capacity, and increase mental alertness. This quantity of caffeine does not produce any harmful changes in fluid balance or lead to dehydration. Athletes who try caffeine will typically notice an immediate difference.

The use of nutrition supplements with aerobic endurance athletes is widespread; however, they vary widely in their efficacy and safety. Many do not have scientific or field evidence to support their mechanisms of action or efficacy of use in athletics. Others are not backed by research, but some athletes swear by them. The sport nutrition professional should pay particularly close attention to the safety and legality of sport supplements since drug testing is becoming more frequent in collegiate, professional, and Olympic athletes. It is always wise to conduct an extensive background check on supplement companies, their manufacturing process, and standards of quality assurance before recommending any supplement to an athlete. Supplements for NCAA athletes and the means of procuring them (whether they are provided by the school or purchased by the athlete himself) should be in accordance with NCAA regulations. Each professional sport governing body recognizes specific certification organizations (such as the National Science Foundation and Informed Choice). Before considering any ergogenic aid, an athlete should become informed about the safety, legality, and efficacy of the supplement. And finally, nutrition supplements are substances meant to be added to a normal or typical eating program and not consumed as a main source of nutrients.

SUMMARY POINTS

- Sport drinks can improve performance by increasing levels of blood glucose, improving carbohydrate oxidation, and reducing perception of fatigue (Sawka et al. 2007).

- A sport drink with a carbohydrate concentration between 6% and 8% is ideal for faster gastric emptying rates (Benardot 2006).

- According to new research, using two sources of sugar, specifically glucose and fructose in a 2:1 ratio, leads to an improvement in performance over use of a single sugar (Currell and Jeukendrup 2008).

- Electrolyte needs vary among athletes. However, regular electrolyte consumption during aerobic endurance exercise, specifically sodium, is important for improving cardiovascular function and performance by replacing lost sodium, continuing the thirst response, and encouraging voluntary drinking (Baker, Munce, and Kenney 2005).

- Branched-chain amino acid supplementation can enhance recovery from exercise by creating a more anabolic protein balance environment postexercise (Carli et al. 1992) and decreasing markers of muscle damage (Greer et al. 2007).

- One highly branched HMW carbohydrate has been found to empty from the stomach twice as fast as low molecular weight carbohydrates, resulting in a 70% increase in muscle glycogen stores 2 hours after glycogen-depleting exercise (Leiper, Aulin, and Soderlund 2000).

- Caffeine can be used as a beneficial ergogenic aid in doses ranging from 3 to 9 mg/kg body weight (Hoffman et al. 2007). The performance effects are usually seen with consumption of caffeine within 60 minutes before exercise but are also noticeable with consumption during prolonged exercise (Yeo et al. 2005).

- Buffering supplements such as sodium bicarbonate and sodium citrate may benefit individuals participating in high intensity, short duration exercise such as track and field events like the 400 and 800 m (Requena et al. 2005), though they may also cause gastrointestinal distress.

9

Nutrient Timing

Chad M. Kerksick, PhD; ATC; CSCS,*D; NSCA-CPT,*D

Timed administration of nutrients facilitates physiological adaptations to exercise and promotes optimal health and performance. Nutrient timing recommendations vary among athletes within a particular sport as well as between sports. These considerations also change for an individual athlete as demands related to travel, competition, and training vary throughout the year. The dynamic nature of nutrient timing makes it important for all athletes and coaches to develop a firm foundation of knowledge regarding energy, macronutrient, fluid, and micronutrient consumption. This chapter gives a step-by-step breakdown of the nutritional considerations that are supported by the scientific literature, helping the reader develop a nutrition plan that will optimally deliver the necessary levels of energy and nutrients to maximally sustain human performance and promote recovery.

This chapter emphasizes when to consume specific foods or supplements. Many research studies have illustrated that the timed ingestion of specific macronutrients and amino acids may significantly affect the adaptive response to exercise. Depending on the type of training, these responses range from improved glycogen resynthesis to maintenance of blood-based fuels, improved performance, and improvements in muscle growth, as well as improved body composition, immune system functioning, and mood.

Historically, the first consideration of nutrient timing involved delivering a source of carbohydrate before or during the exercise bout. In fact, reports indicate that sugary snacks or foods were consumed before the 1928 Olympic marathon. Starting in the 1960s, researchers began to explore the impact of carbohydrate status, and the concept of carbohydrate loading was born. Carbohydrate loading increases the storage of carbohydrate in the liver and muscles (Bussau et al. 2002; Goforth et al. 2003; Kavouras, Troup, and Berning 2004; Sherman et al. 1981; Yaspelkis et al. 1993), and it can help sustain normal glucose (carbohydrate) levels in the blood during prolonged exercise (Coyle et al. 1986; Kavouras, Troup, and Berning 2004). More recently, preexercise ingestion of carbohydrate, amino acids, protein, and creatine (Cr) has been studied for the ability of these substances to further stimulate adaptations to exercise training (Coburn et al. 2006; Cribb and Hayes 2006; Kraemer et al. 2007; Tipton and Wolfe 2001; Willoughby, Stout, and Wilborn 2007) and prevent the breakdown of muscle tissue (Kraemer et al. 2007; White et al. 2008).

Nutrient Timing and Aerobic Endurance Performance

To sustain life, the human body primarily burns three compounds—carbohydrate, fat, and protein—to generate the energy necessary to drive hundreds of chemical reactions. Carbohydrate is the preferred fuel source, but unfortunately, carbohydrate supply in the muscle and liver is limited (Coyle et al. 1986). During prolonged moderate- to high-intensity exercise (65% to 85% $\dot{V}O_2max$), internal carbohydrate stores become depleted (Hawley et al. 1997; Tarnopolsky et al. 2005), often resulting in decreases in exercise intensity (Coyle et al. 1986), breakdown of muscle tissue (Saunders, Kane, and Todd 2004), and a weakened immune system (American College of Sports Medicine, American Dietetic Association, and Dietitians of Canada 2000; Gleeson, Nieman, and Pedersen 2004).

> ➤ $\dot{V}O_2max$—The maximum oxygen the body can utilize per unit of time. Higher values are associated with higher levels of fitness and training.

At rest, intramuscular glycogen levels of trained athletes are adequate to meet the physical demands of events lasting anywhere from 60 to 90 minutes (Dennis, Noakes, and Hawley 1997). Assuming no appreciable amount of muscle damage, a carbohydrate intake of 8 to 10 g/kg body weight per day along with adequate rest can sustain this level of glycogen in the muscle. Another recommendation, which also facilitates adequate maintenance of glycogen levels, is to ingest 55% to 65% of daily caloric intake as carbohydrate. This recommendation, however, assumes that the athlete is consuming an adequate number of calories relative to body size and physical activity level. For athletes who regularly ingest this recommended level of dietary carbohydrate based on adequate caloric intake, simply taking a day or two off (or exercising at reduced volume and intensity) before competition will allow for maximal restoration of **muscle glycogen**. Unfortunately, many athletes do not consume adequate levels of carbohydrate (Burke 2001). Therefore, strategies have been developed to help athletes quickly achieve maximal levels of glycogen in their muscle.

> ➤ muscle glycogen—Stores of carbohydrate exclusively in skeletal muscle; depending on size of muscle, estimated to be around 250 to 300 g carbohydrate. During exercise or times of stress, muscle glycogen is depleted before liver glycogen.

Carbohydrate Loading

Carbohydrate loading is a practice used by athletes to saturate their endogenous stores of muscle glycogen before longer-duration events that typically lead to depletion of glycogen stores. Traditional carbohydrate loading studies conducted on untrained individuals incorporated a three- or four-day depletion phase in which athletes ingested a low-carbohydrate diet and completed a high volume of exercise training to "deplete" the internal stores of glycogen (Bergstrom and Hultman 1966). This phase was followed by a three- or four-day period of high carbohydrate ingestion (>70% carbohydrate or 8 to 10 g carbohydrate per kilogram body weight per day) and a decrease in exercise volume to facilitate supersaturation of muscle glycogen. Using this approach, early studies reported an ability of athletes to maintain their pace of training for significantly longer periods of time (Karlsson and Saltin 1971).

A series of studies in well-trained runners (Sherman et al. 1983, 1981) suggested that a reduction in exercise training volume along with a high-carbohydrate diet (65% to 70% dietary carbohydrate) over a minimum of three days can elevate muscle glycogen levels. These conclusions were well received as a much more practical approach to maximizing muscle glycogen. In eight trained runners, three days of a high-carbohydrate diet (10 g carbohydrate per kilogram body weight per day) while runners completely refrained from exercise maximized muscle glycogen stores (Bussau et al. 2002). Additionally, a high-carbohydrate (8.1 g carbohydrate per kilogram body weight per day or 600 g carbohydrate per day) diet significantly elevated preexercise glycogen stores versus a low-carbohydrate (1.4 g carbohydrate per kilogram body weight per day or 100 g carbohydrate per day) diet given to trained individuals for three days before completion of a 45-minute bicycle ride at 82% $\dot{V}O_2$peak.

Interestingly, a dose–response effect may be evident regarding the amount of carbohydrate that needs to be ingested when no depletion phase occurs to promote maximal levels of muscle glycogen. For example, baseline muscle glycogen was notably higher after ingestion of 10 g carbohydrate per kilogram body weight per day for one to three days when compared to ingesting 8 g/kg body weight per day for three days. Currently, this effect has not been investigated further, because initial carbohydrate loading studies that incorporated depletion phases and longer intakes of high carbohydrate reported higher levels of muscle glycogen (Bergstrom et al. 1967).

Nutrient Intake Before Aerobic Endurance Exercise

The hours before an aerobic endurance exercise bout or competition are an important consideration, because athletes can take many steps to ensure provision of optimal doses of carbohydrate and other fuel sources. This period is further categorized into two phases: (a) 2 to 4 hours preexercise and (b) 30 to 60 minutes preexercise (Dennis, Noakes, and Hawley 1997; Kerksick et al. 2008). Collectively, research involving single carbohydrate feedings before exercise suggests that it is possible to achieve higher levels of muscle glycogen and an improvement of **blood glucose** maintenance **(euglycemia)**, though changes in performance have been equivocal (Coyle et al. 1985; Dennis, Noakes, and Hawley 1997; Earnest et al. 2004; Febbraio et al. 2000b; Febbraio and Stewart 1996). To optimize carbohydrate utilization, preexercise meals should consist largely of high-carbohydrate foods or liquids. This practice becomes even more important when athletes make poor recovery efforts (e.g., low dietary carbohydrate intake, failure to rest or reduce training volume, or both). In this situation, or when an athlete has fasted overnight (i.e., sleeping), a high-carbohydrate meal ingested 4 hours before an exercise bout causes significant increases in both muscle and **liver glycogen** levels (Coyle et al. 1985). See figure 9.1.

➤ blood glucose—The amount of sugar or glucose found in the bloodstream. Assuming 5 L of blood in the average person, approximately 4 to 10 g glucose is found in the bloodstream.

➤ euglycemia—A state in which blood glucose levels are in normal ranges; often considered values between 80 and 100 mg/dl (4.4-5.5 mmol/L).

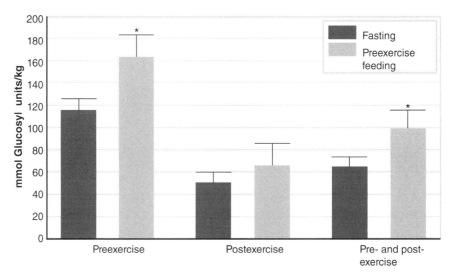

FIGURE 9.1 Impact of preexercise feedings on muscle glycogen levels. Preexercise feeding of a high-carbohydrate meal significantly increased muscle glycogen levels before exercise and also reduced the extent to which these glycogen stores were depleted after exercise. This study provided the first documented evidence that feeding preexercise affects glycogen status. The need to sustain glycogen levels during exercise or competition largely serves as the basis for preexercise nutrient timing and the need for carbohydrate before exercise or competition.

* = Different from preexercise feeding.

Data from Coyle et al. 1985.

➤ liver glycogen—Stored form of carbohydrate exclusively in liver; depending on the size of the liver, has been estimated at around 80 to 100 g carbohydrate. During exercise or times of stress, liver glycogen is the last form of stored carbohydrate to be depleted.

Similarly, when subjects either consumed no carbohydrate or ingested a large carbohydrate meal (~300 g carbohydrate) 4 hours before completing a standardized bout of cycling exercise, participants who ingested carbohydrate were able to significantly reduce the amount of time required to complete the session (Sherman et al. 1989). Other studies have supported these findings, demonstrating that ingestion of a carbohydrate-rich meal (200 to 300 g) in the 3- to 4-hour period before exercise can improve aerobic endurance or work output compared to no carbohydrate ingestion (Neufer et al. 1987; Wright, Sherman, and Dernbach 1991). For this reason, it is commonly recommended that aerobic endurance athletes ingest snacks or meals high in carbohydrate at a dosage of 1 to 4 g carbohydrate per kilogram body mass several hours before exercise (Tarnopolsky et al. 2005).

Ingestion of a high-carbohydrate meal 2 to 4 hours before an exercise bout becomes extremely important when the exercise bout begins in the early morning hours. The time spent sleeping is similar to a fasting period, which will often result in a reduction of liver glycogen stores, affecting carbohydrate availability once the exercise bout begins. From a practicality standpoint, however, ingestion of nutrients 4 hours (or even 2 hours) before an exercise bout may be limited by the start time of the practice, training session, or competition. Morning start times may complicate the decision between optimal fueling and an additional hour or two of sleep. In these situations, it is important that the athlete not overwhelm the storage capacity of the stomach in an attempt to fuel the body (with less digestive time) and end up causing gastrointestinal distress in the process. In this scenario, the athlete needs to overcome the lack of available carbohydrate by working harder to ingest optimal carbohydrate levels during the first hour of exercise. While many food choices can provide carbohydrate, athletes need to experiment during training sessions to figure out what foods work for them without causing gastrointestinal distress.

Although it is widely accepted that ingestion of carbohydrate before an exercise bout is necessary, much controversy and misinformation exist regarding the extent to which the type of carbohydrate can positively or negatively influence the metabolic response to ingestion and subsequent exercise performance. Ingestion of carbohydrate results in a concomitant increase in insulin levels, which increases the uptake of glucose into the body's cells and decreases the level of glucose in the blood. Also, increased insulin levels decrease the breakdown of adipose tissue and increase the rate of **carbohydrate oxidation** when compared to fasted conditions. This physiological response may lead to situations in which blood glucose levels become hypoglycemic (<3.5 mmol/L), leading to reduced exercise intensity and increased feelings of fatigue from exercise.

➤ carbohydrate oxidation—The amount of carbohydrate that can be broken down or utilized in a given time period.

Foster and colleagues (1979) conducted the first study to report a hypoglycemic response to ingesting carbohydrate before (<60 min) exercise. Though this response has not been consistently reported in the scientific literature (Hawley and Burke 1997), it continues to be widely reported anecdotally and is an area of concern for athletes and coaches. Glucose and insulin changes immediately after carbohydrate ingestion are markedly transient. During exercise, though initial hypoglycemia may be reported, this response has not been shown to negatively affect performance in several studies. In fact, most studies report that after 20 to 30 minutes of exercise, glucose levels return to normal with no untoward effects on the athlete. A review by Hawley and Burke (1997) revealed that providing some form of carbohydrate within 60 minutes before exercise has no negative impact on performance and may, in fact, increase performance anywhere from 7% to 20%.

Nonetheless, it is apparent that some athletes do have negative responses to preexercise carbohydrate ingestion, but a consensus is still unavailable on why this response occurs. Further, the extent to which the glycemic index of a carbohydrate source alters glucose and insulin kinetics, glycogen utilization, and subsequent performance has received much consideration. Initially, it was reported that lower-glycemic carbohydrate sources such as fructose may be preferred to avoid the hypoglycemic rebound and subsequently improve performance. However, research does not support this theory. Febbraio and Stewart (1996) showed that ingestion of a high-glycemic meal 45 minutes before 135 minutes of cycling exercise was not responsible for changes in muscle glycogen utilization or performance when compared to a low-glycemic meal or water.

Additional studies have shown that altering the glycemic index of a pre-exercise carbohydrate source has no impact on subsequent performance (Earnest et al. 2004; Febbraio et al. 2000b). Further research indicates that fructose ingestion may be responsible for gastrointestinal distress and may have a negative impact on performance (Erickson, Schwarzkopf, and Mckenzie 1987). For this reason, a common recommendation is that athletes avoid ingesting fructose as a primary carbohydrate source before and during exercise.

In summary, athletes should ingest a diet high in carbohydrate (8-10 g carbohydrate per kilogram body mass per day), especially during the days before competition. High dietary intake of carbohydrate along with a brief reduction in training volume can maximize glycogen stores. Ingesting a carbohydrate meal (200 to 300 g) 2 to 4 hours before exercise helps to maximize glycogen stores and performance. Athletes should be cautious about ingesting too much food volume before exercise and should limit fructose due to the potential for gastrointestinal upset with ingestion of large quantities of fructose.

Nutrient Intake During Aerobic Endurance Exercise

During-exercise nutrient considerations have largely focused on aerobic endurance exercise due to the increased energy demands placed on aerobic endurance athletes. Initially, research efforts focused on carbohydrate administration to sustain blood glucose levels and spare internal stores of glycogen (Febbraio et al. 2000a; Koopman et al. 2004; Nicholas et al. 1995; Widrick et al. 1993). Recent efforts have mixed carbohydrate sources and added varying amounts of amino acids during aerobic endurance exercise to monitor recovery and muscle damage.

Providing Carbohydrate During Aerobic Endurance Exercise

While some studies suggest that carbohydrate ingestion before or during exercise may have negative metabolic consequences (e.g., reactive hypoglycemia) (Foster, Costill, and Fink 1979), an overwhelming majority of the published studies support the contention that carbohydrate ingestion improves (and minimally sustains) performance (Febbraio et al. 2000a; McConell et al. 1999; Nicholas et al. 1995; Widrick et al. 1993). The metabolic demand for carbohydrate can be quite high during exercise. Providing carbohydrate to the muscle before exercise may slow down the rate at which muscle glycogen is broken down (Erickson, Schwarzkopf, and Mckenzie 1987; Hargreaves et al. 1984). But this is not universally accepted, because other studies have reported that the rate of muscle glycogen breakdown is not affected by carbohydrate feedings (Coyle et al. 1985; Fielding et al. 1985). The biochemistry within the body during exercise (specifically the active muscle) suggests that ingestion of carbohydrate at this time may facilitate performance by providing a readily available supply of glucose and therefore sparing muscle and liver glycogen stores (Bosch, Dennis, and Noakes 1993; Coyle et al. 1986, 1985).

Carbohydrate Oxidation Rate   The rate at which carbohydrate is oxidized, whether it comes from blood glucose, liver glycogen, or muscle glycogen, is an important consideration. It has been widely accepted that regardless of the source of carbohydrate (high or low glycemic, with the exception of fructose), the peak rate of carbohydrate oxidation during prolonged moderate-intensity exercise is around 1 g carbohydrate per minute (60 g/hour) (Jeukendrup, Jentjens, and Moseley 2005). Carbohydrate oxidation refers to the amount of carbohydrate that can be broken down or utilized in a given time period. When feeding schedules are altered, the rate of carbohydrate oxidation does not appear to be influenced, leading some to conclude that a limiting factor may be the rate at which carbohydrate is absorbed throughout the digestive system and subsequently made available in the bloodstream (Hawley et al. 1994).

While peak carbohydrate oxidation rates are well established, a research group led by Asker Jeukendrup studied the impact of mixing various forms of carbohydrate in an attempt to increase peak carbohydrate oxidation rates

(Jentjens, Achten, and Jeukendrup 2004; Jentjens and Jeukendrup 2005; Jentjens et al. 2005; Jentjens, Venables, and Jeukendrup 2004; Jentjens et al. 2004; Jeukendrup 2004; Jeukendrup and Jentjens 2000). Different types of carbohydrate have different transport mechanisms; therefore providing more than one type of carbohydrate may increase the amount of carbohydrate in the bloodstream and thus provide more carbohydrate for oxidation as a fuel source. For example, a 21% increase in carbohydrate oxidation (1.2 g carbohydrate per minute) was seen during moderate-intensity exercise after ingestion of a mixture of glucose and sucrose (Jentjens et al. 2005). Similarly, a combination of maltodextrin and fructose resulted in a peak carbohydrate oxidation rate of 1.5 g/minute, which was approximately 40% greater than with ingestion of maltodextrin alone during prolonged cycling at 60% to 65% $\dot{V}O_2$max (Wallis et al. 2005).

Indeed, findings from this research team have regularly shown enhanced carbohydrate oxidation rates, from 1.2 to 1.75 g/minute, with use of a mixture of carbohydrate (Jentjens, Achten, and Jeukendrup 2004; Jentjens and Jeukendrup 2005; Jentjens et al. 2005; Jentjens, Venables, and Jeukendrup 2004; Jentjens et al. 2004). More recently, this same group reported an 8% increase in time-trial performance after a 120-minute ride at 55% maximum power with ingestion of a combination of glucose and fructose during exercise (Currell and Jeukendrup 2008). During exercise, aerobic endurance athletes may benefit from consuming a mixture of carbohydrate types, especially if they start exercise without having consumed a high-carbohydrate meal over the last few hours and therefore are working harder to make up for a lack of available carbohydrate to fuel working muscles.

Frequency and Timing of Carbohydrate Intake   Other research efforts have focused on changing the frequency of feedings or the timing of feedings within an exercise bout to determine if favorable metabolic adaptations or an increase in performance occurs during exercise (Fielding et al. 1985; McConell et al. 1999). Fielding and colleagues (1985) reported that a more frequent intake of carbohydrate (10.75 g every 30 minutes) versus one large feeding (21 g every hour) over a 4-hour cycling ride better maintained blood glucose levels, but this difference did not influence how much muscle glycogen was utilized during the exercise trial. Performance in an exhaustive time trial at the end of the 4-hour exercise bout significantly improved with more frequent ingestion of carbohydrate. A 4-hour exercise session is substantially longer than most training or competitive exercise sessions, with the exception of half-Ironman or Ironman triathlons or ultra-endurance or marathon races. The ability of carbohydrate administration to continue delivering adequate blood glucose for this extended period of time to facilitate improvements in performance is a significant finding favoring enhancing carbohydrate delivery during exercise. In any case, it appears that the frequency or size of carbohydrate feeding does not influence glycogen changes (Fielding et al. 1985) but may affect performance after a long bout of exercise.

In a study by McConell and colleagues (1999) on the impact of carbohydrate supplementation during exercise, aerobic endurance–trained males participated in two time trials in which they cycled to volitional exhaustion. The cyclists consumed either 250 ml of an 8% carbohydrate solution or an artificially flavored and sweetened placebo immediately before and every 15 minutes during exercise. The cyclists given carbohydrate throughout the entire trial increased time to fatigue by 30% (47 minutes) compared to the placebo group.

Febbraio and colleagues (2000a) also reported the benefit of consuming carbohydrate throughout exercise. In this study, cyclists completed a 120-minute bout of cycling at 63% of their peak power under four conditions:

1. Noncarbohydrate placebo 30 minutes before and during exercise
2. Noncaloric placebo 30 minutes before + 2 g carbohydrate per kilogram body mass in a 6.4% solution during exercise
3. 2 g carbohydrate per kilogram body mass in a 25.7% solution before exercise + noncaloric placebo during exercise
4. 2 g carbohydrate per kilogram body mass in a 25.7% solution before exercise + 2 g carbohydrate per kilogram body mass in a 6.4% solution during exercise

Changes in blood glucose oxidation throughout the exercise bout and performance in the time trial were improved only when carbohydrate was provided during exercise. The authors concluded that preexercise ingestion of carbohydrate improves performance only when carbohydrate ingestion continues throughout the exercise bout, and that the ingestion of carbohydrate during 120 minutes of cycling with or without a preexercise carbohydrate feeding can improve subsequent time-trial performance (Febbraio et al. 2000a). See figure 9.2.

Influence of Baseline Glycogen Levels   Both the Febbraio et al. (2000a) study and the study by McConell and colleagues (1999) clearly illustrate the importance of providing carbohydrate throughout exercise to sustain blood glucose and carbohydrate oxidation. The impact of glycogen status before beginning the exercise bout remains an undetermined factor. Widrick and colleagues (1993) had cyclists complete 70 km self-paced time trials under four different conditions: (1) high intramuscular glycogen + carbohydrate beverage; (2) high intramuscular glycogen + noncaloric beverage; (3) low intramuscular glycogen + carbohydrate beverage; (4) low intramuscular glycogen + noncaloric beverage (Widrick et al. 1993). The carbohydrate drink was ingested at the onset of exercise and every 10 km afterward, providing 116 ± 6 g carbohydrate per exercise trial. Carbohydrate

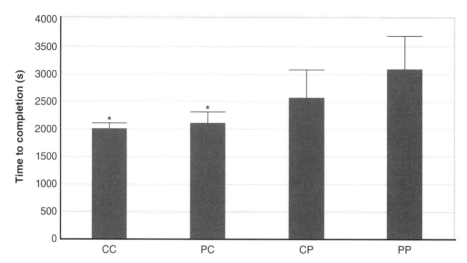

FIGURE 9.2 Impact of preexercise and during-exercise carbohydrate provision. The study showed that providing carbohydrate during exercise was of greatest importance; providing carbohydrate before exercise affected performance only when carbohydrate was provided throughout the exercise bout. CC = carbohydrate before and during exercise; PC = placebo before and carbohydrate during exercise; CP = carbohydrate before and placebo during exercise; PP = placebo before and during exercise.

* = Both CC (constant carbohydrate; 2 g/kg body weight of CHO in a 25.7% CHO beverage 30 min preexercise and 2 g/kg of CHO in a 6.4% CHO solution throughout the time trial) and CP (carbohydrate before the time trial followed by placebo during the time trial; 2 g/kg body weight of CHO in a 25.7% CHO beverage 30 min preexercise and placebo throughout the time trial) were different from either PC or PP (placebo consumed before and during the time trial).

Data from Febbraio et al. 2000a.

administration adequately maintained blood glucose, while blood glucose declined significantly under the noncaloric conditions. Over the final 14% of the time trial (9.8 km), power output and pace were significantly less in the low glycogen + noncaloric condition compared to the other three conditions (figure 9.3). Thus, it appears that baseline glycogen levels are an important consideration before prolonged exercise, because carbohydrate delivery during exercise did not improve performance when muscle glycogen was high but did significantly improve performance when muscle glycogen was low before the beginning of the exercise bout.

As seen throughout this discussion, carbohydrate clearly influences performance. A majority of these studies used prolonged (120 to 150 minutes) exercise bouts at a moderate intensity (65% to 70% $\dot{V}O_2$max). The results of one study suggested that carbohydrate delivery during a high-intensity intermittent running test of trained field players can increase performance. Subjects received either a 6.9% carbohydrate solution or a noncaloric placebo before exercise at a dose of 5 ml/kg body mass, as well as 2 ml/kg body mass every 15 minutes throughout exercise. The athletes who received carbohydrate were able to exercise significantly longer than the placebo group (Nicholas et al. 1995). Another study showed that a carbohydrate-gel

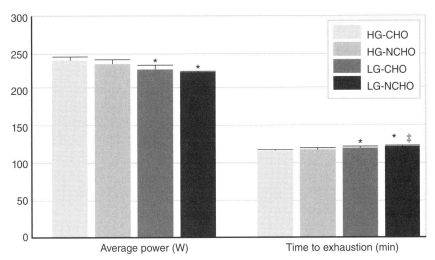

FIGURE 9.3 Impact of preexercise glycogen status and carbohydrate availability on power output and time to exhaustion. Delivery of carbohydrate during exercise did not improve performance when muscle glycogen was high but did significantly improve performance when muscle glycogen was low before the start of the exercise bout, indicating the importance of starting exercise or competition with high glycogen levels.

* = Both LG-CHO (low levels of muscle glycogen preexercise with a carbohydrate beverage consumed before and during exercise) and LG-NCHO (low levels of muscle glycogen preexercise and a non-carbohydrate beverage consumed before and during exercise) had lower average power output and greater time to exhaustion when compared to HG-CHO (high levels of muscle glycogen preexercise and a carbohydrate beverage consumed before and during exercise).

‡ = LG-NCHO time to exhaustion was significantly greater than HG-NCHO.

Data from Widrick et al. 1993.

preparation helped soccer players maintain blood glucose and enhanced performance during a high-intensity intermittent run compared to a placebo (Patterson and Gray 2007).

In summary, a great deal of research supports the notion that carbohydrate ingestion during exercise can sustain blood glucose levels, spare glycogen (Yaspelkis et al. 1993), and promote greater levels of performance (Febbraio et al. 2000a; Nicholas et al. 1995). Several reviews deal with this topic in more detail (Dennis, Noakes, and Hawley 1997; Jeukendrup 2004; Jeukendrup and Jentjens 2000).

Providing Carbohydrate and Protein During Aerobic Endurance Exercise

In recent years, studies have examined the addition of protein to carbohydrate during aerobic endurance exercise. While much of this research is still in its infancy, preliminary findings suggest that the addition of protein or amino acids may facilitate improved performance and may help promote recovery or prevent the amount of damage that occurs to the exercising muscle tissue. In one study, participants completed 3 hours of cycling at 45% to 75% $\dot{V}O_2$max, followed by a time-to-exhaustion trial at 85% $\dot{V}O_2$max.

During each session, participants consumed a placebo, a 7.75% carbohydrate solution, or a 7.75% carbohydrate + 1.94% protein solution. While the carbohydrate group increased time to exhaustion versus the placebo, the addition of protein resulted in even greater performance (Ivy et al. 2003).

Saunders and colleagues (2004) examined the impact of ingesting a carbohydrate + protein combination on performance and changes in muscle damage. Subjects completed an exhaustive bout of exercise at 75% $\dot{V}O_2$max before resting for 12 to 15 hours and then completed a second exhaustive exercise bout at 85% $\dot{V}O_2$max. Throughout both exercise bouts, cyclists ingested a consistent amount of either a 7.3% carbohydrate solution or a 7.3% carbohydrate + 1.8% protein solution every 15 minutes. Immediately after exercise, they ingested identical solutions at a dose of 10 ml/kg body mass. Each group ingested identical amounts of carbohydrate, but energy intake was slightly different (due to the extra calories provided by the added protein). With the combination of carbohydrate and protein, performance (time taken to reach exhaustion) after the first bout of exercise increased by 29% and after the second bout by 40% (figure 9.4). Markers of muscle damage were also 83% lower, suggesting that the carbohydrate + protein combination, or the higher total calorie intake, helped attenuate the muscle

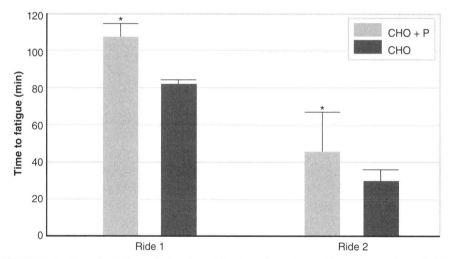

FIGURE 9.4   Time to fatigue during two rides to exhaustion with consumption of either carbohydrate only or carbohydrate + protein. Ride 1 was at 75% $\dot{V}O_2$max. Ride 2 was at 85% $\dot{V}O_2$max, approximately 12 to 15 hours later. Supplementation with carbohydrate and protein every 15 min during exercise resulted in significantly greater performance during two exhaustion rides at 75% and 85% $\dot{V}O_2$max. This was one of the first studies to show that adding protein to a carbohydrate drink may improve performance. However, total calories were not controlled for, so it was unclear whether the increased total calories or addition of whey protein made the difference.

* = Time to exhaustion was significantly greater for the CHO + P (carbohydrate and protein) group when directly compared to the CHO (carbohydrate-only) group.

Data from Saunders, Kane, and Todd 2004.

damage associated with prolonged and exhaustive exercise (Saunders, Kane, and Todd 2004).

The same group reported similar performance increases in a 2007 study in which subjects ingested the carbohydrate + protein combination in a gel composition rather than a liquid solution (Saunders, Luden, and Herrick 2007). Finally, a 2004 study recruited ultra-endurance athletes in order to compare the impact of consuming carbohydrate alone or a combination of carbohydrate + protein for changes in protein turnover and recovery after 6 hours of aerobic endurance exercise (Koopman et al. 2004). With carbohydrate alone, **protein balance** became negative, which suggests that **protein breakdown** (likely muscle) was occurring at a rate greater than **protein synthesis**. When protein was added to the carbohydrate, the overall protein breakdown was lessened, although protein balance remained negative. The authors concluded that combined ingestion of protein and carbohydrate improves net protein balance at rest as well as during exercise and postexercise recovery (Koopman et al. 2004).

➤ protein balance—Generally defined as the balance between protein synthesis and protein breakdown. If rates of protein synthesis are greater than those of protein breakdown, protein balance is positive.

➤ protein breakdown—Generally defined as the breakdown of cellular protein. The overall process occurs through a number of mechanisms and ultimately results in liberation of increased amounts of amino acids into the bloodstream.

➤ protein synthesis—Generally defined as the building of cellular protein. In exercise and nutrition literature, protein synthesis often refers to muscle protein synthesis.

In summary, the results from several studies (Ivy et al. 2003; Koopman et al. 2004; Saunders, Kane, and Todd 2004) provide evidence that combining carbohydrate with protein in a 4:1 ratio before or after prolonged bouts of exercise can facilitate greater performance, while other studies (Koopman et al. 2004; Saunders, Kane, and Todd 2004) show that this combination also reduces muscle damage.

Nutrient Intake and Recovery

Among studies on the various aspects of nutrient timing, postexercise investigations constitute an overwhelming majority of the scientific literature. Collective findings from these studies have provided and continue to provide insight into how nutritional strategies can optimize specific aspects of the recovery process. Throughout this chapter and others, the importance of maintaining maximal glycogen levels is evident. Also, much research interest exists in determining the extent to which providing nutrients in the postexercise period will affect muscle protein balance. Finally, several studies have used prolonged resistance training programs with various nutrient timing strategies to determine the changes in resistance training adaptations such as improved strength and power as well as body composition parameters.

Carbohydrate and Glycogen Resynthesis

The recovery and maintenance of optimal levels of muscle glycogen are a key consideration for almost any type of athlete. An extremely consistent finding in the literature is that athletes who ingest 1.5 g carbohydrate per kilogram body weight within 30 minutes after exercise experience greater muscle glycogen resynthesis than when carbohydrate is delayed by 2 hours (Ivy 1998). While many studies continue to explore the mechanisms associated with these increases, research has revealed that exercise leads to an increase in sensitivity to the hormone insulin, which increases markedly after carbohydrate ingestion (Ivy 1998). Multiple studies have agreed that solid or liquid forms of carbohydrate yield a similar result (Keizer, Kuipers, and Van Kranenburg 1987; Reed et al. 1989; Tarnopolsky et al. 2005). High levels of fructose ingestion are not advised because this form of carbohydrate is associated with lower levels of glycogen resynthesis than other forms of simple carbohydrate (Conlee, Lawler, and Ross 1987). An important consideration, which is highlighted in figure 9.5, is that delaying carbohydrate ingestion by as little as 2 hours can reduce muscle glycogen resynthesis by 50% (Ivy 1998).

If glycogen depletion occurs, which typically results from prolonged-duration (>90 minutes) moderate-intensity exercise (65% to 85% $\dot{V}O_2$max) but can also result from shorter durations of higher intensity or situations in which the athlete began the workout with less than maximal muscle glycogen levels, an aggressive regimen of carbohydrate administration is necessary. A carbohydrate intake of 0.6 to 1.0 g/kg body weight per hour during the first 30 minutes, and again every 2 hours for the next 4 to 6 hours, can adequately replace glycogen stores (Jentjens and Jeukendrup 2003; Jentjens et al. 2001). A 165-pound (75-kg) athlete, for example, should ingest 45 to 75 g carbohydrate within 30 minutes of completing exercise and an identical dose every 2 hours after exercise for the next 4 to 6 hours.

Additional strategies have been investigated, and a slightly more aggressive approach has shown that maximal glycogen resynthesis rates can be achieved if 1.2 g carbohydrate per kilogram body weight per hour is consumed every 30 minutes over a period of 3.5 hours (Jentjens and Jeukendrup 2003; Van Loon et al. 2000). Consequently, the recommendation is that athletes have frequent feedings of carbohydrate in high amounts over the 4 to 6 hours after exercise to ensure recovery of muscle and liver glycogen (Jeukendrup, Jentjens, and Moseley 2005; Tarnopolsky et al. 2005).

An important consideration connected with these studies, however, is the practicality associated with the athlete's immediate need to recover. For

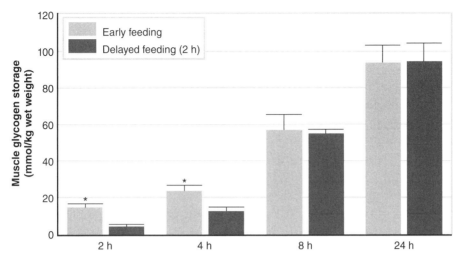

FIGURE 9.5   Postexercise glycogen values after early feeding of carbohydrate or feeding delayed by 2 hours. During short-term recovery (<4 hours), early feeding had a significant impact on recovery of muscle glycogen. If recovery is delayed by several more hours, immediate intake provides no further impact on glycogen recovery if total carbohydrate intake meets recommended guidelines. This demonstrates that early feedings replace glycogen faster; however, this is not as important if the athlete does not need to perform again within 4 to 6 hours.

* = Early feeding resulted in significantly greater muscle glycogen levels than delayed feeding.

Data from Ivy 1998.

example, if an athlete is participating in a sporting activity that requires a follow-up performance within this 2- to 4-hour time period (e.g., track and field and swimming athletes participating in multiple events that often have preliminary heats and semifinal and final heats), then findings from these studies are of the utmost importance. If, however, the athlete does not need to recover in less than 4 hours, other studies illustrate that eating high-carbohydrate meals and snacks at regular intervals can also result in maximal muscle glycogen levels. Research has shown that maximal glycogen levels are restored within 24 hours if optimal levels of dietary carbohydrate are available (typically around 8 g carbohydrate per kilogram body weight per day) and the degree of glycogen depletion is not too severe (Keizer, Kuipers, and Van Kranenburg 1987). Another study suggested a carbohydrate intake of 9 to 10 g/kg body weight per day for athletes completing intense exercise bouts on consecutive days (Nicholas, Green, and Hawkins 1997). Also, it is possible that providing energy in the form of carbohydrate may help to alter inflammatory or proteolytic (breakdown of protein) cascades or other untoward events that will ultimately delay optimal recovery in an exercising athlete.

Carbohydrate With Protein and Glycogen Resynthesis

The addition of protein to carbohydrate has evolved into a dynamic area of research; studies suggest that this combination may help promote even greater recovery of muscle glycogen as well as attenuate muscle damage. Ivy and colleagues (2002) instructed cyclists to complete a 2.5-hour bout of intense cycling before ingesting (1) a low-carbohydrate + protein + fat (80 g carbohydrate + 28 g protein + 6 g fat), (2) a low-carbohydrate + fat (80 g carbohydrate + 6 g fat), or (3) a high-carbohydrate + fat (108 g carbohydrate + 6 g fat) supplement immediately after exercise and 2 hours postexercise. The aim was to determine if the carbohydrate + protein + fat combination promoted greater restoration of muscle glycogen. Glycogen levels were similar between the two carbohydrate + fat conditions (low carbohydrate and high carbohydrate), but muscle glycogen levels were significantly greater in the carbohydrate + protein + fat treatment. The authors concluded that a carbohydrate + protein + fat supplement may be more effective due to a greater insulin response (Ivy et al. 2002; Jentjens et al. 2001; Zawadzki, Yaspelkis, and Ivy 1992), but this guideline has yet to be universally accepted.

Separate studies by Berardi and colleagues (Berardi, Noreen, and Lemon 2008; Berardi et al. 2006) and Tarnopolsky and colleagues (1997) had cyclists complete exercise bouts of 60 and 90 minutes, respectively, on separate occasions before ingesting either carbohydrate + protein or carbohydrate only. Both research teams concluded that carbohydrate ingestion increased muscle glycogen compared to placebo (Berardi et al. 2006; Tarnopolsky et al. 1997). Berardi and colleagues, however, reported greater glycogen levels (Berardi et al. 2006) in addition to increased performance and work output (Berardi, Noreen, and Lemon 2008) when the carbohydrate + protein combination was consumed postexercise. Furthermore, increasing the availability of the essential amino acids, possibly the branched-chain amino acids in particular, may influence the recovery process by optimizing protein synthesis and glycogen synthesis after exercise (Borsheim et al. 2002; Ivy 1998; Ivy et al. 2002; Tarnopolsky et al. 1997; Tipton et al. 1999a; Zawadzki, Yaspelkis, and Ivy 1992). A major consideration for an athlete or coach relative to promoting optimal glycogen levels should be the time available before a subsequent training session or competition.

In summary, clear evidence exists that ingestion of carbohydrate as a single meal (1.5 g carbohydrate per kilogram body weight within 30 minutes after exercise) or as frequent feedings (0.6 to 1.2 g carbohydrate per kilogram body weight per hour every 30 to 60 minutes for up to 3 to 6 hours) can result in rapid restoration of muscle glycogen levels. Furthermore, the addition of protein to carbohydrate has been shown to result in greater glycogen resynthesis (and also greater protein synthesis), but overall the absolute amount of carbohydrate ingested is the primary factor that facilitates recovery of muscle glycogen.

Nutrient Timing, Resistance Training, and Strength and Power Performance

Additional research efforts are now aimed at exploring how providing nutrients (carbohydrate and protein) during resistance exercise may alter muscle protein balance, anabolic hormone changes in the blood, recovery of muscle damage, and modulation of strength or performance (Baty et al. 2007; Bird, Tarpenning, and Marino 2006a, 2006b, 2006c; Haff et al. 2000). This area of research is one that will change significantly; additional efforts are rapidly adding to the current body of knowledge. Nutrient timing strategies can enhance adaptations to resistance training for any athlete who wants to gain strength, power, or size. Males and female athletes of all ages can benefit from the strategies outlined in this chapter.

Nutrient Intake Before and After Resistance Training

For many years, preexercise nutrient administration focused on delivering carbohydrate sources at various points before the start of a bout of exercise. Interestingly, much of this initial research centered on aerobic endurance exercise, specifically cycling. In recent years, researchers have begun to explore the potential of ingesting protein or amino acids or both (sometimes in combination with carbohydrate) before exercise to enhance training adaptations to resistance exercise, modulate the process of recovery from damage known to occur with eccentric contractions, or both.

When carbohydrate (35 g sucrose) and essential amino acids (6 g) were provided in combination either immediately before or immediately after the resistance training bout, ingestion immediately beforehand increased levels of muscle protein synthesis to a greater extent (Tipton et al. 2001). The same authors compared the changes in muscle protein metabolism after ingestion of 20 g whey protein immediately before, or immediately after, a single bout of resistance exercise; they found that irrespective of timing, whey protein ingestion significantly increased the rate of muscle protein synthesis (Tipton et al. 2007). Collectively, results from these two studies suggest that pre- or postexercise whey protein ingestion can stimulate significantly greater levels of muscle protein synthesis. However, when essential amino acids are combined with a carbohydrate source, preexercise ingestion may elicit superior results than postexercise ingestion.

For resistance training athletes, increases in strength or power and in lean mass are often the primary desired outcomes. A study by Kraemer and colleagues (2007) suggested that preexercise ingestion of a multinutrient compound may modulate performance during explosive–powerful movements. In a double-blind format, subjects ingested a 25 kcal multivitamin–mineral supplement containing 3 g creatine and other bioactives (e.g., 70 mg caffeine, 2 g arginine) or an isoenergetic maltodextrin placebo for seven days before reporting for two consecutive days of resistance training (Kraemer et al. 2007). On both exercise days, they ingested the supplement 30 minutes before the exercise bout. When compared to the placebo, the multinutrient supplement significantly improved vertical jump power and the number of repetitions performed at 80% 1RM (1-repetition maximum) while also increasing serum levels of hormones closely linked to muscle hypertrophy and enhanced training adaptations (i.e., growth hormone and free and total testosterone) (Kraemer et al. 2007). Given the results of this study, it is plausible that this supplement combination, if consumed in a similar manner daily during a training season, will help athletes increase training load and potentially training volume, which will help them achieve greater adaptations to training. And greater training adaptations should lead to better performance during competition that requires strength or power movements.

Although acute studies provide detailed information about immediate responses, the additive effect of nutrient provision and several weeks of following a resistance training program are of the greatest practical interest. Several studies have used heavy resistance training programs over 8- to 12-week periods in conjunction with nutrient timing to determine the changes in strength and body composition. Longer-duration studies are more applicable to real-life training cycles in which athletes engage in preseason training and then lighten their training load during the season in favor of skill work and simulation of game-time situations. For example, Coburn and colleagues reported that preexercise supplementation of 26 g whey protein and 6 g leucine resulted in greater increases in maximal strength over a six-week period than 26 g carbohydrate alone (Coburn et al. 2006). Preexercise protein and carbohydrate supplementation significantly increased strength (30.3% and 22.4%, respectively) when compared to only carbohydrate supplementation (3.6%) (Coburn et al. 2006).

Further research has examined the effects of protein-only or carbohydrate + protein taken before and after 8 and 10 weeks of resistance training, respectively. One of these studies compared equal doses of whey protein and soy protein taken before and after each resistance training bout over an eight-week resistance training period. Both forms of supplementation increased strength and lean mass when compared to a placebo, but no differences were found between the two sources of protein (Candow et al. 2006). Similarly, Willoughby and colleagues (2007) had subjects resistance train four days per week for 10 weeks and ingest either 20 g protein or 20 g carbohydrate before and after each exercise bout for a total of 40 g. Impressively, protein supplementation increased body mass, fat-free mass, strength, and several markers of muscle hypertrophy (Willoughby, Stout, and Wilborn 2007). Combined, these studies indicate that providing some combination of protein and carbohydrate before and after resistance exercise is associated with greater improvements in strength, lean mass, body fat percentage, serum levels of important anabolic (muscle building) hormones, and intramuscular markers of muscle hypertrophy.

By supplementing on a consistent basis, along with performing an effective training program, athletes should make greater gains during preseason training. Gaining strength can benefit athletes in various ways in different sports. For instance, a high school basketball player who improves strength in all major leg and buttock muscle groups will be able to hold her defensive position better when guarding her opponent. Likewise, strength gains can help a gymnast integrate more difficult moves into his parallel bar routine. In addition to gaining strength, maintaining a specific range of acceptable body fat is important for certain athletes, especially those in aesthetic sports like figure skating, gymnastics, synchronized swimming, and cheerleading. And finally, while some sports require a small, compact body size, other sports, or more specifically positions within these sports, may require that an athlete put on size so he stands out among the competition for his position. For instance, American football offensive linemen are typically big so they can protect the quarterback from oncoming pass rushers and shield the running back from the defense. Defensive linemen are typically lighter and more agile because they need to move quickly to where they anticipate the ball is going and maneuver through offensive blocks to tackle or cover an offensive player.

Sports vary tremendously in terms of ideal body type; and even within a given sport, body types vary. Therefore, when considering supplements, it is wise to look at the training program goals and first determine what an athlete needs—strength, speed, size, aerobic endurance, agility, better overall skills, or a combination of these—and then decide if supplements can expedite the training goals.

Cribb and Hayes (2006) investigated the impact of nutrient timing strategies over several weeks of supplementation and resistance training. Figure 9.6 shows some of the results. Participants ingested equal quantities of a supplement containing protein, creatine, and carbohydrate either immediately before and immediately after each workout or in the morning and evening of each workout day. Significantly greater increases in lean body mass, 1RM strength, and Type II muscle fiber cross-sectional area, as well as higher muscle creatine and glycogen levels, were seen when the supplements were consumed immediately before and after workouts (Cribb and Hayes 2006). All of these adaptations may allow an athlete to train harder over time, thereby contributing to better performance. However, the benefits gained depend on the athlete—athletes in weight-restricted or aesthetic sports may need to carefully consider whether strength gains are worth the increase in body weight.

In a follow-up to this study by Hoffman and colleagues (2009), participants ingested 42 g of a protein source before and after workouts over the course of several weeks. The authors reported no difference in strength, power, or body composition based on the timing strategies—an effect linked to the already high protein intake of their participants and the lack of any

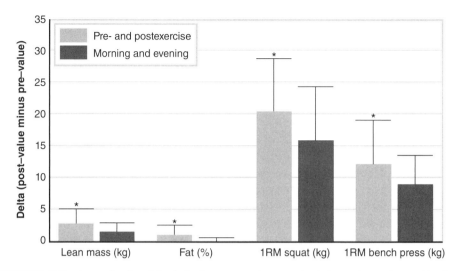

FIGURE 9.6 Impact of nutrient timing on resistance training adaptations. Nutrient ingestion (protein, creatine, and glucose) occurred either in the morning and evening on workout days or immediately pre- and postexercise. Pre–post ingestion was responsible for significant improvements in lean mass, percent body fat, 1RM squat, and 1RM bench press. This was the first resistance training study to focus solely on nutrient timing and show greater body composition adaptations in addition to performance improvements.

* = Different from morning and evening.

Data from Cribb and Hayes 2006.

carbohydrate source as part of the supplementation regimen (Hoffman et al. 2009).

Ingestion of amino acids or a whole protein source (e.g., whey), alone or in combination with carbohydrate, within 30 minutes before a bout of resistance training will significantly increase muscle protein synthesis (Tipton et al. 2007, 2004, 2001). Studies have suggested that when free amino acids are ingested immediately before resistance exercise, the increase in amino acid concentrations and muscle protein synthesis is greater than when they are ingested immediately after exercise (Tipton et al. 2001). However, a complete protein source such as whey protein increases protein synthesis to a similar degree whether it is ingested 1 hour before or 1 hour after a single bout of resistance exercise (Bucci and Lm 2000; Tipton et al. 2007). Adding carbohydrate (e.g., 35 g sucrose) to essential amino acids (e.g., 6 g) immediately before a resistance exercise bout may lead to an even greater anabolic environment, resulting in significantly higher levels of muscle protein synthesis than immediate postexercise ingestion of the same nutrients (Tipton et al. 2001).

Data, however, do exist to suggest that soy protein may not be as adequate a protein source for muscle hypertrophy as milk protein (e.g., whey and casein) (Wilkinson et al. 2007). Nonetheless, ingestion of soy protein has been shown to promote increases in lean mass and strength if this is the only source of protein consumed (Candow et al. 2006). Changes after only one bout of exercise are important; but prolonged studies involving several weeks (8 to 12 weeks) of supplementation and resistance training reveal that any form of nutrients provided before and after exercise leads to significant improvements in body mass, lean mass, body fat percentage, cross-sectional area, strength, and myofibrillar content (Candow et al. 2006; Coburn et al. 2006; Cribb and Hayes 2006; Kraemer et al. 2007; Willoughby, Stout, and Wilborn 2007).

Nutrient Intake During Resistance Training

To date, a limited number of studies have examined nutrient ingestion during resistance exercise or strength and power events. As with the aerobic endurance exercise studies, the data suggest that providing carbohydrate, or a combination of carbohydrate and protein, may help sustain muscle glycogen (Haff et al. 2000), prevent increases in serum cortisol and urinary markers of muscle breakdown (Bird, Tarpenning, and Marino 2006a, 2006c), and promote muscle hypertrophy (Bird, Tarpenning, and Marino 2006b).

Haff and colleagues (2000) had resistance-trained males ingest either a noncaloric placebo or carbohydrate at a dose of 1 g/kg body weight before as well as during (every 10 minutes) a single bout of lower body resistance training. Muscle biopsies during each condition revealed that muscle glycogen levels were 49% higher with carbohydrate compared to no carbohydrate. These results were published in one of the initial reports suggesting that significant decreases in muscle glycogen could occur during resistance exercise and that providing carbohydrate during resistance exercise may promote recovery as well as an overall higher volume of training (Haff et al. 2000). During competition in strength and power sports that last over a long time period and require high caloric expenditures, maintaining higher muscle glycogen levels could potentially attenuate any performance decrements later in the competition that could result in part from decreases in glycogen.

Later, researchers (Bird, Tarpenning, and Marino 2006b, 2006c) examined the extent to which a carbohydrate + protein combination could mitigate changes in protein degradation in the blood and urine during a single bout of resistance exercise. Thirty-two participants completed a 60-minute bout of resistance training while consuming either a 6% carbohydrate solution, a 6% carbohydrate + 6 g essential amino acid solution, or a placebo beverage. Blood cortisol levels (a crude indicator of protein breakdown) increased 105% in the placebo group, while increases in the carbohydrate and the carbohydrate + essential amino acid groups were only 11% and 7%, respectively. Further, urinary levels of 3-methyl-histidine (an additional marker of muscle protein breakdown) decreased by 27% in the carbohydrate + essential amino acid group but increased by 56% in the placebo group (Bird, Tarpenning, and Marino 2006b, 2006c). Beelen and colleagues (2008) presented similar conclusions when participants ingested a bolus of carbohydrate + protein before beginning a 2-hour bout of resistance training and at 15-minute intervals during the training session. The carbohydrate + protein combination lowered the rate of protein breakdown by 8.4 ± 3.6% and increased the protein synthesis rate by 49 ± 22%, resulting in a fivefold increase in protein balance.

While immediate changes (in blood and urine markers) support the ingestion of a carbohydrate + protein combination during a single resistance training bout, the cumulative effect of this practice remained to be determined. Over a 12-week period, Bird and colleagues (2006b) had participants ingest a 6% carbohydrate solution, a 6% carbohydrate solution + 6 g of an essential amino acid solution, or a placebo during resistance training sessions. Serum insulin and cortisol, urinary markers of protein breakdown, and muscle cross-sectional area were measured; and as reported previously, carbohydrate + essential amino acid ingestion decreased protein breakdown by 26% while the placebo group experienced a 52% increase in the same markers. Interestingly, muscle cross-sectional areas of the Type I, IIa, and IIx fibers were increased with carbohydrate + essential amino acid ingestion compared to the placebo. The authors concluded that over a 12-week period ingesting a carbohydrate + essential amino acid combination during regular resistance training optimizes the balance between muscle growth and muscle loss, resulting in significant increases in the size of muscle fibers (Bird, Tarpenning, and Marino 2006b).

Overall, the research supports the conclusion that the intake of nutrients such as carbohydrate alone during resistance training, or a combination of carbohydrate + protein, may help promote greater levels of muscle glycogen, increase muscle cross-sectional area, and decrease protein breakdown (Bird, Tarpenning, and Marino 2006a, 2006b, 2006c; Haff et al. 2000). Athletes do need to be careful about ingesting food during competition or events. Before implementing any supplementation strategy that will be used in competition, it is vital to try it in a practice situation that simulates competition. Some athletes experience gastrointestinal upset from foods they experiment with while training or competing, and the last thing they want to do is to hamper performance because they decided to try something new during competition.

Posttraining Nutrition and Protein Balance

A single bout of resistance training modestly stimulates protein synthesis but also stimulates protein breakdown, resulting in an overall negative protein balance after exercise (Phillips et al. 1999; Pitkanen et al. 2003) in untrained individuals. As training continues, this balance shifts to the point that protein balance after an acute bout of resistance training (without provision of any form of nutrients before or after exercise) is neutral, meaning that no appreciable growth or breakdown of muscle is occurring (Phillips et al. 1999). Providing amino acids (either by infusion or, more practically, through ingestion of amino acids as a dietary supplement, snack, or meal) increases plasma amino acid concentrations at rest or after resistance exercise (Biolo et al. 1997; Borsheim et al. 2002) and also leads to increases in muscle protein synthesis. Combining a modest supply of protein as amino acids (6 to 12 g essential amino acids) with a carbohydrate source (20 to 40 g) after exercise may result in even greater increases in protein synthesis. While providing carbohydrate + essential amino acids immediately before exercise results in greater increases in muscle protein synthesis, the immediate postexercise response is also responsible for remarkable increases in muscle protein synthesis and should be a primary consideration for athletes (Tipton et al. 2001). Consequently, increasing the concentration and availability of essential amino acids in the blood is an important consideration when one is attempting to promote increases in lean tissue and improve body composition with resistance training (Biolo et al. 1997; Tipton et al. 1999a).

A large dose of carbohydrate (100 g) 1 hour after completion of an intense bout of lower body resistance training causes only marginal improvements in the balance between protein synthesis and protein breakdown, resulting in a net negative protein balance (Borsheim et al. 2004). Regarding protein (muscle) changes, no studies have found carbohydrate to be detrimental, but it certainly is not the ideal nutrient (in isolation) to consume after resistance exercise. Its inclusion, however, is important for stimulating glycogen resynthesis and enhancing palatability (Ivy et al. 2002; Tarnopolsky et al. 1997). Of primary interest has been the delivery of free amino acids (often just the essential amino acids) in dosages ranging from 6 to 40 g. These dosages have consistently been shown to stimulate rates of muscle protein synthesis (Borsheim et al. 2002; Miller et al. 2003), while adding carbohydrate to them may enhance this effect (Tipton et al. 2001; Tipton and Wolfe 2001). Immediately after competition, depending on the sport, the amount of time an athlete plays, and other variables, carbohydrate supplementation is important for restoring glycogen, and protein may potentially enhance glycogen resynthesis and facilitate the muscle repair process.

Consuming amino acids after resistance training (whether immediately after or up to 3 hours later) can increase muscle protein synthesis and blunt the increases commonly seen in protein breakdown (Borsheim et al. 2002; Miller et al. 2003; Pitkanen et al. 2003). The optimal time point for supplementation has not yet been demonstrated, but most sport nutrition researchers suggest that the sooner nutrients (whether just carbohydrate, just protein, or a combination) can be provided, the better (Ivy et al. 2002; Tipton and Wolfe 2001). When amino acids were provided with or without carbohydrate immediately, 1 hour, 2 hours, or 3 hours after exercise, similar increases in protein balance were reported (Borsheim et al. 2002; Ivy et al. 2002; Tipton et al. 1999b, 2001; Tipton and Wolfe 2001).

Although individual results from these studies and others differ, the majority of the research has continued to demonstrate that providing amino acids during the postexercise time period significantly increases muscle protein synthesis. Levenhagen and colleagues (2001) found that ingestion of 10 g protein + 8 g carbohydrate + 3 g fat, either immediately or three hours after 60 minutes of moderate-intensity cycling exercise, elevated leg muscle glucose uptake and whole-body glucose utilization threefold and 44%, respectively. Furthermore, peripheral (leg muscle) and whole-body rates of protein synthesis have been shown to increase threefold and 12%, respectively. Finally, Tipton and colleagues (2001) supplemented participants with 35 g sucrose + 6 g essential amino acids immediately before or immediately after a single bout of resistance exercise. They reported significantly greater levels of protein synthesis under both conditions, but rates were higher when the nutrients were ingested immediately before the exercise bout.

To summarize, at present there is no universal recommendation about the dosage and ratio of essential amino acids and carbohydrate to apply in order to maximally increase protein balance. Studies using similar research methodologies and analytical techniques to measure protein kinetics during resistance exercise have used several nutrient combinations during the 2-hour postexercise period. Six grams of essential amino acids alone, 6 g essential amino acids + 6 g nonessential amino acids, 12 g essential amino acids alone, 17.5 g whey protein, 20 g casein protein, 20 g whey protein, 40 g of a mixed amino acid solution (essential and nonessential amino acids), and 40 g essential amino acids all have resulted in an increase in protein synthesis and protein balance (Biolo et al. 1997; Tipton et al. 1999b; Tipton and Wolfe 2001).

Much research has addressed the impact of different types and dosages of protein (as either free amino acids or whole protein sources) on changes in muscle protein balance after resistance exercise. Results from these studies have led to practical recommendations that athletes ingest some form of nutrients as soon as possible after completing an exercise bout, with an absolute requirement that this occur within 2 hours (Ivy 1998). Optimal dosages are also still unknown; however, a carbohydrate + protein combination in a 4:1 carbohydrate-to-protein ratio during this time period is widely accepted as a general guideline. This recommendation translates to ingesting 1.2 to 1.5 g carbohydrate (e.g., dextrose, sucrose) per kilogram body weight, as well as 0.3 to 0.5 g essential amino acids or whole protein per kilogram body weight (Borsheim et al. 2002; Rasmussen et al. 2000; Tipton et al. 1999a).

Posttraining Supplementation and Training Adaptations

The postexercise considerations discussed thus far center on restoring muscle glycogen and the immediate changes in muscle protein synthesis during exercise, specifically resistance training. While optimal levels of muscle glycogen are extremely important to athletes participating in prolonged events that challenge muscle glycogen stores, their importance for an athlete who resistance trains for 45 to 90 minutes to promote maximal strength and body composition changes is not as great. The immediate change in muscle protein synthesis after a bout of resistance training is much more important for a resistance training athlete than glycogen resynthesis, but the results from only one exercise session do not always extrapolate to what would occur after several weeks of resistance training and supplementation.

Researchers have investigated the impact of varying combinations of carbohydrate and protein after each exercise bout (1 to 3 hours postexercise) during resistance training over the course of several weeks (Candow et al. 2006; Cribb and Hayes 2006; Cribb, Williams, and Hayes 2007; Cribb et al. 2007; Hartman et al. 2007; Kerksick et al. 2007, 2006; Tarnopolsky et al. 2001; Wilkinson et al. 2007; Willoughby, Stout, and Wilborn 2007). As before, the individual results from these studies differ, but the collective findings support the rationale for postexercise administration of carbohydrate and protein to facilitate improvements in body composition and strength. Figures 9.7 and 9.8 show the changes in body composition and strength performance from one study using postexercise supplementation. Overall, results from these studies suggest that when 20 to 75 g protein is ingested alone or in conjunction with similar amounts of carbohydrate

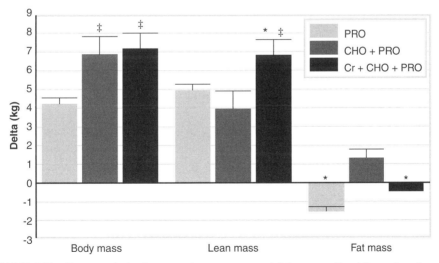

FIGURE 9.7 Changes in body mass, lean mass, and fat mass after 10 weeks of resistance training with postexercise supplementation. These results show that long-term consistent nutrient administration after resistance exercise may favorably affect body composition.

* = Significantly different from CHO + PRO. ‡ = Significantly different from PRO.

Data from Cribb and Hayes 2006.

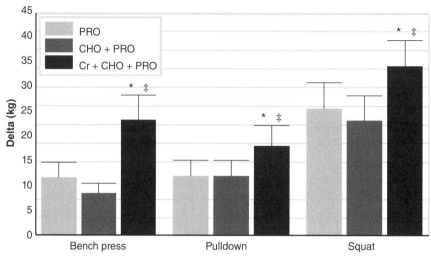

FIGURE 9.8   Delta value for changes in 1RM values for bench press, lat pulldown, and squat exercises after 10 weeks of resistance training with postexercise supplementation.

* = Significantly different from CHO + PRO. ‡ = Significantly different from PRO.

Data from Cribb and Hayes 2006.

during resistance training, increases in strength and body composition can result. Summary tables listing results from these studies are available in a comprehensive review devoted to the topic of nutrient timing (Kerksick et al. 2008).

Whey and Casein

As with carbohydrate, researchers have investigated the impact of various protein sources on digestive and amino acid kinetics and resistance training adaptations (Boirie et al. 1997; Dangin et al. 2001; Kerksick et al. 2007, 2006). In two studies, French researchers were the first to report on the differences in digestive and absorptive properties of the two primary forms of milk protein, whey and casein. Their studies illustrated that whey protein is digested and absorbed into the bloodstream at a much greater rate than casein protein. This difference was associated with the much greater effect of whey protein, compared to casein protein, on increasing synthesis of protein. On the flip side, casein protein appeared to be responsible for preventing the breakdown of muscle tissue while whey protein did not appear to have any influence over this parameter. When the two types of protein were compared in a head-to-head fashion, casein protein appeared to result in a greater overall improvement in whole-body protein balance (Boirie et al. 1997; Dangin et al. 2001). Comparison of identical amounts of protein shows that whey protein contains a greater amount of the essential amino acids than casein protein; for this reason, whey protein is much more highly favored.

Wilkinson and colleagues (2007) compared 18 g of a milk protein source to an equal dose of a soy protein source for their ability to increase net muscle protein accretion and protein balance after a single bout of resistance training. They concluded that the milk protein source was responsible for a greater increase in both net protein and muscle protein accretion when compared to soy and that a milk protein source would likely be responsible for an increase in lean mass when combined with resistance training. Kerksick and colleagues (2006) examined the influence of a "fast" protein source (40 g whey protein + 5 g glutamine + 3 g branched-chain amino acids [isoleucine, leucine, valine]) compared to a blend of fast and slow proteins (40 g whey + 8 g casein), ingested postexercise over a 10-week period of resistance training. Subjects who ingested the blend of fast and slow protein showed significantly greater increases in muscle mass (+1.8 kg) than those who ingested the fast proteins (−0.1 kg). An additional study by this group demonstrated that daily ingestion of a 60 g blend of whey and casein protein over 12 weeks resulted in gains in lean body mass (+0.8 to +1.3 kg) similar to those seen in the previous investigation (Kerksick et al. 2007).

Creatine

Researchers have also examined adding creatine monohydrate to carbohydrate + protein combinations in subjects participating in a regular resistance training program for up to 10 to 12 weeks (Cribb, Williams, and Hayes 2007; Cribb et al. 2007; Kerksick et al. 2007; Tarnopolsky et al. 2001). Creatine monohydrate is a popular dietary supplement that has been heavily researched for its ability to increase performance and facilitate positive training adaptations (Buford et al. 2007; Kreider 2003). Tarnopolsky and colleagues (2001) had previously untrained male participants follow an eight-week resistance training program while ingesting on a daily basis, 30 minutes after their assigned workout, either 10 g creatine + 75 g carbohydrate or 10 g protein + 75 g carbohydrate. The creatine + carbohydrate combination resulted in significantly greater gains in body mass (5.4% increase from baseline) than the protein + carbohydrate combination (2.4% increase from baseline). Fat-free mass, muscle fiber area, 1RM, and isokinetic strength improved in both groups but were not different between the groups. Cribb and colleagues (2007) had participants resistance train for 11 weeks while consuming an isocaloric amount of creatine + carbohydrate, creatine + whey protein, whey protein only, or carbohydrate only. When compared to the carbohydrate-only group, all other groups showed greater improvements in maximal strength and muscle hypertrophy, but no differences were seen with the addition of creatine to the supplement (Cribb et al. 2007).

In contrast, two studies suggest that the addition of creatine to a supplement may promote greater increases in muscle hypertrophy during resistance training over the course of several weeks (Cribb, Williams, and Hayes

2007; Kerksick et al. 2007). Over a 10-week period, participants underwent a heavy resistance training program and ingested one of the following iso-caloric supplements: protein, protein + carbohydrate, or creatine + protein + carbohydrate. The investigators found that in contrast to their previous results, the addition of creatine appeared to elicit greater improvements in strength and muscle hypertrophy than the consumption of protein alone or protein + carbohydrate (Cribb, Williams, and Hayes 2007). Similarly, Kerksick and colleagues (2007) had participants complete 12 weeks of resistance training and ingest a blend of either colostrum or whey or casein protein with or without creatine. While all groups showed increases in strength and muscle mass, the groups ingesting creatine with a protein blend (regardless of the exact composition of the protein source) experienced greater gains in body mass and fat-free mass. The mixed results from these studies suggest the need for additional research; however, a majority of the available studies do indicate that adding creatine monohydrate to a postexercise regimen of carbohydrate and protein can maximally stimulate improvements in strength and body composition (Cribb, Williams, and Hayes 2007; Cribb et al. 2007; Kerksick et al. 2007).

Professional Applications

Timed administration of nutrients facilitates physiological adaptations to exercise and promotes optimal health and performance. Nutrient timing recommendations vary for athletes within a particular sport as well as between sports. Considerations will also vary for an individual athlete as demands related to travel, competition, and training change throughout the year. The dynamic nature of nutrient timing makes it important for all athletes and coaches to develop a firm foundation of knowledge regarding energy, macronutrient, fluid, and micronutrient consumption.

Based on the current research on nutrient timing, these are some recommendations that athletes can put into practice before, during, and after training and competition.

Before

- Athletes can maximize glycogen stores by following a high-carbohydrate diet (600 to 1,000 g or ~8 to 10 g carbohydrate per kilogram body weight per day) (Bussau et al. 2002; Goforth et al. 2003; Tarnopolsky et al. 2005).

- A carbohydrate-rich meal 4 hours before exercise may increase performance, work output, or both (Neufer et al. 1987; Sherman et al. 1989; Wright, Sherman, and Dernbach 1991). In general, athletes should ingest 1 to 4 g carbohydrate per kilogram body weight 1 to 4 hours before aerobic endurance exercise or competition (Tarnopolsky et al. 2005).

- The type of carbohydrate consumed 60 minutes before exercise does not appear to have any negative effects on performance or glycemic status and in many cases may increase performance (Hawley and Burke 1997).

- The glycemic index of a meal eaten before prolonged exercise does not appear to negatively affect performance or utilization of muscle glycogen (Earnest et al. 2004; Febbraio et al. 2000b; Febbraio and Stewart 1996).
- When combined with a regular resistance training program, ingestion of a combination of carbohydrate + protein, amino acids, or both before and after training leads to improvements in strength, power, body mass, lean mass, and intramuscular markers of muscle growth (Coburn et al. 2006; Cribb and Hayes 2006; Kraemer et al. 2007; Willoughby, Stout, and Wilborn 2007).

During

- For exercise or events lasting longer than 60 minutes, athletes should consume a source of carbohydrate that provides 30 to 60 g carbohydrate per hour, typically by drinking 1 to 2 cups (8 to 16 fluid ounces) of a 6% to 8% carbohydrate solution (6 to 8 g carbohydrate per 100 ml of fluid) every 10 to 15 minutes (Jeukendrup, Jentjens, and Moseley 2005).
- Mixing different forms of carbohydrate has been shown to increase muscle carbohydrate oxidation (Jentjens, Achten, and Jeukendrup 2004; Jentjens and Jeukendrup 2005; Jentjens et al. 2005; Jentjens, Venables, and Jeukendrup 2004; Jentjens et al. 2004), an effect associated with an improvement in time-trial performance (Currell and Jeukendrup 2008).
- Glucose, fructose, sucrose, and maltodextrin can be used in combination, but large amounts of fructose are not recommended due to the greater likelihood of gastrointestinal problems.
- A carbohydrate-to-protein ratio of 4:1 has been shown to increase aerobic endurance performance during both acute exercise and subsequent bouts of aerobic endurance exercise (Ivy et al. 2003; Saunders, Kane, and Todd 2004) and may help to prevent muscle damage (Saunders, Kane, and Todd 2004).
- Ingesting carbohydrate alone, or in combination with protein, during resistance exercise can increase muscle glycogen stores (Haff et al. 2000) and facilitate greater training adaptations after acute (Beelen et al. 2008; Bird, Tarpenning, and Marino 2006a, 2006c) and prolonged periods of resistance training (Bird, Tarpenning, and Marino 2006b).

After

- Postexercise consumption of carbohydrate should occur within 30 minutes but minimally within 2 hours at a dose of 1.5 g carbohydrate per kilogram body weight to stimulate glycogen resynthesis (Ivy 1998).
- If an athlete does not need to rapidly replenish glycogen for repeated heats, trials, or events, a diet that provides high levels of dietary carbohydrate (8 to 10 g carbohydrate per kilogram body weight per day)

is adequate to promote peak levels of muscle glycogen (Jentjens and Jeukendrup 2003; Tarnopolsky et al. 2005).

- Ingesting amino acids, primarily the essential amino acids, immediately after exercise until 3 hours postexercise can stimulate sharp increases in protein synthesis (Borsheim et al. 2002; Rasmussen et al. 2000; Tipton et al. 1999b). The addition of carbohydrate to protein may increase postexercise muscle protein synthesis rates even more, but the effect may be maximized when this combination is ingested immediately before resistance training (Tipton et al. 2001).

- Maximal improvements in muscular strength and body composition during resistance training over several weeks can be achieved by ingestion of a combination of carbohydrate + protein after exercise (Kerksick et al. 2006; Tarnopolsky et al. 2001; Willoughby, Stout, and Wilborn 2007).

- The addition of creatine (0.1 g creatine per kilogram body weight per day) to a carbohydrate + protein supplement may facilitate even greater adaptations to resistance training (Cribb, Williams, and Hayes 2007; Kerksick et al. 2007), but this finding is not universal (Cribb et al. 2007).

Arguably one of the most important aspects of recovery and subsequent performance for the aerobic endurance athlete is the maintenance of maximal muscle glycogen levels. Though maximizing internal glycogen stores (e.g., liver and muscles) will not necessarily enhance work output or speed, it will enable athletes to maintain their pace of training for a longer period of time. At rest, average intramuscular glycogen levels of trained athletes are adequate to meet the physical demands of events lasting anywhere from 60 to 90 minutes—significantly less than the amount of time needed to complete a marathon or an ultra-endurance event. Athletes can do three main things to maximize glycogen levels: (1) consume carbohydrate immediately after training to refuel for the next exercise session, (2) load carbohydrate before an event, and (3) consume carbohydrate during exercise.

To ensure maximum glycogen before an event, an athlete should consume 8 to 10 g carbohydrate per kilogram body weight per day and get adequate rest (do little training or no training) before competition. To optimize carbohydrate utilization, preexercise meals should be largely composed of high-carbohydrate foods or liquids. This practice becomes even more important when the athlete makes poor recovery efforts (e.g., low dietary carbohydrate intake, failure to rest or reduce training volume, or both). In addition to a high-carbohydrate diet and rest, consuming a high-carbohydrate meal (200-300 g) several (4 to 6) hours before exercise helps to maintain maximal muscle and liver glycogen levels.

Athletes who do not ingest an optimal amount of carbohydrate preexercise need to overcome the lack of available carbohydrate by working harder to ingest optimal carbohydrate levels during the first hour of exercise. While many food choices can provide carbohydrate, athletes need to experiment during training sessions to figure out what foods work for them without causing gastrointestinal distress. Consuming a variety of types of sugar, maltodextrin, sucrose, and fructose, for example, may be more beneficial than consuming one type of sugar. This may enhance the amount of carbohydrate that the body can use in a given time period. In addition to consuming different types of carbohydrate, athletes may benefit from ingesting carbohydrate at frequent intervals throughout exercise rather than a large dose before exercise.

Addition of protein to carbohydrate consumed during aerobic endurance exercise will not necessarily enhance performance but may boost recovery and minimize muscle damage to the exercising muscle tissue. Ingestion of protein with and without carbohydrate before or during resistance training sessions is a new area of research, but preliminary results suggest greater improvements in strength, lean mass, body fat percentage, serum levels of important anabolic (muscle building) hormones, and intramuscular markers of muscle hypertrophy.

After aerobic endurance exercise, athletes should consume 1.5 g carbohydrate per kilogram body weight within 30 minutes of completing exercise, or 0.6 to 1.0 g carbohydrate per kilogram body weight per hour during the first 30 minutes and again every 2 hours for the next 4 to 6 hours, to adequately replace glycogen stores. Delaying delivery of nutrients by just 2 hours may cut muscle glycogen resynthesis in half. The postexercise carbohydrate can be either solid or liquid but should not be high in fructose because this form of carbohydrate is associated with lower levels of glycogen resynthesis than other carbohydrate sources.

Athletes may benefit from adding protein to their postexercise carbohydrate meal. The addition of protein has been shown to result in greater glycogen resynthesis (and also greater protein synthesis) compared to carbohydrate only. Though optimal dosages are still unknown, a carbohydrate + protein combination in a 4:1 carbohydrate-to-protein ratio during this time period is widely accepted as a general guideline for aerobic endurance athletes; typical dosages are 1.2 to 1.5 g carbohydrate per kilogram body weight and 0.3 to 0.5 g essential amino acids or whole protein per kilogram body weight. After regular resistance training, a common practice supported by research is to ingest a high-quality protein source (e.g., whey, casein, egg) in a dose that provides 10 to 12 g of the essential amino acids as soon as possible but certainly within 1 hour after completion of training. Some studies show this practice leads to greater improvements in body composition, and ingesting this protein dose with 30 to 40 g carbohydrate both before and after exercise may also be effective in stimulating positive resistance training adaptations.

Table 9.1 provides an example of what all these timing recommendations would look like in practice for a 180-pound (82-kg) athlete performing regular aerobic endurance or resistance exercise. It is important for all athletes to consider their own training goals and adjust the nutrient timing plan to support those goals.

TABLE 9.1 Simplified Timing Recommendations for Aerobic Endurance and Resistance Athletes

	Aerobic endurance exercise*	Resistance training*
PREEXERCISE		
Everyday diet		
Recommendation	8-10 g CHO/kg	5-8 g CHO/kg 1.2-1.5 g PRO/kg
Intake	654-810 g CHO/day	409-654 g CHO/day 98-123 g PRO/day
Foods	Complex carbohydrates, pastas, starches, breads	Complex carbohydrates, pastas, starches, breads Lean proteins (chicken, beef, turkey, skim milk, egg)
2 to 4 h before		
Recommendation	4 g CHO/kg	
Intake	200-300 g CHO	No recommendation
Foods	Whole wheat bagel or toast, oatmeal, cereal, 24 fl oz sport drink	
30 to 60 min before		
Recommendation	1.2-1.5 g CHO/kg	
Intake	60-80 g CHO	No recommendation
Foods	Small energy or food bar, sport drink	
DURING EXERCISE		
Recommendation	6-8% CHO solution; add protein to 4:1 ratio	6% CHO solution + 6 g essential amino acids (EAAs)
Intake	1.5-2 cups (12-16 fl oz) every 15-20 min	22.5-30 ml after every set
Foods	Sport drink, gel packet with water	Sport drink, gel packet with water
POSTEXERCISE		
Recommendation	1.5 g CHO/kg within 30 min *or* 0.6-1 g CHO/kg in 30 min and again every 2 h	30-40 g carbohydrate and ~20-25 g protein delivering 8-12 g EAAs
Intake	123 g within 30 min *or* 49-82 g in 30 min and again every 2 h	30-40 g carbohydrate and ~20-25 g protein delivering 8-12 g EAAs
Foods	Sport drinks, bagels, fruits	Sport drinks, bagels, fruits, whey protein

*Note: All values are developed using a 180-pound (82-kg) athlete. CHO refers to carbohydrate; PRO refers to protein.

SUMMARY POINTS

- Appropriate incorporation of science-based nutrient timing strategies takes a great deal of work and dedication on the part of the athlete and sometimes the coach or parent. Because this area of research is relatively new, the science and therefore the recommendations can change over relatively short periods of time.

- The internal supply of carbohydrate is limited and will likely become depleted during any form of exercise at a moderate to high intensity continued for at least 60 to 90 minutes. For this reason, ingestion of high-carbohydrate meals at regular intervals during the postexercise period is recommended to maximally stimulate increases in muscle glycogen. During exercise, athletes should consume 10 to 15 fluid ounces (300-450 ml) of a carbohydrate–electrolyte solution that delivers 6 to 8 g carbohydrate for every 100 ml fluid (6% to 8% carbohydrate solution) every 15 to 20 minutes to sustain blood glucose levels.

- Many different forms of carbohydrate are acceptable, but fructose is not easily digested and thus not recommended due to its known relationship with gastrointestinal distress and low rates of glycogen resynthesis. Combining different forms of carbohydrate for ingestion during exercise is encouraged and may increase the rate of carbohydrate oxidation.

- A small amount of protein (0.15 to 0.25 g/kg body weight) added to carbohydrate at all time points, especially postexercise, is well tolerated and may promote greater restoration of muscle glycogen and rates of muscle protein synthesis. Maximal muscle protein synthesis can occur when 6 to 20 g of the essential amino acids is ingested along with an easily digestible form of carbohydrate within 3 hours of completing a resistance training workout. Over the course of several weeks, postexercise ingestion of a carbohydrate + protein supplement supports greater resistance training adaptations such as maximal strength and lean mass accretion.

- Milk protein sources (e.g., whey and casein) exhibit different digestion kinetics resulting in differences in delivery of amino acids into the bloodstream, which may affect accretion of lean tissue during resistance training.

- Adding creatine to nutrients in conjunction with regular resistance training may facilitate greater improvements in strength and body composition as compared to no creatine.

- Athletes should focus primarily on adequate availability and delivery of energy through appropriate proportions of the macronutrients (carbohydrate, protein, and fat) before spending significant financial resources on additional single ingredients (e.g., creatine monohydrate, essential amino acids). Irrespective of timing, regular snacks or meals should consist of adequate levels of carbohydrate and protein to maximally sustain required work outputs and prompt recovery.

10

Energy Expenditure and Body Composition

Paul La Bounty, PhD, MPT, CSCS
Jose Antonio, PhD, CSCS, FACSM, FISSN, FNSCA

Of the many physical attributes that can be modified, body composition is of paramount importance for most athletes regardless of the sport they participate in or their gender. Most athletes have one of two goals when attempting to change their body composition:

- Increase lean tissue mass (i.e., skeletal muscle)
- Decrease fat mass

A desire to improve body composition may be due to a wish to improve athletic performance; however, many athletes and fitness enthusiasts seek to improve body composition for aesthetic reasons alone. In addition to performance and cosmetic issues, excessive body fat, particularly visceral (i.e., abdominal) fat, most likely plays a role in the development of deleterious conditions such as heart disease, insulin resistance, non-insulin-dependent diabetes, sleep apnea, certain cancers, and osteoarthritis (Bray 2003; Moayyedi 2008; World Health Organization 2000; Reaven 2008; Vgontzas 2008).

Athletes, though, tend to be interested in the consequences of excessive body fat related to sport performance; in most sports, the inability to maintain an optimal body composition can negatively influence the athlete's performance. For example, increased body fat without a concomitant increase in lean muscle mass may decrease acceleration, jumping ability, and overall power in activities in which one's body weight needs to be moved through space (Jeukendrup and Gleeson 2004). In sports that require a high power–to–body mass ratio (e.g., gymnastics), excess body fat is not desirable. Therefore, athletes often devote significant effort to improving or maintaining body composition. Body composition can be modified through diet, exercise, nutritional supplements, various drugs, and surgery. This chapter focuses on two basic nutritional strategies that can affect body composition: hypercaloric diets to gain weight (with an emphasis on lean muscle mass accretion) and hypocaloric diets with the goal of decreasing body weight, particularly body fat. In addition, the chapter discusses various nutritional supplements and their effects on body composition.

Energy Balance

One of the ways people can achieve weight loss and fat loss is by modifying nutritional intake, primarily the amounts and types of calories consumed. The easiest way for athletes to change their body composition is to alter the energy balance equation. The energy balance equation, when in equilibrium, states that energy intake (i.e., food consumption) equals energy expenditure through normal metabolic processes and activity or exercise. When in a state of energy balance, a person is consuming a **eucaloric diet**. Due to fluctuations in body weight, this equation is not always in perfect balance. If more food is consumed than calories are expended, a positive energy balance is created and weight gain is likely to occur. Conversely, if fewer calories are consumed than needed for normal daily activities and metabolism, an energy deficit is created (figure 10.1). A diet inducing an energy deficit is termed a hypoenergetic or hypocaloric diet. A diet inducing a positive energy balance is known as a hyperenergetic or hypercaloric diet.

> ➤ eucaloric diet—Diet that includes the number of daily kilocalories needed to maintain existing weight; achieved by consumption of the number of kilocalories equal to an individual's total energy expenditure (TEE).

Thermic Effect of Food

Total caloric intake, as well as the macronutrient ratio of ingested nutrients, plays a role in weight gain and loss. The energy released from the catabolism of carbohydrate, protein, and fat is approximately 4, 4, and 9 kilocalories (kcal) per gram, respectively (Livesey 2001). Often overlooked, however, is that the process of digesting, absorbing, transporting, and storing the various macronutrients is associated with the expenditure of energy (i.e., kilocalories). This process, known as the thermic effect of food or diet-induced thermogenesis (DIT), causes a release of energy in the form of heat. The thermic effect of food actually increases one's metabolism above the normal baseline energy expenditure for a period of time (possibly several hours) after a meal (Tappy 1996).

As a result of the thermic effect of food, each macronutrient produces less net usable energy for the body after it is ingested (as compared to its

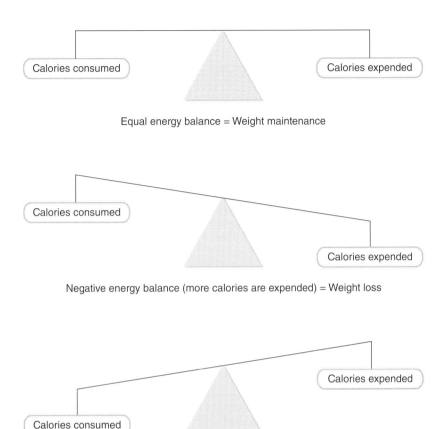

Equal energy balance = Weight maintenance

Negative energy balance (more calories are expended) = Weight loss

Positive energy balance (more calories are consumed) = Weight gain

FIGURE 10.1   The energy balance equation.

energy content on the training table before a meal). Furthermore, certain macronutrients require more energy than others (i.e., have a higher thermic effect) in order to be digested, absorbed, transported, and stored. Specifically, the thermic effect of the caloric content of fat, carbohydrate, and protein is approximately 0% to 3%, 5% to 10%, and 20% to 30%, respectively (Tappy 1996). In other words, fat has a relatively low thermic effect, protein has the highest thermic effect, and carbohydrate is in the middle. Some scientists would like to revamp the current food labels to reflect the actual net kilocalories that are gained after subtraction of the kilocalories required to digest and store the macronutrients (i.e., net metabolizable energy, NME) (Livesey 2001). If the current system were changed, the energy balance equation would be more accurate and meaningful (Livesey 2001).

It is important to keep the thermic effect of food in mind when formulating a nutritional plan to enhance weight gain or weight loss, because all calories are not the same biologically. For example, if a person consumed 300 kcal of extra protein every day for a year as opposed to 300 kcal of extra sucrose (i.e., table sugar) for the same length of time, it could be theorized that the effect on weight gain would not be the same because of the differing thermogenic properties of these macronutrients. When athletes embark on a hypocaloric diet to lose body weight, they will invariably lose some lean body mass. By increasing the proportion of protein ingested during a hypocaloric diet, the athlete realizes two benefits. First, the higher protein content will help to preserve lean body mass; and secondly, more calories will be burned because of the high thermogenic properties of protein.

Deleterious Effects of Energy-Restricted Diets

Athletes in weight-restricted sports such as mixed martial arts, wrestling, boxing, gymnastics, figure skating, and diving may need to lose body weight or improve body composition or both. Reasons for wanting to lose weight may range from enhancing performance to qualifying for a lower weight class or may involve aesthetic considerations. Regardless of why an athlete desires to lose weight, the athlete or trainer should focus on losing excessive body fat and attempting to minimize the loss of lean muscle tissue.

An important phenomenon to consider is that when an individual loses body fat, lean muscle mass typically decreases concomitantly. In fact, one study demonstrated that after six weeks of consuming a very-low-calorie diet, obese subjects lost ~11.5 kg (25.3 pounds) (Eston et al. 1992); however, of that weight, approximately 63% was from fat and the remaining 37% was from fat-free mass. Other studies using short-term caloric-restricted diets have also reported varying losses of fat-free mass (Krotkiewski et al. 2000; Valtuena et al. 1995; Zahouani, Boulier, and Hespel 2003). In rare instances, an athlete may want to lose both muscle and fat (e.g., a very lean elite wrestler needing to drop into a lower weight class). For the most part, however, fat loss, not lean muscle, is the primary goal. In these cases, some muscle may need to be sacrificed to achieve the goal. Interestingly, Mourier and colleagues (1997) demonstrated that the combination of a hypocaloric diet and branched-chain amino acid consumption led to greater decreases in body weight and visceral fat loss than either a high-protein or a low-protein hypocaloric diet.

Hypocaloric Diets

When athletes need to lose weight, one of the first things they often do is adopt an energy-restricted diet **(hypocaloric diet)**. Hypocaloric diets can modestly or severely reduce total calorie intake. On the extreme end of dieting, some people adopt diets commonly referred to as very-low-calorie diets. With athletes, depending on the sport, performance can begin to suffer if caloric intake becomes too low.

> ➤ hypocaloric diet—Diet in which fewer kilocalories are consumed than are needed to maintain existing body weight; also known as an energy-restricted or hypoenergetic diet.

The **very-low-calorie diet (VLCD)** as defined by the National Heart, Lung, and Blood Institute is a specific type of diet containing less than 800 kcal/day (Gilden Tsai and Wadden 2006). Generally, the diet consists of relatively large amounts of dietary protein (70 to 100 g/day or 0.8 to 1.5 g protein per kilogram "ideal body weight"), relatively modest carbohydrate (80 g/day), and minimal fat (15 g/day) (Gilden Tsai and Wadden 2006). However, the VLCD generally meets 100% of the Recommended Dietary Allowance (RDA) of all essential vitamins and minerals (Gilden Tsai and Wadden 2006). These diets are often consumed in a liquid form (National Task Force and National Institutes of Health 1993) and are generally advocated only for people who are obese (body mass index [BMI] ≥30) and are working with a psychologist, dietitian, or exercise physiologist (Gilden Tsai and Wadden 2006).

> ➤ very-low-calorie diet (VLCD)—A type of hypocaloric diet, usually in a liquid form, in which 800 or fewer kilocalories are consumed on a daily basis.

Typically, VLCD are 12 to 14 weeks in duration; then a diet consisting of whole food is slowly reintroduced over the next two to three months in an attempt to stabilize the individual's weight (Gilden Tsai and Wadden 2006). The average weight loss on a VLCD is approximately 1.5 to 2.5 kg (~3-5 pounds) per week for an average weight loss of 20 kg (44 pounds) after 12 to 16 weeks (National Task Force and National Institutes of Health 1993). However, it is not easy to maintain this reduction in weight, as seen in a study in which 113 men and 508 women adhered to a VLCD for 12 weeks (as part of an overall 26-week weight loss program) and lost approximately 25.5% and 22.6% of their original weight, respectively (Wadden and Frey 1997). All participants were followed up two years later, and only 77.5% of the men and 59.9% of the women had maintained losses of 5% or more of body weight (Wadden and Frey 1997).

A similar type of diet, the **low-calorie diet (LCD)**, allows for approximately 1,000 to 1,500 kcal/day of conventional food. Gilden Tsai and Wadden (2006) conducted a meta-analysis on the effectiveness of the VLCD and the traditional LCD with regard to weight loss. The authors concluded that initial weight loss was greater with the VLCD. However, in contrast to what had been shown in an earlier meta-analysis (Anderson et al. 2001), Gilden Tsai and Wadden concluded that after a year's time, the actual weight loss with the VLCD was not significantly different from that achieved with the traditional LCD. These authors reported that the earlier meta-analysis had not actually compared VLCD and LCD studies head to head but had "extrapolate[d] information across investigations, in which only one or the other diet was used" (p. 1289). Equally important, Gilden Tsai and Wadden noted the conclusion of the National Heart, Lung, and Blood Institute's expert panel that LCD should be advocated over VLCD. From a practical standpoint, a LCD is much more realistic for most people to adhere to on a day-to-day basis.

➤ low-calorie diet (LCD)—A type of hypocaloric diet, usually containing traditional food, in which ~1,000 to 1,500 kcal are consumed on a daily basis.

Due to the deleterious effects of energy-restricted diets on lean muscle mass as already discussed, VLCD are not recommended for athletes (except very rarely in weight-restricted sports when making weight is a critical issue). If VLCD are prescribed for athletes, performance may be severely limited because a drastic reduction in overall kilocalories decreases glycogen stores in skeletal muscle (Eston et al. 1992; Krotkiewski et al. 2000). Furthermore, VLCD have been reported to decrease both absolute strength and muscular endurance (Eston et al. 1992). These potentially harmful effects may diminish the ability to train intensely and adequately recover from exercise. Of these two types of diets, a LCD is a better approach for athletes attempting to lose weight. Because the caloric deficits are not as severe, lean muscle mass is better maintained; and glycogen levels, although compromised, would not be as depleted and would not affect training intensity to the same extent as with a VLCD regimen.

High-Carbohydrate, Low-Fat Diets

Regarding weight loss, the optimal ratio of carbohydrate to protein to fat has been debated for some time, and consensus is currently lacking. Relatively high-carbohydrate, low-fat diets have been popular in athletic populations for years. However, these diets, particularly in nonathletic populations, have lost some of their popularity over the last few years due to the introduction of various high-protein, low-carbohydrate diets.

Studies lasting 12 months or less suggest that low-carbohydrate diets may be more advantageous than high-carbohydrate diets for short-term improvements in body composition (Brehm and D'Alessio 2008) (high-protein diets are discussed later in the chapter). The current long-term data (>12 months) suggest that weight loss is similar in those consuming low-fat, high-carbohydrate diets and those consuming higher-protein, lower-carbohydrate diets (Kushner and Doerfler 2008). Debate continues as to the type of carbohydrate in the diet (i.e., high glycemic index, high glycemic load, low glycemic index, or low glycemic load) that is optimal for weight loss.

Although a handful of weight loss studies have involved athletes and trained individuals (Horswill et al. 1990; Mourier et al. 1997), in most cases these studies have used overweight or obese nonathletic subjects. Thus much of the research information pertaining to weight loss can only be extrapolated to athletic populations. Many studies using relatively high-carbohydrate, low-fat hypocaloric diets have manipulated the type of carbohydrate consumed to determine its impact on weight loss. In 2004, the CARMEN study (Carbohydrate Ratio Management in European National diets) revealed that individuals who consumed either a low-fat, high simple carbohydrate group (LFSC) or a low-fat, high complex carbohydrate group (LFCC) lost similar amounts of both body weight and fat mass (0.9 kg and 1.8 kg; 1.3 kg and 1.8 kg, respectively) while maintaining lean mass (Saris et al. 2000).

Similarly, Sloth and colleagues (2004) demonstrated that when everything was equal except for the type of carbohydrate consumed (low or high glycemic index), individuals had lost approximately the same amount of body weight (−1.9 kg and −1.3 kg, respectively) and fat mass (−1.0 kg and −0.4 kg) at the conclusion of the 10-week study. Furthermore, the two groups lost approximately the same amount of fat-free mass (i.e., −0.8 kg) (Sloth et al. 2004). Das and colleagues (2007) obtained comparable results for weight loss and body composition with diets consisting of either a low (40% carbohydrate, 30% fat, 30% protein) or high (60% carbohydrate, 20% fat, and 20% protein) glycemic load. The authors reported that at the end of the study there were no significant differences between the two groups in body weight, body fat, resting metabolic rate, hunger, or satiety. After 12 months, the percent changes in body weight were −7.81% and −8.04% and in body composition were −17.9% and −14.8% in the low and high glycemic load groups, respectively (Das et al. 2007). Results for weight loss were similar in another study comparing hypocaloric diets while varying the type (low vs. high glycemic index) of carbohydrate ingested (Sichieri et al. 2007).

Conversely, de Rougemont and colleagues (2007) reported that in a five-week study, individuals in the group that ingested a low glycemic index diet lost significantly more weight (−1.1 kg vs. −0.3 kg) than the group that consumed a high glycemic index carbohydrate diet. Regarding fat loss, neither group lost a significant amount of fat (0.17 vs. 0.04 kg) during the five-week intervention, and there was no significant difference between the groups (de Rougemont et al. 2007). Bouche and colleagues (2002) also demonstrated in a five-week study that a low as compared to a high glycemic index diet led to a significant decrease in fat mass (0.7 kg), as well as a statistical trend toward gaining lean mass, without actually changing body weight.

Although not all research agrees, it should be noted that other positive effects of a low glycemic index diet have been reported. Specifically, an increase in satiety (Ball et al. 2003), a decrease in lipid profile (low-density lipoprotein and total cholesterol) (de Rougemont et al. 2007), and enhanced insulin and glucose control (Brynes et al. 2005; Stevenson et al. 2005) have been observed with a low- versus a high-glycemic diet. Athletes often are encouraged to ingest high-glycemic carbohydrate to enhance glycogen resynthesis after exercise, which may also have an effect on weight loss and lean muscle mass changes during a period of dieting. Unfortunately, much of the published research in this area is conflicting. Thus more research is needed to allow conclusions about whether a high or a low glycemic index diet is more efficacious for improving body composition and weight loss.

Fat ingestion remains an area of scientific investigation, and at this point specific recommendations with regard to fat intake remain elusive. Concerning body composition, Strychar (2006) has reported that a reduction in overall fat ingestion in a weight loss program is beneficial, but the optimal percentage is not fully agreed upon by scientists. Nevertheless, the 2009 position stand of the American Dietetic Association, Dietitians of Canada, and the American College of Sports Medicine on nutrition and athletic performance gives some guidance pertaining to fat intake (Rodriguez et al. 2009). One point made in the position stand is that "Fat intake should be sufficient to provide the essential fatty acids and fat-soluble vitamins, as well as contribute energy for weight maintenance" (p. 709). Another is that "Fat intake should range from 20% to 35% of total energy intake. Consuming ≤20% of energy from fat does not benefit performance" (p. 710). Fat is an important part of athletes diets because it is a source of energy, fat-soluble vitamins, and essential fatty acids (Rodriguez et al. 2009). For more information on fat intake and athletic performance, refer to chapter 4.

In conclusion, hypocaloric diets such as VLCD and LCD can lead to significant weight loss. However, for athletes these diets are not generally advised because performance and recovery may suffer (Eston et al. 1992; Krotkiewski et al. 2000). Hypocaloric diets that are relatively high in carbohydrate and low in fat have been shown to decrease body fat and improve body composition. However, the optimal amount of fat in the diet to promote weight loss is still unclear. Furthermore, whether or not high- or low-glycemic carbohydrates or the glycemic load affects weight loss remains debated. One should take into account that individuals engaging in high-intensity training have different needs than sedentary or minimally active adults. Specifically, intense activity is primarily fueled by skeletal muscle carbohydrate (which is burned for energy during the process of glycolysis). For this reason, individuals engaged in high-intensity training need higher levels of carbohydrate.

High-Protein Diets

High-protein diets, often with concomitant carbohydrate restriction, have gained a lot of attention and become quite popular as a means to lose weight, improve body composition, curb hunger, and improve certain blood lipid profiles and insulin sensitivity (Brehm and D'Alessio 2008; Halton and Hu 2004; Kushner and Doerfler 2008; Noble and Kushner 2006). Published research findings demonstrate that diets higher in protein most likely aid in weight loss due to the satiating and thermic effect of protein (Brehm and D'Alessio 2008). In fact, Johnston and colleagues (2002) demonstrated that the thermic effect of a meal containing relatively high protein (30%

of energy as complex carbohydrate, 10% as simple sugar, 30% as protein, and 30% as fat), on average, was nearly two times greater than that of a high-carbohydrate meal containing equal calories (50% of energy as complex carbohydrate, 10% as simple sugar, 15% as protein, and 25% as fat).

An additional suggestion is that individuals who consume higher-protein diets are more likely to eat less at subsequent meals due to satiating effects (Halton and Hu 2004). Specifically, eating a high-protein meal has resulted in consuming 12% (Barkeling, Rossner, and Bjorvell 1990) and 31% (Latner and Schwartz 1999) fewer calories at the next meal. One reason higher-protein diets may be more satiating than high-carbohydrate diets is that protein, as opposed to fat and carbohydrate, is a relatively strong stimulator of the satiating gastrointestinal hormone cholecystokinin (CCK) (Johnston, Day, and Swan 2002). Elevated CCK levels have been shown to inhibit food intake in both rats and humans (Bray 2000).

Researchers in Denmark showed that when participants on a high-protein diet (46% carbohydrate, 25% protein, 29% fat) or a high-carbohydrate diet (59% carbohydrate, 12% protein, 29% fat) ate ad libitum (i.e., as much as they wanted), those on the high-protein diet consumed significantly fewer calories over the course of the study (Skov et al. 1999). Moreover, the high-protein diet group lost significantly more weight than the participants on the high-carbohydrate diet. Specifically, participants on the high-protein and high-carbohydrate diets lost 8.9 kg and 5.1 kg of body weight and 7.6 kg and 4.3 kg of fat, respectively (Skov et al. 1999). Layman and colleagues (2003) examined the effects of two different hypocaloric (~1,700 kcal/day) isoenergetic diets with varying carbohydrate-to-protein ratios on body composition. One of the diets had a carbohydrate-to-protein ratio of 3.5 (providing 68 g protein per day), and the other had a carbohydrate-to-protein ratio of 1.4 (providing 125 g protein per day). The two diets resulted in similar weight loss, but the diet that contained a greater percentage of protein led to greater fat loss, better lean muscle preservation, and ultimately improved body composition (Layman et al. 2003).

According to Brehm and D'Alessio (2008), among studies lasting up to 12 months, randomized, controlled trials repeatedly demonstrate that high-protein diets are comparable, and possibly superior, to low-protein diets when it comes to weight loss, preservation of lean body mass, and improvement in several cardiovascular risk factors. Therefore, diets that moderately increase protein and modestly restrict carbohydrate and fat may have beneficial effects on body weight and body composition (Brehm and D'Alessio 2008; Halton and Hu 2004).

Interestingly, as Kushner and Doerfler (2008) point out in a review, long-term data continue to indicate that total weight loss does not differ significantly between low-carbohydrate dieters and low-fat dieters. Therefore, although not all research agrees, high-protein, low-carbohydrate diets may be better for weight loss and body composition in the short term; but long-duration studies suggest that the traditional lower-fat, higher-carbohydrate diets may be just as effective. Even though diets higher in protein and lower in carbohydrate seem promising, scientists point out that the long-term effects of a high-protein diet on overall cardiovascular and metabolic health need to be studied (Kushner and Doerfler 2008). However, to date, the majority of "high-protein" studies that evaluated the potential effects on cardiovascular risk profile actually show an improvement or reduced risk in comparison to traditional American diets.

In conclusion, it appears that diets moderately higher in protein and slightly lower in carbohydrate may be beneficial when it comes to weight loss and improving body composition. Furthermore, increasing protein intake during weight loss at varying calorie intakes will prevent a negative nitrogen balance, which may also help lessen the loss of lean muscle tissue and ultimately resting energy expenditure (Stiegler and Cunliffe 2006). However, adequate carbohydrate intake is also critical for several aspects of athletic performance and high-intensity exercise. Therefore, with physically active individuals, it is often unwise to advocate drastically decreasing carbohydrate intake because this may adversely affect muscle glycogen stores and performance (Cook and Haub 2007). Hypocaloric diets that restrict carbohydrate intake are probably not prudent during the competitive season if the sport relies on heavy carbohydrate usage, as do long- and middle-distance running, swimming, basketball, wrestling, and

Tips to Decrease Body Fat

1. If possible, attempt to reduce body fat in the off-season or pre-season.
2. Keep a record of all food and drink intake (record the amount and type of food consumed and feelings, times, and places associated with food intake).
3. The easiest way to decrease body fat is to alter your energy balance equation (i.e., create a negative energy balance).
4. For most athletes, reduce calories by approximately 500 per day.
5. Reduce caloric intake by reducing the amount of calories derived from fat in your diet. Maintain or slightly increase protein intake (protein recommendations are 1.5 to 2.0 g/kg of body weight per day) when following a hypocaloric diet.
6. Assess body composition frequently to confirm that weight lost is coming from stored body fat and not lean muscle mass.
7. Make weight loss gradual to ensure maximum fat loss and preservation of lean tissue. For most athletes, a loss of one pound per week is best.

others. However, variations of these diets may be beneficial in promoting weight loss for athletes in the off-season. An important point is that weight loss should take place in a competitive athlete's off-season when possible. Since competitive performance is not a part of the off-season, attaining an ideal body weight and body composition through changes in dietary intakes at this time will not directly affect competitive performance.

Combining Diet and Exercise for Weight Loss

The research on whether the combination of aerobic exercise and a hypocaloric diet leads to (statistically significant) improvements in body composition versus a calorie-restricted diet alone remains somewhat equivocal. Neiman and colleagues (2002) demonstrated that aerobic exercise (i.e., walking at 60-80% of maximal heart rate) plus an energy-restricted diet did not lead to greater weight loss than a hypocaloric diet alone in obese individuals. Similarly, 30 minutes of moderate-intensity cycling performed three times a week for 16 weeks by sedentary men did not lead to greater improvements in body mass or body composition than a calorie-restricted diet alone (Cox et al. 2003). Kraemer and colleagues (1997) have also reported that neither weight loss nor percent body fat during moderate caloric restriction was enhanced by the addition of aerobic exercise. Several other studies have also shown that the addition of aerobic exercise to a hypocaloric diet did not significantly enhance body composition or weight loss above that observed with dieting alone (Dengel et al. 1994a, 1994b; Strasser, Spreitzer, and Haber 2007).

Unfortunately, many researchers making this comparison did not control energy deficits. In other words, in some of the investigations, the diet plus exercise group created a greater energy deficit than the diet-only group. Thus, it is difficult to make accurate comparisons from and interpretations of these studies or to draw conclusions about whether diet alone or diet plus exercise is superior for weight loss and body composition improvements. However, one study, by Redman and colleagues (2007), did control energy deficits. Participants were randomized into one of three groups for six months:

- A control group placed on a weight maintenance diet
- A group placed on a 25% calorie restriction
- A group placed on caloric restriction (12.5% deficit) and aerobic exercise (12.5% deficit)

The authors reported that both energy-restricted groups lost approximately 10% of their overall body weight, 24% of their fat mass, and 27% of their visceral fat (Redman et al. 2007). They concluded that exercise plus caloric restriction was just as effective as caloric restriction alone with respect to body composition and fat mass. Both groups lost approximately 2 to 3 kg of fat-free mass, but the groups did not significantly differ from each other (Redman et al. 2007). However, the investigators also pointed out that the individuals who lost the weight with the addition of exercise realized added benefits such as enhanced aerobic fitness and improved cardiovascular health. To realize these health benefits, the recommendation is that modest dietary restriction be combined with physical activity.

Resistance training (as compared to aerobic training) combined with a hypocaloric diet may be more promising with regard to maintaining lean tissue and decreasing fat mass. It has been shown that after weight loss, individuals who performed resistance training, but not aerobic exercise, were able to preserve both fat-free mass and resting energy expenditure (Hunter et al. 2008). Frimel and colleagues (2008) also demonstrated preservation of lean muscle mass when a progressive resistance training program was combined with a hypocaloric diet (as opposed to just dieting alone). Interestingly, Demling and DeSanti (2000) studied the effects of a 12-week moderate hypocaloric, high-protein diet combined with resistance training on body composition, using two different protein supplements (whey and casein protein hydrosylates), and compared this combination to a hypocaloric diet alone. At the end of the study, all three groups lost ~2.5 kg of body weight (Demling and DeSanti 2000). However, the individuals using diet alone, diet and exercise plus casein, and diet and exercise plus whey protein decreased body fat from 27% to 25%, 26% to 18%, and 27% to 23%, respectively (Demling and DeSanti 2000). The average fat loss was 2.5, 7.0, and 4.2 kg in the three groups, respectively. Equally important, lean mass did not improve in the diet-alone group but increased by 4 and 2 kg in the casein and whey groups, respectively (Demling and DeSanti 2000). The information reported in this study is welcomed by athletes who need to lose body fat. Assuming that all athletes engage in resistance training (as they should) to improve functional strength on the playing field, this study also provides scientific support indicating that resistance training during dieting will assist the athlete in preserving lean muscle mass.

However, in some studies, resistance training combined with aerobic exercise and a hypocaloric diet did not lead to enhanced weight loss or improved body composition over diet alone (Kraemer et al. 1997). In addition, a four-week study that added resistance training to VLCD consisting of ~812 kcal/day did not lead to the preservation of fat-free mass or resting energy expenditure (Gornall and Villani 1996). However, this is most likely attributable to the fact that the VLCD provided only 40 g protein a day. The minimal amount of protein supplied in the diet was most likely not able to prevent excessive protein degradation (Stiegler and Cunliffe 2006).

Hypercaloric Diets

On the other end of the spectrum of body composition modification is the need or desire to gain weight, particularly lean muscle mass. Interestingly, if excess calories (i.e., a **hypercaloric diet**) are consumed by untrained individuals, even without resistance training, both fat mass and muscle mass accretion can occur (Forbes 2000). Moreover, initial body composition may play a role in the type of weight (fat vs. muscle) that is gained on a hyperenergetic diet. Forbes (2000) stated in a review that the weight gain of thin people is composed of 60% to 70% lean tissue (in overfeeding studies lasting at least three weeks). Conversely, in obese individuals, only 30% to 40% of the weight gain was lean tissue.

> ➤ hypercaloric diet—Diet in which more kilocalories than needed to maintain existing body weight are consumed; also known as an energy-rich or hyperenergetic diet.

If gaining lean mass is the primary goal, two things must occur. First, an appropriate stimulus must be exerted on the skeletal muscles to enhance hypertrophy. This is generally achieved through performance of a well-designed, periodized resistance training program. Secondly, more calories need to be consumed than are expended. The types of calories consumed may also influence the type of weight gained. As a general rule, to optimize muscle mass gain while also minimizing fat mass accretion, the increased caloric intake should come predominately from protein–amino acids and carbohydrate, with only minimal increases in fat (particularly saturated fat) consumption.

The combination of an appropriate anabolic stimulus (resistance exercise) and ingestion of adequate substrate (protein) results in a positive nitrogen balance. Positive nitrogen balance occurs when protein synthesis exceeds protein degradation (i.e., breakdown). It is also important to remember that for protein synthesis to occur in skeletal muscle, all 20 amino acids, in proper amounts, must be present (Jeukendrup 2004). Thus, an adequate supply of amino acids must be consumed in the diet. The sidebar lists some general recommendations for enhancing lean body mass. Around 0.25 to 1.5 pounds a week is a realistic weight gain goal. However, the percentage of actual lean muscle tissue that can be gained is highly variable.

Of all sports, few place as much emphasis on gaining muscle mass as bodybuilding. Lambert and colleagues (2004) have suggested a macronutrient ratio for bodybuilders of about 55% to 60% carbohydrate, 25% to 30% protein, and 15% to 20% fat. This recommendation would allow enough protein to optimize muscle growth, as well as sufficient carbohydrate to allow for optimal energy for high-intensity resistance training, and still provide enough fat to maintain adequate testosterone levels in the blood (Lambert, Frank, and Evans 2004). Protein synthesis requires the use of adenosine triphosphate (ATP), so an energy-deficient diet may decrease protein synthesis. As a result, a slightly hyperenergetic diet, with an approximately 15% increase in energy intake above what is required to maintain weight, is recommended to optimize muscle protein synthesis (i.e., hypertrophy) (Lambert, Frank, and Evans 2004).

Tips to Increase Lean Muscle Mass

1. Consume a hypercaloric diet, approximately 10% to 15% above what is needed to maintain existing body weight.

2. Spread out your daily caloric intake over five or six meals.

3. Engage in a periodized resistance training program.

4. Consume ~40% to 50% carbohydrate, ~30% protein, and ~20% to 30% fat. For additional kcals, consume high protein, high fat foods.

5. Ingest adequate protein every day (approximately 1.5-2.0 g/kg per day).

6. Regularly consume whey protein, various amino acids (such as the branched-chain amino acids), casein protein, and carbohydrate, particularly timed around your workouts (i.e., pre-, during-, and post-workout meals).

7. Consider supplementing with creatine.

An earlier study, although of the elderly, also found an increase in muscle mass when an increase in energy intake was combined with resistance training. Meredith and colleagues (1992) investigated the effects of consuming an extra 560 kcal (~60 g carbohydrate, ~25 g fat, and ~24 g protein) per day in elderly individuals. This dietary protocol, when combined with resistance training, resulted in a significantly greater thigh muscle mass as measured by magnetic resonance imaging (MRI) than in participants who did not consume the extra kilocalories. Note, though, that this investigation was conducted in an elderly population, and it has not yet been proven that younger, physically active adults would experience the same physiological adaptations.

Timing of the intake of macronutrients around a resistance training session may play a role in muscle hypertrophy and improving body composition. Tipton and colleagues (2001) demonstrated that a preworkout intake of a carbohydrate plus essential amino acid solution was more efficacious in promoting postworkout protein synthesis than ingesting the same mixture immediately after the session. The same group (2007) then compared the effects of whey protein consumed before and after a resistance training bout to determine if the timing of intact, whole proteins would have a similar effect on protein synthesis as in the earlier study. Both the pre- and postworkout whey protein meals increased protein synthesis to an extent that was different but not significantly so (Tipton et al. 2007). A plethora of other investigations have also demonstrated the importance of the timing of protein intake and its effects on maximizing the anabolic stimulus of a resistance exercise bout (Borsheim et al. 2002; Rasmussen et al. 2000; Tipton et al. 2003, 2004). For a complete discussion on the timing of protein and carbohydrate intake, refer to chapter 9.

How much protein should an athlete consume in order to promote increases in lean muscle mass? At this time, all experts do not agree. However, the International Society of Sports Nutrition published a position stand on protein and exercise (Campbell et al. 2007) that included the following findings:

- Vast research supports the contention that individuals engaged in regular exercise training require more dietary protein than sedentary individuals.

- Protein intakes of up to 2.0 g/kg per day for physically active individuals are not only safe but may improve the training adaptations to exercise training.

- When part of a balanced, nutrient-dense diet, protein intakes at this level are not detrimental to kidney function or bone metabolism in healthy, active people.

It should be noted, however, that Rennie and Tipton (2000), also experts in protein metabolism, suggest in their review article that active individuals may not need additional protein. Specifically, they state, "There is no evidence that habitual exercise increases protein requirements; indeed protein metabolism may become more efficient as a result of training" (p. 457).

Although these seemingly contradictory statements can be confusing, the bottom line is that a slight increase in protein consumption does not appear to be harmful in healthy adults and may enhance training adaptations like muscle hypertrophy. Therefore, athletes may consider slightly increasing lean protein consumption when attempting to increase lean muscle mass and improve body composition. As discussed in chapter 3, a protein intake of 1.5 to 2.0 g/kg body mass is recommended. Athletes attempting to gain lean body mass should opt for the upper levels of this range. In conclusion, in order to increase body weight, one must consume a hyperenergetic diet. However, to emphasize lean muscle mass accretion, the hypercaloric diet should be combined with resistance training and a protein intake adequate to support protein synthesis.

Sport Supplements to Improve Body Composition

A few dietary supplements have been shown to increase lean body mass and decrease fat mass or percentage body fat. This section focuses on studies in which the clinical end point is an actual change in body composition. Numerous studies have measured acute changes in muscle protein synthesis and degradation; these are not discussed here because body composition alterations were not addressed or were not part of the study design (Biolo et al. 1995; Borsheim, Aarsland, and Wolfe 2004; Tipton et al. 2003, 2007, 1999a, 1999b, 2001). Note that in each of the studies discussed, the sport supplements were consumed in conjunction with a resistance training program.

Creatine

Creatine, which may be one of the more commonly used dietary supplements, has been shown to promote significant gains in lean body mass. As a stand-alone supplement, creatine has more supportive evidence with regard to enhancing gains in lean body mass than the rest of the supplement category combined. In fact, one of the most consistent side effects of creatine supplementation has been increases in body weight (in the form of lean body mass). This has been observed in several populations, including males, females, the elderly, and many groups of American and international athletes (Branch 2003; Brose, Parise, and Tarnopolsky 2003; Chrusch et al. 2001; Gotshalk et al. 2002; Kelly and Jenkins 1998; Kreider et al. 1998; Stone et al. 1999; van Loon et al. 2003; Vandenberghe et al. 1997).

Many of the studies performed to date indicate that short-term (about one week) creatine ingestion increases total body mass by approximately 0.8 to 1.7 kg (~1.8 to 3.7 pounds) (Terjung et al. 2000). Longer-term creatine supplementation (about two months) in conjunction with resistance training has been shown to increase lean body mass by approximately 2.8 to 3.2 kg (~7 pounds) (Earnest et al. 1995; Kreider et al. 1996; Stout, Eckerson, and Noonan 1999). Even though creatine supplementation has support with regard to increasing body mass, there was a time when some questioned whether the gains were due to increased water retention or to actual lean tissue accretion. Two landmark studies confirmed that creatine supplementation, in conjunction with a resistance training program, elicited an increase in protein content (specifically, contractile protein content).

In the first of these clinical investigations (Volek et al. 1999), adaptations at the cellular level were determined in 19 healthy resistance-trained men who were matched and then randomly assigned in a double-blind fashion to either a creatine or placebo group. Groups performed periodized heavy resistance training for 12 weeks. Participants took creatine or placebo capsules (25 g/day) for one week followed by a maintenance dose (5 g/day) for the remainder of the training. After 12 weeks, increases in body mass and fat-free mass were significantly greater in creatine (6.3% and 6.3%, respectively) than placebo (3.6% and 3.1%, respectively) subjects. Furthermore, biopsy data revealed that compared with placebo subjects, creatine subjects demonstrated significantly greater increases in Type I (35% vs. 11%), IIa (36% vs. 15%), and IIab (35% vs. 6%) muscle fiber cross-sectional areas. Muscle total creatine concentrations were unchanged in placebo subjects. Muscle creatine was significantly elevated after one week in creatine subjects (22%), and values remained significantly greater than in placebo subjects after 12 weeks. This study clearly demonstrated that increases in protein content, specifically across all three types of muscle fibers, were in part responsible for gains in body mass (Volek et al. 1999).

Elsewhere, Willoughby and Rosene (2001) investigated oral creatine ingestion and its effects on myofibrillar protein content (a marker of the amount of intracellular protein). Untrained male subjects ingested 6 g creatine per day or a placebo in conjunction with heavy resistance training for 12 weeks. At the end of the intervention, those ingesting creatine significantly increased fat-free mass (~7 pounds) in comparison with the placebo group (~1 pound). One of the most interesting findings from this study related to what was occurring at the cellular level of the skeletal muscle. Myofibrillar protein content was significantly greater in the creatine group than in the placebo group, despite the fact that the two groups performed identical resistance training programs. More specifically, the authors reported significant increases in the content of two isoforms of myosin heavy chain protein (the major constituent of contractile skeletal muscle) (Willoughby and Rosene 2001). Taken together, these studies appear to indicate that the increases in lean body mass seen with creatine supplementation are due to augmentation of skeletal muscle fiber hypertrophy (possibly due to the activation of satellite cells) and not solely water retention.

Other Sport Supplements

The consumption of protein, amino acids, and various combinations of different proteins and amino acids is an effective way to promote further gains in muscle fiber size when combined with a proper exercise training regimen. In fact, the prevalence of studies that have used combinations of carbohydrate, creatine, protein, and amino acids makes it difficult to pinpoint the exact mechanisms governing the adaptive response. Nevertheless, it is clear from a practical standpoint that if a supplement combination safely enhances body composition and muscle fiber size, it is beneficial to the athlete or end user, regardless of how it works.

Anderson and colleagues (2005) compared the effect of 14 weeks of resistance training, combined with timed ingestion of isoenergetic protein versus carbohydrate supplementation, on muscle fiber hypertrophy and mechanical muscle performance. Supplementation was administered before and immediately after each training bout, and in addition in the morning on nontraining days. Muscle biopsy specimens were obtained from the vastus lateralis muscle and analyzed for muscle fiber cross-sectional area. After 14 weeks of resistance training, the protein group showed hypertrophy of Type I (18%) and Type II (26%) muscle fibers, whereas no change above baseline occurred in the carbohydrate group (Andersen et al. 2005). Another investigation showed that protein supplementation during resistance training, independent of source (whey or soy), increased lean tissue mass and strength over isocaloric placebo and resistance training (Candow et al. 2006). Yet another study demonstrated that supplementation with creatine plus carbohydrate, whey protein, and creatine plus whey protein resulted in significantly greater 1RM (1-repetition maximum) strength improvements and muscle hypertrophy than carbohydrate alone (Cribb et al. 2007).

Elsewhere, researchers ascertained the effects of varying kinds of protein supplementation on body composition and other exercise performance variables during 10 weeks of resistance training (Kerksick et al. 2006). Thirty-six resistance-trained males followed a four day per week split body part resistance training program for 10 weeks. Three groups of supplements were randomly assigned to subjects in a double-blind manner: 48 g/day of a carbohydrate placebo; 40 g/day of whey protein plus 8 g/day of casein; or 40 g/day of whey protein plus 3 g/day of branched-chain amino acids and 5 g/day of L-glutamine. The whey plus casein group experienced the greatest increases in DEXA (dual-energy X-ray absorptiometry) lean mass and DEXA fat-free mass. Thus, the combination of whey and casein protein promoted the greatest increases in fat-free mass after 10 weeks of heavy resistance training (Kerksick et al. 2006).

Evidence clearly demonstrates that supplementation with creatine mono-hydrate (and various combinations of creatine + protein or carbohydrate or both) has a significant anabolic effect leading to positive changes in body composition. Supplementing with protein or combinations of protein, carbohydrate, and amino acids also has an anabolic effect. This is shown with both whole-body measures such as lean body mass augmentation and cellular measures of muscle fiber hypertrophy. Chapter 7 discusses supplements for strength and power in more detail.

Professional Applications

When attempting to optimize body composition, athletes seek to either increase muscle mass or lose body fat. While a plethora of scientific studies provide details on how to lose or gain body weight, some of these approaches are not appropriate for athletes. For instance, athletes who ingest a hypocaloric diet (eating fewer calories than needed) will lose weight, but a significant proportion of the weight lost will be from lean tissue if the protein intake is not sufficiently adjusted and if the resistance training program is not maintained. Similarly, a hypercaloric diet (eating more calories than needed) will cause weight gain, but a large proportion of the weight gain may be in the form of body fat if the athlete's resistance training and conditioning programs are not adjusted accordingly.

Athletes attempting to lose weight can do one of two things—either increase their physical activity or decrease their caloric intake. Assuming that athletes are already engaged in weight training, sport skills training, and conditioning, the option of increasing physical activity must be balanced against the risk of exhibiting symptoms of overtraining syndrome. Therefore, decreasing caloric intake is often recommended for athletes wishing to lose weight. However, this must be done carefully, since decreasing energy intake may also place the athlete at greater risk for overtraining and for losing hard-earned muscle mass. To maximize fat loss and prevent the loss of lean muscle mass, it is important that dieting athletes participate in a periodized resistance training program. In addition, as calories are reduced, the reduction should primarily come from carbohydrate and fat, and protein intake should not be limited to a large extent. While this will help to maximize fat loss and preserve muscle mass, training intensity and exercise performance may suffer due to the reduced carbohydrate intake. For this reason, weight loss programs should be undertaken in the off-season (so that competitive performance is not sacrificed) whenever possible.

Athletes attempting to gain weight (in the form of lean muscle mass) should adhere to two simple rules: (1) Follow a periodized resistance training program and (2) consume more calories than are expended. These two simple rules serve as the blueprint for gaining lean muscle mass. More specifically, the increased caloric intake should predominately come from protein–amino acids and carbohydrate, with only minimal increases in fat. This will optimize gains in muscle mass while also minimizing fat mass accretion. To what extent should calories be increased above maintenance levels? Approximately 15% above maintenance levels is a good place to begin. For instance, if a female basketball player wishes to gain lean muscle mass and her caloric intake is 2,100 calories to maintain her current weight, then the advice would be to increase her caloric intake to 2,415 calories. However, it is very important to monitor body composition during this time to make sure that weight gain is primarily manifesting itself as lean muscle mass and not body fat. In addition to changes in caloric intake, creatine monohydrate supplementation has been shown to promote significant gains in lean body mass and should also be considered.

SUMMARY POINTS

- When attempting to lose weight (in the form of body fat), it is important for athletes and physically active individuals to decrease caloric intake but keep protein intake at 1.5 to 2.0 g/kg body weight per day.

- When athletes are attempting to gain weight (in the form of lean muscle mass), ingesting approximately 15% calories above maintenance levels is a good place to begin.

- Whether the goal is to lose body fat or increase lean muscle mass, it is imperative that athletes follow a well-designed, periodized resistance training program.

- Whether the goal is to lose or gain weight, it is very important to monitor changes in body composition so that the dietary plan and resistance training program can be adjusted if nondesirable changes are occurring (i.e., weight loss is occurring with too much loss of lean tissue mass; weight gain is occurring with too much gain of body fat).

- Chapters 11 and 12 discuss how to determine nutritional needs and how to develop a nutrition plan.

- Certain sport supplements (such as creatine and protein) have been shown to assist with favorably altering body composition.

Nutritional Needs Analysis

Marie A. Spano, MS, RD, LD, CSCS, CSSD, FISSN

Before working with each athlete to develop an individual nutrition plan, it is essential that the sport nutrition professional assesses the athlete's current body composition, weight history, diet history, and current diet. In addition, if current lab work or bone density scans are available, these are valuable tools that can aid in developing a plan tailored specifically to the athlete.

Though weight and weight history both provide a glimpse into an athlete's nutrition status and any weight struggles he may have or may have had in the past, an accurate body composition measure tells a lot more than the scale does. By tracking body composition changes over time, the sport nutrition professional can determine if the athlete is maintaining or moving toward a body composition range that is both healthy and beneficial for the specific sport. In addition, body composition changes can help in assessment of whether the athlete is gaining, maintaining, or losing lean mass.

In addition to assessing body composition, it is imperative that the sport nutrition professional analyze the athlete's diet. The best way to do this is to have the athlete keep a food record for a minimum of three days. An accurate, detailed food record can be analyzed through use of a number of nutrition programs to gauge average intake of both macronutrients and micronutrients from food.

Measuring Body Composition

Coaches and athletes alike often place at least some emphasis on **body composition**. This is especially true in sports in which speed and aerobic endurance are critical for success (e.g., running), sports with weight classes (e.g., wrestling), and aesthetic sports (figure skating, gymnastics, diving, etc.). Because measures of body composition can affect how athletes feel about their body (potentially promoting eating-disordered behavior), as well as how a coach designs an athlete's workout program, it is critical that accurate tools be used to measure body composition and that a professional well versed in body composition interpret the results (in the context of health and the athlete's sport) for the athlete.

> ➤ body composition—An assessment of fat mass as compared to lean tissue.

Research settings use many methods of body composition: dual-energy X-ray absorptiometry (DEXA), underwater weighing, skinfold calipers, bioelectrical impedance analysis (BIA), dilution techniques, air displacement plethysmography (Bod Pod), near-infrared interactance, magnetic resonance imaging (MRI), and magnetic resonance spectroscopy (MRS). These differing techniques vary in the body components measured, which may include fat, fat-free mass, bone mineral content, total body water, extracellular water, total adipose tissue and its subdepots (visceral, subcutaneous, and intramuscular), skeletal muscle, select organs, and ectopic fat depots (Lee and Gallagher 2008).

Field measures commonly used include body mass index (BMI), skinfolds, and BIA because these tools are most convenient. Athletes in university settings and athletes with access to professional training facilities may also have their body composition measured by more accurate methods commonly used in research settings such as DEXA, Bod Pod, and underwater weighing.

Field Methods

Field methods for assessing body composition are those that are portable and easy to use for assessment of several people in a short time period. How do these measures compare, and what are the major differences between them? First, it is important to take a look at the most common field measures that sport nutritionist professionals use. Body mass index is a simple calculation: weight in kilograms / height in meters². The resulting number categorizes the person as underweight, normal weight, overweight, or obese. Body mass index is a very convenient way to measure obesity rates in a population but should not be used by itself to categorize an individual. Table 11.1 shows the BMI categories used by the World Health Organization.

The National Health and Nutrition Examination Survey (NHANES), a survey research program started in 1959 and directed by the Department of Health and Human Services (a federal government agency), measures BMI in the physical examination component of the survey (both physical exams and interviews are used). The NHANES assesses the health and nutrition status of adults and children in the United States and tracks changes over time to determine the prevalence of disease and risk factors for disease

TABLE 11.1 World Health Organization's Body Mass Index Categories

Classification	BMI (kg/m²)
Underweight	<18.50
Normal range	18.50-24.99
Overweight	≥25.00
Obese	≥30

This chart has been simplified to show the major categories.

From World Health Organization. BMI Classification. www.who.int/bmi/index.jsp?introPage=intro_3.html

(United States Department of Health and Human Services and Centers for Disease Control and Prevention 2009, 2010).

Measuring BMI is noninvasive and requires only an accurate scale and stadiometer (for measuring height). The downside to BMI is that it does not assess actual body composition or distinguish between fat and muscle tissue. Since muscle has greater density than fat and weighs more than fat per volume of tissue, BMI tends to overestimate body fat levels in muscular individuals (Witt and Bush 2005). It can also overestimate body fat in individuals with large body frames (Ortiz-Hernández et al. 2008). For example, a professional running back who is 5 feet 9 inches (1.75 m), weighs 210 pounds (95.5 kg), and has 8% body fat would have a BMI of 31.2. This BMI classifies him as obese. However, at 8% body fat, the athlete is not obese or overfat. The example illustrates a limitation of using BMI in athletes.

Though BMI may overestimate body fat in muscular individuals, it may underestimate body fat in other populations (Chang et al. 2003; Jones, Legge, and Goulding 2003). A study conducted using NHANES data showed that BMI cannot accurately diagnose obesity, especially in men and the elderly as well as people with intermediate BMI ranges, and therefore, BMI should only be used to assess population-based rates of obesity and not an individual's status (Romero-Corral et al. 2008). Body mass index is a tool best used to estimate population-based rates of weight correlated to height and not a tool designed to assess obesity or underweight in single individuals in a clinical setting in the absence of other clinical measures (Piers et al. 2000).

Trainers and coaches commonly turn to **skinfold calipers** for assessing body composition. Skinfold calipers measure skinfold thickness at various sites on the body. The technician takes measures by grasping a fold of skin and subcutaneous fat with the thumb and forefingers and pulling the fold away from the underlying muscle, then pinching it with the caliper and taking the reading within 2 seconds.

➤ skinfold calipers—A tool for measuring skinfold thickness, which can then be used to estimate body fat.

A three-site skinfold is commonly done and includes the chest, abdomen, and thigh on men and triceps, suprailiac, and thigh on women (figure 11.1). The five most common sites assessed include triceps, subscapular, suprailiac, abdomen, thigh (McArdle, Katch, and Katch 2005). Chest and biceps are additional sites that are sometimes used. The skinfold measures (which should be taken two or three times at each site and then averaged) are then incorporated into equations to predict percent body fat. These are the main advantages of skinfold calipers:

- They are easy to use (once the person is well trained in the technique).
- They do not require much time per person.
- They are noninvasive and inexpensive.

However, there are also several disadvantages. These include interperson variability (if body fat is measured by one person and then months later by another person) and less accuracy when less expensive calipers are used. In addition, over 100 different equations are used to estimate body fat from calipers, and people measure different sites among the seven. All of these factors can lead to errors in reliability, validity, or both. An accurate measure of body composition using skinfold calipers is within ±3% to 5% error of **hydrostatic weighing** (McArdle, Katch, and Katch 2005).

> ➤ hydrostatic weighing (underwater weighing)—A method of measuring body composition whereby the subject is submerged into a tank of water and body composition is determined based on total body density using Archimedes' principle of displacement (the weight of displaced fluid can be found mathematically). Underwater weighing assumes that the densities of fat mass and fat-free mass are constant, lean tissue is more dense than water, and fat tissue is less dense than water.

Bioelectrical impedance measures the impedance to the flow and distribution of a radiofrequency, alternating current (Lukaski et al. 1985). Both water and electrolytes influence the impedance of the applied current; therefore BIA measures total body water and then indirectly determines fat-free mass from this measure (Lukaski et al. 1985). Bioelectrical impedance is convenient, cost-effective, and quick; and operation requires little knowledge. However, it cannot accurately measure short-term changes in body composition nor can it accurately assess body composition in obese individuals (in whom it may underestimate body fat) and very lean individuals (in whom it may overestimate body fat) (Sun et al. 2005). Finally, small changes in fluid balance can affect the measurements (Saunders, Blevins, and Broeder 1998).

> ➤ bioelectrical impedance—A way of assessing body composition by measuring the flow of a small electrical current through the body. This measures total body water, which can be used to determine total fat free mass.

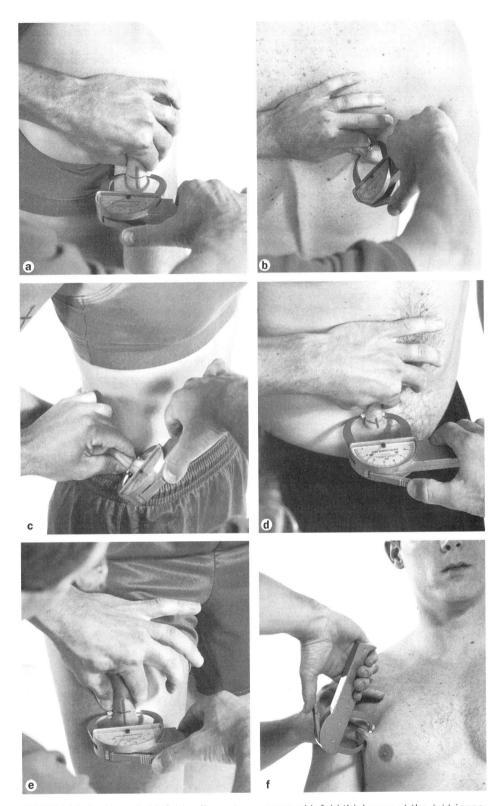

FIGURE 11.1 Use of skinfold calipers to measure skinfold thickness at the *(a)* triceps, *(b)* subscapular, *(c)* suprailiac, *(d)* abdominal, *(e)* upper thigh, and *(f)* chest.

Laboratory Measures

Laboratory measures for assessing body composition are typically more accurate than field measures but also more costly and time-consuming; therefore they are used in the lab versus in a field setting. The **Bod Pod** uses air displacement plethysmography to measure body density (from mass and volume). The Bod Pod obtains body mass from a weighing scale and obtains body volume by first measuring the interior of the empty chamber and then taking this measure again with the person inside. Densitometric principles are used to derive body composition measures from body density (McCrory et al. 1998). This method divides the body into two compartments, fat and fat-free mass. The dense, fat-free mass compartment consists of protein, water, mineral, and glycogen whereas the fat compartment consists of fat.

> ➤ Bod Pod—An egg-shaped device that an athlete sits in for assessment of body composition. It uses air displacement plethysmography to measure body density (from mass and volume).

The Bod Pod is noninvasive and easy to use, and the measurement takes only about 5 minutes. These are other benefits of the Bod Pod:

- It is comfortable for the person being measured (unless the individual is claustrophobic).
- It offers resting metabolic rate (RMR) and total energy expenditure (TEE) measures.
- Operation does not require a technician license.
- The machine is mobile (can be rolled to other locations).
- It can accommodate individuals up to 7 feet tall (2.1 m) and 550 pounds (250 kg).

As a newer technology, Bod Pod has been compared to other, well-established methods of measuring body composition. In a study comparing Bod Pod to DEXA, 160 men (32 ± 11 years) had their body composition measured with both machines. Percent body fat measures were 19.4 ± 6.8 and 21.6 ± 8.4 for DEXA and the Bod Pod, respectively. The two methods were highly correlated, but the mean difference of 2.2% was significant ($p < 0.01$). The difference between the two instruments was also greater as body fatness increased (Ball and Altena 2004). This study showed that differences will exist depending on the method used to assess body composition. Therefore, if an athlete is being tested with different measures over time, differences in body composition observed may not be completely accounted for by increases or decreases in body fat.

In a group of Division I female collegiate track and field athletes ($N = 30$), Bod Pod measures were compared to hydrostatic weighing, DEXA, and skinfold calipers. In this study, Bod Pod significantly overestimated body fat in comparison to hydrostatic weighing, and Bod Pod values also differed significantly from those obtained by DEXA. Body fat measured by skinfolds did not differ significantly from body fat measured by Bod Pod. If skinfold values do not differ significantly in this population, using this method would be a more cost-effective way to measure body composition than Bod Pod (Bentzur, Kravitz, and Lockner 2008). Another study also found the use of skinfold calipers equivalent to Bod Pod. In this particular study, percent body fat values as obtained by Bod Pod were validated against hydrostatic weighing in 30 high school boys. Body fat was also measured with near-infrared interactance, BIA, and skinfold calipers and compared to hydrostatic weighing. Both near-infrared interactance and BIA produced significant constant error and total error. Bod Pod produced acceptable total error values but significantly higher constant error than hydrostatic weighing, indicating that it is an acceptable choice for measuring body composition but no better than the use of skinfold calipers.

Dual-energy X-ray absorptiometry (DEXA) works by emitting X-rays (containing low radiation dosage) at two discrete energy levels, which are collimated into a beam and directed into the body posteriorly to anteriorly (Lukaski 1993). DEXA is based on the basic principle that a beam of X-rays passed through a complex material attenuates the beam in proportion to the composition, thickness, and individual components of the material. Therefore, when energy from an X-ray source passes through the human body, it experiences greater reduction in intensity when it interacts with bone than it does with soft tissue (Lukaski 1993). DEXA is quick, noninvasive, accurate, and reproducible. As with all methods of assessing body composition, there are benefits and drawbacks to DEXA. When compared to a four-compartment model, DEXA estimates of fat mass, percent body fat, and fat-free mass were significantly different in older individuals, indicating that this tool may not be the best method for measuring body composition in this age group (Moon et al. 2009, Tvlavsky et al. 2008).

Regardless of the method used to assess body composition in athletes, it is important to also monitor changes in body composition over time, along with body weight, when altering an existing nutrition or exercise program. By measuring body composition, along with body weight, the coach or trainer can effectively determine what type of weight (i.e., muscle, fat, or water) is actually being lost or gained.

Recording and Analyzing Food Intake

Before analyzing an athlete's diet, the sport nutrition professional needs to know what the athlete is eating on a daily basis. Methods commonly used to examine what an athlete is eating include dietary recalls and diet records. Though diet records (clients keep a running record of the specific foods and beverages they have consumed, including the amounts of each and how the food is prepared) are preferable to recalls because people often forget what they eat, diet records have limitations as well. The mere act of keeping a diet record makes people change their typical eating habits. In addition, some people are embarrassed by their food or drink consumption and therefore leave out crucial details due to shame. For instance, an American football player who drinks 18 beers on a weekend night might record only six of those beers. Another tool some people use is a camera phone. They snap a picture of their meal and send it to their sport nutritionist. However, a photo does not provide complete details regarding how a food was prepared or quantities of food consumed. Despite the drawbacks of dietary recalls and food records, these tools are among the best available for helping the sport nutrition professional assess an athlete's dietary intake. Form 11.1 on page 219 is a template athletes could use for a three-day dietary recall.

Some sport nutrition professionals can examine diet records and quickly spot areas of low intake (e.g., no dairy would signal a potential shortfall in both calcium and vitamin D). However, a computerized analysis program can accurately assess every component of the diet.

Food intake is typically analyzed through a food analysis program or with use of a food frequency questionnaire. A food analysis program requires a 24-hour dietary recall, three-day diet record, or a seven-day diet record (the more days analyzed and averaged, the more accurate the analysis of dietary intake). Food analysis programs can help determine a person's intake of macronutrients, micronutrients, and certain food components such as omega-3 fatty acids. A food frequency questionnaire asks how often a person eats certain foods (how many times per day, week, month, or year, for instance). Researchers commonly use food frequency questionnaires to measure the frequency and total intake of certain foods and correlate intake with disease risk. For instance, epidemiology studies have examined populations with a high intake of red meat and their risk of developing colorectal cancer in comparison to populations that consume less red meat (Sinha et al. 1999).

A variety of software programs, both on the computer and made for phones, analyze food intake. In addition, some Web sites allow people to track their food intake. Finally, specific software programs have been developed for dietitians to use to analyze their clients' food intake.

The basic programs that are free and that allow individuals to track their food intake can help an athlete stay within a certain calorie or macronutrient range. However, all of these programs are limited, and all rely on the user to have a basic knowledge about macronutrients and calorie needs. The best approach is to work with a sport nutrition professional who can look beyond macronutrients and calories and into the many other factors that influence health, athletic performance, and recovery.

Software Programs for Individuals

People who are not nutrition or research professionals can use several software programs to track their food intake, and new programs are being developed all the time. Many software programs have benefits, aside from just calculating calorie intake, to keep users engaged. These may include charting changes in weight over time (see figure 11.2), comparing calories burned through physical activity with dietary intake, and providing sample diets for specific calorie levels (1,200, 1,500, 1,800, 2,000, 2,200, etc.). Though all of these programs are geared toward weight loss and therefore are more applicable to the recreational athlete, athletes who have struggled with eating disorders or those trying to gain or maintain weight may find these basic programs helpful in keeping them accountable. Professional athletes are beyond calorie counting and need more detailed and individualized recommendations to improve performance and enhance recovery. Table 11.2 provides more information on various software programs that are available.

Professional Software Programs

Nutrition professionals in university settings also commonly use software programs for research purposes. The differences between free Internet-based software programs and professional programs may be vast. Professional programs typically have a very large database of foods, and they analyze food intake for more than just calories and macronutrient levels. Professional programs can also tally up a client's intake of specific fatty acids, micronutrients, caffeine, and other diet variables. Professional software programs also differ from most free programs in that they provide more detailed, thorough reports that often come in a number of different formats (pie charts, line graphs, etc.; see figure 11.3). These programs are designed

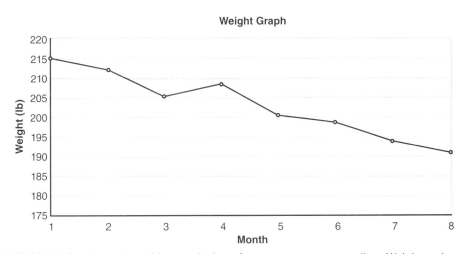

FIGURE 11.2 Several nutrition analysis software programs as well as Web-based programs produce a variety of graphs that help motivate and encourage people to reach their goals. This graph charts weight over time, which can help athletes who need to gain or lose weight to reach an appropriate weight for their sport and overall health.

TABLE 11.2   Internet and PDA—Based Software Programs

Program	Internet or PDA?	Fee?	Capabilities
www.fitday.com (basic membership)	Internet	Free	Tracks food, exercise, weight, and goals
www.sparkpeople.com	Internet	Free	Provides food tracker, personalized meal plans, customized fitness plan, recipes, articles, message boards
www.mypyramidtracker.gov	Internet	Free	Government based; tracks diet and physical activity, energy balance; provides analysis of both food intake and physical fitness
www.calorieking.com	Internet, Windows, Mac, Palm	Yearly fee	Allows nutrition professionals to log on to see what their clients are eating
www.dieticianmobile.com	iPhone and iPod	Payment for application via iTunes	Offers meal planning, access to recipes based on favorite foods, grocery lists, charts and graphs to track progress, diet tracking
www.dietorganizer.com/ Blackberry/index.htm	Windows, Windows Mobile, Palm, Blackberry, mobile phone, Mac	One-time fee	Records food intake (database has over 1,000 foods), tracks weight and graphs results, allows addition of new foods
www.nutrihand.com (basic)	Internet	Free basic service	Tracks meals and medical information; user can upload data from a glucometer, choose from several meal plans, create shopping lists, view and print several reports
www.nutrihand.com (premium)	Internet	Monthly cost	Offers all basic services plus thousands of meal plans that can be customized; creates fitness plans
www.nutrihand.com (professional)	Internet	Yearly cost	Allows nutrition professionals to create personalized plans and analyze client meals, fitness, and medical data; contains thousands of plan templates with nine caloric levels, nine health conditions, and six cuisines

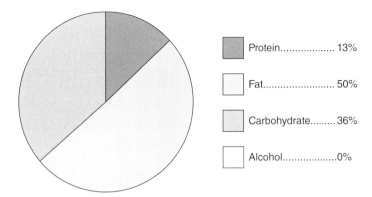

FIGURE 11.3   Professional nutrition analysis software programs often produce a variety of graphs that help sport nutrition professionals communicate the results to their clients. This pie chart shows the macronutrient breakdown of an athlete's diet. In this example, the athlete can clearly see that half of the caloric intake is coming from dietary fat. After making recommended changes to the athlete's diet, the sport nutrition professional can follow up and collect a three-day diet record again and then produce another, similar pie chart to show how the changes in the athlete's diet helped achieve a more balanced approach that better fuels performance.

for the nutrition professional or researcher who needs in-depth analysis of a client's or subject's intake.

- **FoodWorks** is a Windows-based software program designed for professionals working in nutrition research, nutrient database development, dietetics, client counseling, fitness and weight control, food service, recipe development, health care, and nutrition education. FoodWorks can analyze meals, recipes, and menu cycles and lets the user choose from four dietary standards: Dietary Reference Intakes (DRIs), dietary values, Canadian RNI, and Food and Agriculture Organization of the United Nations/World Health Organization. FoodWorks also lets clients create diet recalls and submit them to their nutrition professional for analysis. The program offers many different printouts. For more information, see www.nutritionco .com/FoodWorks.htm.

- **Nutriinfo.com** offers a Web-based weight management program that can be accessed from any computer. Clients enter information about their food intake, exercise, blood sugar levels, and other information on their account; and the health professional can view the client's input and dietary analysis on an administration page. For more information, see http:// nutriinfo.com/index.html.

- **Dine Healthy 7** (Dine Systems Inc.) is an exercise and dietary analysis software program. The food database contains generic, fast food, and brand-name items. The diet analysis includes 122 nutrients and food components, such as trans fats, cholesterol, and polyunsaturated fats, and compares food choices to Dietary Approaches to Stop Hypertension (DASH), renal recommendations, or specific recommendations set up by the nutrition professional. The exercise analysis includes over 500 sports and leisure and recreational activities and calculates calories burned for specific periods of time spent on these activities. This program also helps with planning meals and diets and analyzing recipes, as well as providing recommendations on healthy eating and exercise. Additionally, it offers "Food Explorer," which allows the user to compare multiple foods side by side. The research behind Dine Healthy was funded by the National Heart, Lung, and Blood Institute; the National Cancer Institute; and the National Institute of Digestive Disorders and Kidney Disease.

- **ESHA Food Processor Standard and SQL** analyze food intake with a food database of over 35,000 foods and provide a variety of graphs and reports. Both programs also have recipe planning features, exercise tracking, and customized recommendations. SQL differs from the Standard version in that it contains allergen identifiers, over 400 exercises, information on both the glycemic load and glycemic index, multiday diet recall, Hazard Analysis & Critical Control Points (HACCP) guidelines, and Canadian Food Guide values. Logos and letterhead can be added to reports to customize these as coming from a specific business. Food Processor also contains **FoodProdigy**, an online companion that allows clients to document their diet intakes and activities from their personal computer. The nutrition professional can then enter a key code that provides access to a client's dietary intake.

- **Pure Wellness** can be incorporated into a company's Intranet or Internet site with passwords for employee use. This program allows people to post food logs, as well as produce progress reports, health assessments, and more, directly on the company's Web site. For more information, see www.purewellness.com.

- **NutriBase** has an extensive food database that includes some brand-name foods and restaurant items as well. NutriBase also includes over 600 recipes for a variety of special needs (e.g., vegetarian, diabetic, heart healthy, hypertension, bodybuilding), meal plans at varying calorie levels, therapeutic meal plans, and a free CD-based program clients can use to track their dietary intake and then send via Internet to their nutrition professional for analysis. NutriBase also lets users create meal plans by building meals (from a combination of food items and recipes) and then mixing these meals to build meal plans. Meals, recipes, and meal plans are exportable to other NutriBase users. NutriBase has a variety of report options that can be customized to include only specific nutrients, comments, recommendations, the nutritionist's name or byline, and more. Palm PDA users can record their food and exercise intake directly on their handheld device and sync this to their PC and into NutriBase. For more information, see www.nutribase.com.

- **Nutritionist Pro** has a database of over 32,000 foods and ingredients, including brand-name foods, fast foods, ethnic foods, and clinical nutrition products. Clients can also enter their own foods into the database. Diet analysis can evaluate dietary intake or food frequencies against specific nutrient requirements. Nutritionist Pro also contains over 750 recipes and a recipe analysis feature. For more information, see www.nutritionistpro.com.

Keeping a food log or diary can help enhance weight loss efforts in overweight and obese individuals. In one four-center randomized trial with 1,685 total participants, keeping a daily food record led to twice as much weight loss as not keeping a record (Hollis et al. 2008). Aside from making individuals accountable for their food intake, food diaries entered into a diet analysis program and reviewed by a nutrition professional can provide in-depth insight into micronutrient intake, which is essential for troubleshooting nutrition-related problems such as anemia and hyponatremia. In addition, a **diet analysis** can help pinpoint areas where an athlete may need to alter intake for health reasons.

➤ diet analysis—A comparison of one's typical dietary intake to research-based recommendations based on one's sport and training level as well as the DRIs.

Nutrient analysis programs provide a picture of one's overall nutrition intake—information that can be examined in relation to health and athletic performance. Analyzing an athlete's diet for a few days every month while tracking her weight and body composition changes can help the professional determine what dietary changes are needed to achieve the desired body composition. As a part of this process, working with the athlete to set goals for the nutrition program can be effective. Form 11.2 on page 222 can help athletes identify and track progress on their nutrition goals. Because food fuels athletic performance and an athlete's lean body mass and fat mass affect speed, power, and agility, dietary assessment programs and body composition analysis tools are both very useful components in an athlete's training program.

Before making specific, individualized sport nutrition recommendations to any athlete, it is imperative that the sport nutrition professional gather as much information as possible. Weight, weight history, dieting history (including disordered eating or eating disorders), body composition, dietary intake, supplement intake, lab values, and a bone density assessment all provide very useful information for creating a sport nutrition plan. The following are two examples, using hypothetical athletes, of how a sport nutrition professional would use assessment techniques and an understanding of the athlete's unique situation to develop an effective nutrition plan.

Professional Applications

Anthony

A junior transfer football player, Anthony, was sent to the sport nutritionist for help with losing weight. Anthony's body composition, as tested by skinfold calipers, was high for a linebacker at 24% (his body fat should be about 15%, according to averages for his position). He was asked to keep a three-day diet record (including one weekend day) and come back to the nutritionist a week later. After these dietary records were run through a computerized diet analysis program, it was very clear what Anthony's problem areas were. He consumed 40% of his calories from fat, ate too much fried food, drank quarts of juice every day, and averaged 12 beers on each weekend night. In addition, a plot of his weight history made it evident that his dietary habits had changed in college. Anthony's weight through high school had remained around 220 pounds but had increased steadily in the past two years to his current weight of 245 pounds. He said that his mother had cooked all of his meals during high school and that everything was planned out back then, whereas now he felt his days were haphazard; he grabbed food here and there and didn't always make the best choices. In addition, Anthony was overwhelmed by the number of food choices on campus—he had the option to eat basically anything, anytime he wanted.

In addition to gaining weight, Anthony mentioned that he felt tired all of the time and sometimes reached for an energy drink in the middle of the day for the caffeine + sugar pickup. He knew he shouldn't do this but was at a loss about how to change his lifestyle and diet so he could feel better. Anthony often stayed up late, until 1 or 2 a.m., yet had a 7 a.m. class three days a week. Operating on little sleep, he would go to class and then come home and sleep for hours, wake up and consume an energy drink, and go to practice. After practice, he showered, and twice a week had night class after which he ate dinner at about 9 p.m. On the weekends, his sleep and eating schedule was even more erratic. The night before games he tried to go to bed at 11 p.m. but couldn't fall asleep. On nongame nights he might stay up until 3 or 4 a.m. partying.

The sport nutritionist worked with Anthony to help him see where his lifestyle habits were contributing to poor eating choices. In addition, she covered the effect of alcohol on delaying recovery and potentially hampering his gains in the weight room as well as his 600+ calorie per day juice intake. Anthony agreed to a few simple changes in his schedule, lifestyle, and eating habits, including going to bed by midnight on weeknights, scheduling classes no earlier than 9 a.m. next semester, and sleeping at least 8 hours per night. In addition, Anthony agreed to substitute a low-calorie beverage for the juice, cut his beer intake in half and consume that on only one night per weekend, limit his fried food to one time per week, cut out energy drinks, and work with the strength coach to increase his morning cardio sessions. Although he felt tired at first and had headaches for a few days after cutting out the energy drinks, Anthony continued to work hard to drop the extra body fat he had gained during college. His hard work and dedication paid off, as his playing time increased.

Samantha

A freshman gymnast named Samantha went to see the sport nutritionist at her university because she was concerned about trying to maintain a low weight to compete on a national level. In addition, she had recently experienced a stress fracture in her foot. Measurement of the gymnast's body composition by DEXA revealed that her body fat was 10% and her bone density was slightly below the average for her age. The sport nutritionist quickly realized that at 10% body fat, Samantha may have menstrual cycle irregularities; but she waited to see Samantha's food recall before making any assumptions. This athlete was very fearful of gaining any weight because her coach maintained strict weight and body fat percent guidelines for each athlete on the team. A 24-hour recall revealed that Samantha was eating the same things every single day:

Breakfast – ½ cup oatmeal

Snack – flavored coffee

Lunch – salad

Snack – fat-free frozen yogurt

Dinner – salad with grilled chicken and diet soda

The sport nutritionist saw several weak points in Samantha's diet. Her caloric intake was way too low (less than 1,000 calories/day); she lacked most if not all vitamins and minerals (on a low-calorie diet the likelihood of missing vitamins and minerals is even greater); and she fell very short on calcium, vitamin D, and magnesium—which are all necessary for building bone density and which all play a role in muscle functioning as well. Samantha's diet was also short on protein, carbohydrate, and quality fat. At this point, the sport nutritionist was certain that Samantha was probably amenorrheic or oligomenorrheic.

After talking with Samantha and getting an idea of her weight history, the sport nutritionist found out that this young woman had weighed 15 pounds more in high school, had felt more energetic, and had been doing better at her sport. In addition, when she lost the first 10 pounds, she stopped her menstrual cycle—putting her at risk for bone loss.

Samantha knew that she could be doing long-term damage to her body but was afraid of losing her scholarship. She said that when she came to school, she had been bigger than all of the other gymnasts and that all of them ate very little food and had little body fat. Samantha was concerned that her coach would be unhappy if she gained any weight. She didn't think she had an eating disorder per se but couldn't see how she could get out of her current eating behavior. The sport nutritionist asked Samantha if she would be willing to see a licensed clinical professional counselor in the community, explaining that the counselor regularly worked with clients who had a fear of gaining weight and faced challenges with body image and eating. The sport nutritionist reassured Samantha that she wouldn't tell her coach and that several athletes had worked with the counselor on the very same issues. Over the next year, Samantha worked hard at changing her body image and slowly adding calories and nutrients to her diet. Though her issues didn't resolve immediately, she continued to work with the dietitian and counselor and was moving in a positive direction.

SUMMARY POINTS

- Before working with an athlete to develop an individual nutrition plan, it is essential that the sport nutrition professional assess (at a minimum) the athlete's current body composition, weight history, diet history, and current diet.

- A variety of available body composition assessment tools differ in the particular body components measured, including fat, fat-free mass, bone mineral content, total body water, extracellular water, total adipose tissue and its subdepots (visceral, subcutaneous, and intramuscular), skeletal muscle, select organs, and ectopic fat depots.

- The most common field measure used to assess body composition in athletes is skinfold calipers. Once a person is trained, skinfold calipers are easy to use; the method is also quick, noninvasive, and inexpensive.

- Body mass index should not be used as a tool for assessing body composition in athletes; BMI does not assess actual body composition or distinguish between fat and muscle tissue.

- Laboratory measures for assessing body composition are typically more accurate than field measures, but they are also more costly and time-consuming and therefore used in the lab versus in a field setting. Typical lab measures include Bod Pod, DEXA, and underwater weighing.

- By comparing an athlete's diet analysis (as computed from a nutrition software program) with lab work and bone density scans, the sport nutrition professional can assess whether or not a physician should be involved to prescribe a specific nutrient that the athlete is deficient in (vitamin D or iron, for instance) or whether the sport nutrition professional can help the athlete make up for missing nutrients through dietary intake or dietary supplements.

Three-Day Diet Recall

Instructions: Please be as specific as possible when filling this out. For example, write down condiments and amounts of foods versus just a general description. Do not change what you are currently doing because you are keeping a record.

The goal of a three-day recall is to get a good look at what you are currently eating as a starting point for making dietary improvements.

Nondescript example: Cheeseburger and soda

Better example: McDonald's regular-size cheeseburger with lettuce and tomato slices. One packet mayonnaise. 12 ounces Dr. Pepper.

DAY 1

Date: _____

Meal or snack and time	Food (how prepared, etc.)

FORM 11.1   Three-day diet recall.   *(continued)*

From National Strength and Conditioning Association, 2011, *NSCA's Guide to Sport and Exercise Nutrition,* B.I. Campbell and M.A. Spano (eds.), (Champaign, IL: Human Kinetics).

Form 11.1 *(continued)*

DAY 2

Date: _____

Meal or snack	Food (how prepared, etc.)

From National Strength and Conditioning Association, 2011, *NSCA's Guide to Sport and Exercise Nutrition,* B.I. Campbell and M.A. Spano (eds.), (Champaign, IL: Human Kinetics).

DAY 3

Date:_____

Meal or snack	Food (how prepared, etc.)

Setting Goals

Instructions: As you are filling out this form, think about why you want to make a change and what motivates you.

1. My goals are:

   a.

      Date I'd like to achieve this by:

      Action plan (my plan to reach my goal; this part to be filled out during nutrition consultation):

   b.

      Date I'd like to achieve this by:

      Action plan (my plan to reach my goal; this part to be filled out during nutrition consultation):

   c.

      Date I'd like to achieve this by:

      Action plan (my plan to reach my goal; this part to be filled out during nutrition consultation):

2. What is motivating me to make changes to my diet?

3. How will these changes affect my performance and recovery?

4. How will I track my progress? (This part to be filled out during nutrition consultation.)

FORM 11.2 Goal setting sheet for a nutrition plan.

From National Strength and Conditioning Association, 2011, *NSCA's Guide to Sport and Exercise Nutrition,* B.I. Campbell and M.A. Spano (eds.), (Champaign, IL: Human Kinetics).

12

Consultation and Development of Athlete Plans

Amanda Carlson Phillips, MS, RD, CSSD

The science of sport nutrition has uncovered nutrition and supplement strategies that improve aerobic endurance, speed, strength, focus, and concentration; reduce fatigue; and enhance recovery. However, this body of scientific research is futile if athletes do not change their behavior. Therefore, it is important to create a feasible plan that athletes can easily incorporate into their lifestyle so that sound nutrition changes are made.

Those working with athletes can use a performance nutrition continuum model (figure 12.1) to build programs using an integrated approach. The concepts behind this approach are *assess, educate,* and *implement.* Across each concept is the need to evaluate, isolate, innovate, and then integrate across all levels of the athlete's training.

Providing nutrition advice and orchestrating a sport nutrition program are different. A sport nutrition program has many layers that need to work together. The surface layers encompass education and general guidance, and the center includes specific recommendations that are backed by science and integrated into the athlete's daily routine.

The goal of any nutrition program is to provide athletes with knowledge so that good nutrition practices become second nature, as well as to give them the tools to implement this knowledge. A good plan makes nutrition easy and incorporates foods to choose on days off as well as before, during, and after practices and then around games, matches, or races. Nutrition should become a component of the athlete's training program.

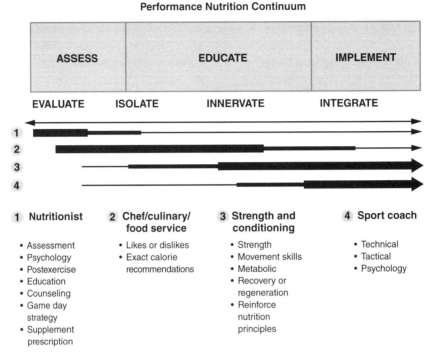

FIGURE 12.1   Many professionals may be involved in implementing a sport nutrition program across all stages of the performance nutrition continuum. The nutritionist, food service staff, strength and conditioning professional, and sport coach are all involved to a greater or lesser degree with each stage of the program. The thickness of the arrows in this figure shows the degree of involvement of each professional.

Providing Nutrition Knowledge

Many fitness professionals (certified personal trainers, conditioning coaches or professionals, athletic trainers, and strength coaches) are very knowledgeable about athletes' physiology, the demands of a sport, and the role of nutrition in performance; however, most are not qualified or legally allowed to deliver detailed nutrition information. Those who are qualified as **registered dietitians** can deliver nutrition information. Given that there are many specializations a dietitian can focus on, it is important that the dietitian has a background in sport nutrition.

➤ registered dietitian (RD)—A food and nutrition expert in the United States who has completed a four-year college degree program in nutrition in addition to an accredited dietetic internship providing at least 900 hours of supervised nutrition practice. After completing both of these, the candidate must pass an exam given by the Commission on Dietetic Registration in order to become a RD (American Dietetic Association n.d.).

Many certifications and certifying bodies (e.g., American College of Sports Medicine, NSCA, National Athletic Training Association) require that fitness professionals demonstrate a certain level of knowledge of basic nutrition before achieving certification status. This knowledge should equip them with the skills necessary to provide general nutrition recommendations and suggestions to athletes. However, athletes should be referred to a registered dietitian when medical nutrition therapy (for a disease state or eating disorder) is required or when the level of nutrition recommendations moves beyond general guidelines and into personalized recommendations. The sidebar lists several common nutrition certifications available in the United States and internationally.

Sport Nutrition Certifications

Board Certified Specialist in Sports Dietetics (CSSD)

The American Dietetic Association (ADA) has taken steps to help distinguish qualified dietitians most knowledgeable in the area of sport nutrition by creating a specialty certification, CSSD. The CSSD is offered by the Commission on Dietetic Registration (CDR) for registered dietitians who have specialized experience in sport dietetics. Being board certified as a Specialist in Sports Dietetics designates specific knowledge, skills, and expertise for competency in sport dietetics practice. CSSDs apply sport nutrition science to fueling fitness, sport, and athletic performance. Specialty certification differentiates sport dietitians from dietitians who are less qualified to provide sport nutrition services. Credibility, visibility, and marketability of sport dietitians are enhanced by specialty certification. Dietitians must meet strict eligibility requirements in order to sit for the CSSD exam. Minimum requirements for specialty certification are established and approved by the CDR. In order to be eligible to become a Board Certified Specialist in Sports Dietetics, candidates must meet the requirements specified by the CDR (www.cdrnet.org/certifications/spec/sports.htm).

Certified Sports Nutritionist From the ISSN (CISSN)

The International Society of Sports Nutrition (ISSN) offers the CISSN exam, incorporating core competencies in basic exercise physiology, integrated physiology, bioenergetics, nutrition, and sport psychology. The CISSN exam is not restricted to registered dietitians (Antonio et al. 2005). In order to sit for the CISSN exam and obtain this certification, people must meet the requirements laid out on the ISSN Web site: www.theissn.org.

(continued)

(continued)

International Sports Sciences Association Sports Nutrition Certification

The sport nutrition certification from the International Sports Sciences Association (ISSA) emphasizes the importance of recommending a sound diet and nutrition regimen while teaching sport nutrition concepts. For more information, see ISSA's Web site: www.issaonline.com.

ACE Lifestyle & Weight Management Consultant Certification

This certification is offered through the American Council of Exercise. The ACE Lifestyle & Weight Management Consultant Certification provides knowledge to develop sound, balanced weight management programs that bring together the three critical components of long-term weight management success: nutrition, exercise, and lifestyle change. The organization's Web site gives information on the eligibility criteria needed to sit for this exam: www.acefitness.org/getcertified/certification_lwmc.aspx.

It is important to remember that sport nutrition certifications do not override state or federal guidelines regarding nutrition practice.

The reason for this blurred scope of practice is that sport nutrition is a unique multidisciplinary field requiring many professionals to work together. Athletic trainers, strength and conditioning coaches, coaches, athletic directors, and food service providers all must come together in order to provide the most effective service, information, and guidance to the athlete (Santana et al. 2007). At the same time, professionals should be aware of the appropriate scope of practice for their credentials and of national or state laws that limit the types of assessment and counseling they can do (American Dietetic Association n.d.). The sidebar describes one example of this type of law.

Maintaining Confidentiality

When working with an athlete, the sport nutritionist is gathering, assessing, and analyzing personal health information. The confidentiality of medical information is protected by law in many countries, and professionals need to be aware of the applicable laws and handle medical information in a way that complies with those laws. In the United States, the **Health Insurance Portability and Accountability Act (HIPAA)** was created to provide a national standard for handling medical information. The key to the privacy act is to ensure that a person's protected health information is not inap-

Nutrition Legality: The Louisiana Example

Like many states in the United States, Louisiana has clear definitions regarding the scope of nutrition practice. Only a licensed dietitian or nutritionist can perform nutrition assessment and counseling. However, other disciplines can provide nutrition education as long as the information is general and accurate and is offered to a person or group without individualization; for example, the educator cannot answer questions specific to a client's or participant's diet or nutrition status.

Nutrition assessment is "the evaluation of the nutritional needs of individuals and groups based on appropriate biochemical, anthropometric, physical and dietary data to determine nutrient needs and to recommend to the primary health care provider appropriate nutritional intake including enteral and parenteral nutrition regardless of setting, including but not limited to ambulatory settings, hospitals, nursing homes, and other extended care facilities" (Louisiana Board of Dietetics 2009).

Nutrition counseling is "the provision of the individual guidance on appropriate food and nutrient intake for those with special needs, taking into consideration health, cultural, socioeconomic, functional, and psychological facts from the nutrition assessment." Nutrition counseling may include advice to increase or decrease nutrients in the diet; to change the timing and size of and composition of meals; to modify food textures, and in extreme instances to change the route of administration." Nutrition education "imparts information about food and nutrients, dietary lifestyle factors, community nutrition resources, and services to people to improve their knowledge" (Louisiana Board of Dietetics 2009).

It is critical that athletic staff know the laws of the state they are working in to determine the legality of their own scope of practice. If a member of the athletic staff is not a registered dietitian and is asked for specific nutrition information and advice, it is important for her to find a registered dietitian well versed in sport nutrition that she can trust and collaborate with. It is also important to check the credentials and qualifications of staff who are providing nutrition recommendations. These licensure laws exist to ensure that people are receiving specific nutrition information from qualified professionals.

propriately distributed to others. The act broadly defines protected health information as individually identifiable information maintained or transmitted by a covered entity in any form or medium (Michael and Pritchett 2002). The current law includes modifications that have been made since it was first passed:

1. Doctors, hospitals, and health care providers are allowed to share patient information with family members or others involved in the individual's care without patient permission.

2. Health care providers must distribute a notice of their privacy practices to individuals no later than the date the service is provided. A health care provider with a direct treatment relationship must make a good faith effort to obtain the individual's written acknowledgment of receipt of the notice. The requirement allows patients to request any additional restrictions on uses and disclosures of their health information or confidential communications. Health care providers may design an acknowledgment of the process best suited to their practices.

3. Patients must grant permission for each nonroutine circumstance in which the patient's personal health information is used or disclosed.

4. Covered entities must obtain authorization to use or disclose protected health information for marketing purposes.

5. Covered entities may use and disclose protected health information in the form of a limited dataset for research, public health, and health care operations. A limited dataset does not contain any direct identifiers of individuals but may contain other demographic or health information needed for research.

Practitioners can review additional information at the U.S. Department of Health and Human Services Web site: www.hhs.gov/ocr/hipaa.

> ➤ Health Insurance Portability and Accountability Act (HIPAA)—Legislation that provides a national standard in the United States for handling medical information.

At times, an athlete's nutrition information is used in a collaborative effort with other members of the athlete's performance team. Sharing this information would fall under point 1 of the HIPAA modifications. However, in other cases the sport nutritionist may be working with an athlete apart from the athlete's inner circle of coaches and strength and conditioning specialists. At these times, HIPAA points 2 and 3 come into play. The sport nutritionist should let the athlete know what he plans to do with the athlete's personal health information and receive permission from the athlete to communicate this information to other staff members when necessary. It is always best to err on the side of caution with the athlete's private information by getting a signed document. The disclosing of a current weight or body fat percent to a coach, strength coach, or agent could result in a fine, a breach of contract by the athlete, or a negative perception about the athlete's lack of progress that may lead to untoward decisions about the athlete's playing time. Always disclose to the athlete what needs to be shared and why, and then get a signed document stating that the athlete acknowledges the disclosure of that information.

Developing the Athlete's Nutrition Plan

The athlete's nutrition plan (figure 12.2) should include specific plans for both training days and game, competition, or race days. It is critical to incorporate plans for nutrition, hydration, and recovery that the athlete can follow on a day-to-day basis. It is also important to design a protocol of pre-, during-, and postworkout nutrition to ensure adequate and timely protein and carbohydrate intake to enhance recovery from the training sessions. The third phase of program development is game or race day strategy. The game day strategy should focus on what is needed to fuel and hydrate the body and recover from the stress of competition. As the nutrition plan development begins, the sport nutritionist should take into consideration the athlete's desire to improve fueling for performance but also look at the athlete holistically. The best nutrition programs go beyond grams of carbohydrate, protein, and fat. The relationship that has been developed between the athlete and coaching staff sets the athlete up for successful nutrition improvement. Even with the help of a coach, nutritionist, trainer, and others, athletes may find themselves facing the same pitfalls as non-athletes: poor planning and poor implementation.

An athlete may want basic advice or a specific nutrition plan. A more specific nutrition plan that fits into an athlete's lifestyle (e.g., relying on fast food, cooking, cultural food preferences) and meets the athlete's needs is more beneficial than basic advice. However, the athlete must be ready

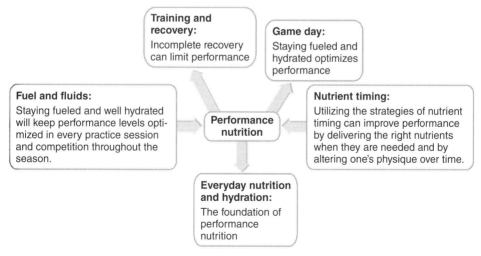

FIGURE 12.2   An athlete's nutrition plan should have good everyday nutrition as its base and include nutrition plans for training and recovery as well as competition.

to receive and implement such a plan. A sport nutritionist can utilize the **stages of change model** to determine how ready an athlete is for making changes and whether or not to provide a detailed plan. From a nutrition standpoint, the ADA's nutrition care process is a good model to follow in working with an individual or team. The ADA adopted the nutrition care process and model in 2003 in hopes of implementing a standardized process for providing high-quality care to patients. This same model is applicable to the development of a nutrition plan for athletes. These are the phases of the nutrition care process (Lacey and Pritchett 2003):

1. Nutrition assessment
2. Nutrition evaluation
3. Nutrition intervention and education
4. Nutrition monitoring and evaluation

> ➤ stages of change model—An approach to assessing a client's readiness to change. The stages are precontemplation, contemplation, preparation, action, maintenance, and relapse.

Step 1: Assessment

Athlete assessment is the first step in creating an effective plan. This is the time to get to know the athlete and understand his situation and his objective data. You can sit down with the athlete one-on-one or develop a questionnaire for the athlete to fill out by hand or electronically. You should gather the following information:

1. Anthropometric data: These include measured height, weight, body fat, and circumference.

2. Biochemical data: Lab values can provide more detailed data; however, it is important to note the physiological state of the athlete when the blood is drawn. Both dehydration and intense training can cause changes in blood volume that can skew the interpretation of blood work. In addition, food and beverage intake can alter certain blood tests (cholesterol, triglycerides, etc.).

3. Sport, position, and point in season or phase of training: Prescribing correct nutrient and hydration recommendations will depend on the specific sport, position within the sport, and point in the athlete's season. Different positions within the same sport can have vastly different nutrient needs. The soccer goalie has dramatically different nutrient needs than a forward on the same team. Long-distance runners have extremely different needs during the maximum-mileage weeks in comparison to the point in their training when they are in a building phase. The concept of altering athletes' food intake to correlate with where they are in their seasons is referred to as nutrition periodization, a term that corresponds with the concept of training periodization. A football player in the beginning of the off-season will have decreased caloric needs as compared to those during the preseason with two-a-day practices. It is critical to individualize the athlete's recommendations beyond just the sport.

4. **Nutrition knowledge:** A basic assessment of the athlete's foundational nutrition knowledge will provide a good idea about where to start with education and what concepts to focus on. Knowledge will empower the athlete and give her a greater understanding of nutrition recommendations.

5. **Stage of change:** The transtheoretical model (Prochaska, Norcross, and DiClemente 1994) is useful for determining a nutrition counseling strategy (Dandoval, Heller, and Wiese 1994). The goal is to help athletes get from stage to stage and help them permanently adopt a new positive behavior or extinguish a behavior that does not enhance performance. Moving too quickly through the stages or developing plans for athletes who are not ready will lead to noncompliance.

6. **Current dietary habits and intake:** A 24-hour or three-day diet recall will provide a snapshot of the athlete's current diet. In addition, questions about food habits should be asked. Questions that will elicit information about the athlete's nutrition habits include the following: How often do you grocery shop? How often do you eat out? How much water do you drink per day? How many meals do you eat per day? What do you typically snack on? How many days per week do you eat breakfast? What dietary supplements do you use, in what doses, and when do you take them? How consistent are you with these dietary supplements? Do you take anything (food or supplement) pre-, during-, or postexercise?

7. **Allergies, dislikes, intolerances, cultural or religious considerations.**

8. **Medications.** It is critical to check for drug–nutrient interactions so that the practitioner can determine if the prescription or over-the-counter drugs interact with nutrients in food or supplements. For instance, an athlete who is taking blood thinners to prevent clots post-surgery needs to watch vitamin K intake through food and supplements and also be aware of any supplements that may increase bleeding time.

9. **Injuries.** Acute injuries may affect training and activity load, but overtraining injuries may be a sign of poor nutrition intake.

10. **Goals and time line.** Understanding the athlete's goals and time line will help shape the strategy for education and coaching. A National Football League draftee may be working on a tight time line to prepare for the draft; an elite figure skater may be looking for a plan to peak for a competition that is nine months away.

Step 2: Evaluation

This step involves the analysis of the assessment.

1. Determine the athlete's calorie needs. A way to do this is to measure the athlete's resting metabolic rate or use an energy expenditure equation and then account for activity. If the athlete is looking to gain or lose weight, add or subtract 500 to 1,000 calories per day from the basal metabolic rate (BMR) + activity total. This should produce a 1- to 2-pound (about 2-4 kg) weight loss or gain per week. Degree of weight loss or gain will depend on the athlete's genetic makeup, daily caloric deficit, number of rest and recovery days per week, and the type of training phase she is in (American College of Sports Medicine [ACSM], American Dietetic Association, and Dietitians of Canada 2000).

2. Address the athlete's goals or issues (e.g., cramping, weight management, fatigue, soreness). When identifying something to work on with the athlete, be sure to state the issue consistently: (a) problem, (b) **etiology**, (c) signs and symptoms (Rosenbloom 2005). For example: "Female tennis player has extreme fatigue and cramping toward the end of matches and practices, which is hindering performance. This is related to low daily energy intake that is not meeting nutrition needs, inadequate fluid intake during matches, and the lack of a carbohydrate/electrolyte drink while playing." Setting up the issues in this way will provide a clear path to additional recommendations beyond general needs for the athlete.

> ➤ etiology—The cause or causes of a disease.

3. Figure out the athlete's carbohydrate, protein, and fat needs depending on sport, position, and stage of training. It is important to create guidelines for everyday, specific recovery needs and also for game or event days. There are two ways to express these values: grams per kilogram body weight or percent of total calories. Utilizing grams per kilogram body weight gives the athlete a more exact recommendation and is advised; but critical thinking is key, and percentage of total calories is secondary to the athlete's total energy intake. For example, a 60-kg (132-pound) female aerobic endurance athlete at the high end of her training would fall into the 7 to 10 grams per kilogram range which would put her at 420 to 600 g carbohydrate ingestion per day. However, if her total caloric intake is 2,800 calories per day, this would be 60% to 85% of her total calories. While 60% makes sense, 85% of calories coming from carbohydrate is too much. That is why it is important to check macronutrient guidelines when you translate research-based recommendations into reality.

4. Determine the athlete's nutrient timing needs for training and for competition days. To do this, first look at the athlete's physique and training goals. Athletes who need to gain strength or size should incorporate a specific

strategy for pre- and postworkout nutrition and possibly during-workout nutrition (depending on the duration and intensity of their training). For example, an athlete who needs to gain strength and size during his training for the NFL combine needs to consume calories during his 4-hour intense training sessions in addition to his pre- and postworkout nutrition. After looking at physique and training goals, it is important to assess an athlete's performance and how he feels during training and performance and to consider this in conjunction with his current diet and supplement regimen. For instance, if a marathon runner tells you that his coach recently increased his mileage to 70 miles per week and he has felt "crummy" ever since the change, you will want to pay close attention to overall calorie intake, macronutrient distribution, and postexercise carbohydrate consumption (in addition to timing of his postexercise intake). Like all nutrition strategies, nutrient timing recommendations should be made on an individual basis and should be given to athletes within a context they can understand. You should not only tell athletes total grams of carbohydrates they need to consume after a 20-mile run but also help them translate this into quantities of the foods or sport nutrition products they typically consume.

The sidebars show general recommendations that can be adapted for individual athletes based on the results of the assessment process.

Daily Nutrient Recommendations

Carbohydrate: 5 to 7 g/kg per day for general training needs and 7 to 10 g/kg per day for increased needs due to aerobic endurance training or for strength and power athletes who perform multiple training sessions per day (Burke et al. 2001; ACSM 2000).

Protein: 1.2 to 2.0 g/kg per day depending on sport and intensity of training (ACSM 2000; Phillips 2006; Campbell et al. 2008).

Fat: The remainder of calories. The amount of fat should be at least 1 g/kg per day and no less than 15% of total calories (ACSM 2000).

Hydration: 2.7 L/day for women and 3.7 L/day for men (Institute of Medicine 2004). Determine an exact amount of fluid for the athlete to consume. Recommending a range of 0.5 to 1 ounces (15-30 ml) per pound of body weight per day (depending on activity throughout the day) gives greater direction for fluid intake.

The need for multivitamins, fish oil, or ergogenic aids must be determined from analysis of the individual's dietary intake, overall training program, and health. These recommendations should be made under the supervision of a dietitian or doctor and need to be in accordance with the athlete's rules on banned substances.

Nutrient Timing Recommendations for Training

Recovery Nutrition

Pretraining or practice: The optimal carbohydrate and protein content of a preexercise meal is dependent on a number of factors, including exercise duration and fitness level.

- General guidelines are 1 to 2 g carbohydrate per kilogram and 0.15 to 0.25 g protein per kilogram 3 to 4 hours before exertion (Kerksick et al. 2008).

- Preexercise ingestion of essential amino acids or whey protein with carbohydrate acutely increases muscle protein synthesis (Tipton 2001, 2007). Similarly, preexercise ingestion of small amounts of protein and carbohydrate has resulted in greater increases in strength and muscle hypertrophy compared to postexercise ingestion of the same nutrients (Esmarck et al. 2001; Kerksick et al. 2008).

- Relative to hydration, the recommendation is 17 to 20 ounces fluid (510-600 ml, water or sport drink) in the 2 hours before training and then an additional 10 ounces (300 ml) 10 to 20 minutes before training (Casa et al. 2000).

During training or practice: Fluid intake is critical during training and practice.

- It is important to make sure athletes understand that they need to drink enough fluid to prevent no more than a 2% decrease in body weight during their training (Casa et al. 2000).

- If exercise duration increases beyond 60 minutes, a sport drink containing carbohydrate and electrolytes is beneficial. This carbohydrate source should supply approximately 30 to 60 g of carbohydrate per hour and can typically be delivered by drinking 1 to 2 cups of a 6% to 8% carbohydrate solution (8 to 16 fluid ounces, 240-480 ml) every 10 to 20 minutes (Sawka et al. 2007; Jeukendrup, Jentjens, and Moseley 2005).

- Mixing different forms of carbohydrate has been shown to increase muscle carbohydrate oxidation, from 1.0 g carbohydrate per minute to levels ranging from 1.2 g to 1.75 g per minute—an effect associated with an improvement in time-trial performance. Therefore, glucose, fructose, sucrose, and maltodextrin can be used in combination, but large amounts of fructose are not recommended due to the greater likelihood of gastrointestinal problems (Kerksick et al. 2008).

- The addition of protein to the during-workout beverage is debated in the literature, but it has been shown that carbohydrate added to protein at a ratio of 3:1 or 4:1 (carbohydrate:protein) increases aerobic endurance performance during both acute exercise and subsequent bouts of aerobic endurance exercise (Kerksick et al. 2008).

- Carbohydrate alone, or in combination with protein, during resistance exercise increases muscle glycogen stores, offsets muscle damage, and facilitates greater training adaptations after acute and prolonged periods of resistance training (Kerksick et al. 2008).

- A beverage that tastes good to the athlete is essential for maintaining hydration.

After training or practice: This is a critical period. Many athletes do not eat anything in the postworkout period. Simply adding a meal, chocolate milk, or a snack facilitates the recovery process. Making specific recommendations will give athletes exact guidelines to follow, providing a more customized solution. The postworkout nutrition beverage or food should consist of both carbohydrate and protein (Kerksick et al. 2008). Athletes often tolerate liquid better than solid food because they may experience appetite suppression with intense exercise.

- Use a repletion factor of 1.2 to 1.5 g/kg body weight depending on the amount of glycogen depletion and the intensity of exercise (Kerksick et al. 2008; ACSM 2000).

- Ratio should be 2:1 to 4:1 of carbohydrate to protein.

- Protein: 0.3 to 0.4 g/kg.

- Carbohydrate: 0.8 to 1.2 g/kg.

- Engineered supplements, like protein shakes and bars, are especially useful after a workout because they are convenient. However, less expensive alternatives like chocolate milk are also effective in helping with recovery (Karp et al. 2006).

- It is advisable for athletes to consume a combination of carbohydrate and protein within the first 30 minutes after the completion of training. They should eat again about 1 hour later. Give recommendations in exact grams of protein and carbohydrates, and provide an example (like 8 ounces [240 ml] of chocolate milk); but taking in some fuel is ultimately better than consuming nothing (Kerksick et al. 2008).

Recommendations for Competition Day Nutrition

If athletes have been following the daily and recovery recommendations, when the day of the event or game arrives they should be well prepared. The focus of nutrition on game or event day is to get the body fueled and hydrated without upsetting the stomach. Athletes should practice their game day nutrition plan so that they are familiar with it and know it is well tolerated and do nothing new on the day of the event. General recommendations are as follows:

The Training Table: Eating Around Competition

- Afternoon or evening competition: Largest meal should be 3 to 4 hours before event.
- Morning competition: Athletes should eat about 2 hours before competition.

Carbohydrate needs (Kerksick et al. 2008):

1 hour before = 0.5 g carbohydrate per kilogram body weight

2 hours before = 1 g carbohydrate per kilogram body weight

3 hours before = 1.5 g carbohydrate per kilogram body weight

4 hours before = 2 g carbohydrate per kilogram body weight

Other nutritional needs:

Protein needs = 0.15 to 0.25 g protein per kilogram (Kerksick et al. 2008).

Fat = Some healthy fat (monounsaturated or polyunsaturated oils) several hours precompetition.

Fluid = The National Athletic Trainers' Association's position paper recommends 17 to 20 fluid ounces (510-600 ml) of water or sport drink 2 to 3 hours before exercise and an additional 10 ounces (300 ml) 10 to 20 minutes before exercise (Casa et al. 2000).

If athletes have problems tolerating food before events, sport drinks and gels may be better options.

Keys to Success in the Pregame Scenario

- Plan ahead.
- Don't experiment on the day of the event.
- Know the restaurants in the area.
- Pack a cooler full of snacks and beverages.

Step 3: Intervention and Education

One might assume that athletes, especially highly trained athletes, have a vast knowledge of their own physiology and the nutrient demands of their sport and that coaches or others who work with them on a daily basis also have that knowledge. Often, this is not the case (Zawila, Steib, and Hoogenboom 2003). When working with an athlete and developing her plan, start with the basics (general education) and then build into personalization and customization. Supplements are often the first thing athletes focus on because they are marketed as performance-enhancing aids (When is the last time you saw an ad for a product that helps an athlete recover?). However, athletes should focus first on their foundation nutrition and hydration, then add performance-based nutrition strategies, and finally take a look at how supplements might help them (figure 12.3). After all, nothing can help make up for years of eating a nutrient-poor diet. Just as athletes must develop foundational basics of their particular sport first, it is very difficult to fine-tune nutrition recommendations when the foundation knowledge is not present.

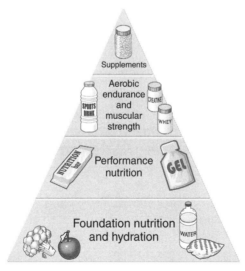

FIGURE 12.3   A pyramid diagram showing the essential parts of a sport nutrition program. Athletes should focus on basic nutrition and hydration; and supplements, if used, should be a small addition to an already solid plan.

A sport nutritionist creates and implements a strategy to improve the problems identified during the assessment. The intervention should have the following components:

1. Education.

2. Nutrition and hydration plan for all phases of training and competition cycle.

3. Specific recommendations in grams per kilogram versus percent of calories (Burke et al. 2001).

4. A plan to help alleviate the problem(s) identified during the diagnosis.

5. Discussion of supplement safety; many athletes are unaware that supplements may contain ingredients not identified on the label or that there may be an issue with the accuracy in labeling. It is important to check the respective governing body (National Collegiate Athletic Association, NFL, Major League Baseball, World Anti-Doping Agency, etc.) to become aware of banned substance lists. It is then important to find third-party testing organizations that the particular governing body supports. Finally, it is critical to remind athletes that the responsibility falls upon them and that if they take a supplement containing a banned substance, they will be held responsible and be reprimanded according to their governing body's specific rules. Useful Web sites for researching supplements include www.nsf.org, www.informed-choice.org, and www.informed-sport.com.

6. Set up realistic systems that will lead to success: exact formulas and products or foods for during- and postworkout and competition, coordination with food service to ensure that proper foods are selected or arranged for athletes or teams.

7. Set short-term and long-term goals.

8. Educate those who have personal relationships with the athlete (spouses, family members, others working with the athlete). All plans need to take into consideration any food intolerances, allergies, religious beliefs, cultural influences, strong likes and dislikes, ability to cook, access to food, restaurants commonly visited, and socioeconomic status as the plan is being developed.

9. Develop a "perfect day" for the athlete in simple terms. The perfect day example in table 12.1 is for a gymnast who needs to eat a more nutrient-rich diet. Sample days can be used to help athletes see patterns of eating, nutrient timing (when they should eat in proximity to training), and how they can incorporate good, healthy foods into their diet. The sport nutritionist should explain that this is an example; ideally athletes will vary the types of foods they consume within each general category. For instance, instead of eating a plum with raw almonds every day for a snack, the athlete should consider a variety of nuts and fruit so as to get a wide variety of nutrients and antioxidants into the diet.

TABLE 12.1   "Perfect Day" Nutrition Plan

Time	Meal
5 a.m.	Wake up
5:15 a.m.	Whole wheat toast with natural peanut butter, yogurt
6:00-7:15 a.m.	Workout
7:30 a.m.	Postworkout shake with carbohydrate and protein
9:30 a.m.	Oatmeal with berries and walnuts; egg whites scrambled with vegetables, low-fat cheese, and olive oil
12:30 p.m.	Turkey sandwich on whole wheat with large spinach salad and low-fat dressing
3:30 p.m.	Plum with raw almonds
6:30 p.m.	Grilled salmon, brown rice, steamed vegetables, large green salad with low-fat dressing
9:30 p.m.	Low-fat cottage cheese and 1/2 cup berries

Step 4: Nutrition Monitoring and Evaluation

An athlete who comes to see the nutritionist one time to get a plan and then never returns will not realize the same degree of success as one who is properly monitored. There are many ways to monitor athletes:

- Weight monitoring: Daily or weekly body weights are tracked depending on the needs and mind-set of the athlete. Some athletes respond well to daily body weight measurement whereas others become fixated on the number on the scale. This is up to the discretion of those working with the athlete (Dionne and Yeudall 2005).

- Body fat monitoring: Monthly body fat measures are a good way to track changes in lean body mass versus fat mass.

- Hydration monitoring: Weigh athletes before and after sessions to assess hydration practices.

- Habit monitoring

- Energy monitoring

- Intake monitoring

- Personal contact and relationship building: It is important for the sport nutritionist to set up communication with the athlete. Staying in touch with athletes is critical to their success. Formal appointments or checkups can be effective, though sometimes time-consuming. Use of technology can be extremely helpful. E-mail checkups are quick and easy, and a simple text message can be a great reminder to help keep the athlete on track. As much as possible, the sport nutritionist should attend the athlete's practice, games, training sessions, or strength and conditioning sessions.

The more the sport nutritionist is integrated into all parts of the athlete's life and sport, the greater impact she will have. It is also important for the sport nutritionist to set realistic time lines to help athletes achieve their goals. For example, a healthy weight gain or weight loss is typically no more than 2 pounds (about 4 kg) per week (ACSM 2000). Using simple tools to allow the athlete to check in with their habits can be extremely helpful. The performance nutrition assessment in form 12.1 is a very simple way to help athletes evaluate their own nutrition progress.

Members of the athlete's training team should be informed of the athlete's nutrition performance plan as necessary. Sharing this information helps to gain reinforcement or support for the athlete's progress from the coaching staff. In addition, this information, when shared appropriately, allows for a continued focus on the behavior change process.

Eating Disorders and Disordered Eating

Involvement in organized sport and general athletic activities offers many positive benefits, both physically and mentally; however, the pressure of athletic competition may compound an existing cultural emphasis on thinness. The result is an increased risk for athletes to develop disordered eating patterns and possibly an eating disorder (McArdle, Katch, and Katch 2005;

Performance Nutrition Assessment

Instructions: If the athlete thinks he or she is not doing well with a task, then mark a 1. If the athlete thinks he or she is doing great with a task, mark a 5.

Eating clean	1	2	3	4	5
Eating often	1	2	3	4	5
Keeping hydrated	1	2	3	4	5
Recovery	1	2	3	4	5
Mind-set	1	2	3	4	5

FORM 12.1   This performance nutrition assessment is a good tool to use at the beginning of a consultation and at consultations down the line. It helps athletes think about their diet and how they are doing and helps the sport nutritionist see what an athlete actually thinks of his diet in comparison to what he is really doing.

Sundgot-Borgen and Tortsveit 2004). A study evaluating Norwegian athletes showed that 13.5% of the athletes studied had subclinical or clinical eating disorders in comparison with 4.6% of the general population controls (Sundgot-Borgen and Tortsveit 2004).

Athletes in many sports face a paradox in that the behavior necessary to achieve a body weight for success in their sport (semi-starvation, purging, compulsive exercising) adversely affects health, fuel reserves, physiological and mental functioning, and the ability to train and compete at the level they desire. Reduced carbohydrate intake will affect the body's fuel stores, and a decrease in protein intake may lead to a decrease in lean tissue. An overall lack of micronutrients resulting from a low energy intake may make growth, repair, and recovery from exercise difficult and also put the athlete at an increased risk for injury (McArdle, Katch, and Katch 2005).

Eating disorders are traditionally associated with female sports, but disordered eating patterns and eating disorders do occur in male athletes as well, specifically those in sports with an aesthetic component or sports that require making weight or emphasize being small and lean. Men represent 6% to 10% of individuals with eating disorders (Baum 2006; McArdle, Katch, and Katch 2005; Glazer 2008). In male athletes, 22% of the eating disorders are in those participating in antigravitation sports such as diving, gymnastics, high jump, and pole vaulting; 9% in aerobic endurance sports; and 5% in ball game sports. In female athletes, 42% of eating disorders are in athletes competing in aesthetic sports, 24% in aerobic endurance sports, 17% in technical sports, and 16% in ball game sports (Sundgot-Borgen and Tortsveit 2004). An additional study on the prevalence of eating disorders among males found that 52% of 25 lower weight category collegiate wrestlers and 59 lightweight rowers reported bingeing; 8% of the rowers and 16% of the wrestlers showed pathologic eating disorder index profiles (Thiel 1993).

This particular study is consistent with the remainder of the literature, in which estimates of the prevalence of eating disorders range between 15% and 62% among female athletes; the greatest prevalence is among athletes in aesthetic sports such as ballet, bodybuilding, diving, figure skating, cheerleading, and gymnastics (McArdle, Katch, and Katch 2005).

Eating disorders are classified in the *Diagnostic and Statistical Manual of Mental Disorders (DSM-IV)* on the basis of the symptoms they present. An eating disorder can be classified as anorexia nervosa, bulimia nervosa, or eating disorder not otherwise specified; however, many of those with a diagnosis in one category demonstrate behaviors across the diagnosis continuum. Clinical eating disorders and disordered eating behaviors exist on a continuum, which makes it important to monitor disordered eating patterns for progression toward eating disorders.

There is a fine but solid line between eating disorders and disordered eating. An eating disorder is a serious mental illness that interferes with an athlete's normal daily activities; disordered eating represents a temporary or mild change in an athlete's eating behaviors. Disordered eating patterns can arise if an athlete is trying to make a weight goal, is under stress, or is intending to change her appearance or performance by making dietary changes. As long as these patterns are short-lived and do not persist, they do not necessarily need to be treated by a psychiatrist or psychologist (but such behaviors should be monitored). However, it is important to note the behavior because prolonged disordered eating patterns can lead to a diagnosed eating disorder (Becker et al. 2008; Dionne and Yeudall 2005).

For individuals with an eating disorder, the focus on food becomes so strong that the constant sense of stress and anxiety around eating requires professional intervention. Definitions and criteria for common eating disorders are shown in the sidebar. Eating disorders are often the result of an emotional issue or issues. Therefore, it is critical to make the appropriate referrals to a medical professional and registered dietitian when one is working with an athlete who has an eating disorder. It is also important to reach out to more qualified professionals in cases of an eating disorder and lend support to their proposed treatment plan (Becker et al. 2008; Dionne and Yeudall 2005).

The complexity, time intensiveness, and expense of managing eating disorders necessitate an interdisciplinary approach. This may include staff from the following disciplines: medicine, nutrition, mental health, athletic training, and athletics administration. An interdisciplinary approach may make it easier for symptomatic athletes to ask for help and may enhance their potential for full recovery. It is equally important to establish educational initiatives for preventing eating disorders.

Diagnostic Criteria for Eating Disorders

The following are modified definitions of eating disorders as specified in *DSM-IV* (American Psychiatric Association 1994).

Anorexia Nervosa

Restricting type: The athlete has not regularly engaged in binge eating or purging behavior.

Binge or purge type: The athlete has regularly engaged in binge eating or purging behavior.

- Refusal to maintain body weight at or above a minimally normal weight for height and age (less than 85% of what is expected)
- Intense fear of gaining weight or becoming fat, even though one is underweight
- Body image disturbances, including a distortion in the way one's body weight or shape is experienced, undue influence of body

weight or shape on self-evaluation, or denial of the consequences associated with the current low body weight

- In postmenarchal females, amenorrhea (absence of at least three consecutive cycles)

Bulimia Nervosa

Purging type: The athlete has regularly engaged in self-induced vomiting or the misuse of laxatives, diuretics, or enemas.

Nonpurging type: The athlete has used inappropriate compensatory behaviors such as fasting or excessive exercise but has not regularly engaged in self-induced vomiting or the misuse of laxatives, diuretics, or enemas.

- Recurrent episodes of binge eating: (1) Eating an amount of food in a discrete period of time (within any 2-hour period) that is significantly larger than what most people would eat in a similar period of time and set of circumstances; (2) a sense of a lack of control over eating during the episode

- Recurrent inappropriate compensatory behavior in order to prevent weight gain (i.e., self-induced vomiting; misuse of laxatives, diuretics, enemas, or other medications; fasting; and excessive exercise)

- Behaviors occurring on average at least two times per week for three months

- Self-evaluation excessively influenced by body shape and weight

- Occurrence of the behavior not exclusively during episodes of anorexia nervosa

Eating Disorder Not Otherwise Specified (EDNOS)

This diagnosis includes disorders of eating that do not meet criteria for any specific eating disorder. Disordered eating patterns are often seen in athletes of all sports as they try to make weight, improve performance, or go through phases of an extreme change in dietary intake and nutrition behavior. EDNOS can look similar to either anorexia or bulimia or may have the following signs:

- Repeatedly chewing and spitting out, but not swallowing, large amounts of food

- Recurrent episodes of binge eating in the absence of the inappropriate compensatory behaviors that are characteristic of bulimia nervosa (this is categorized as binge eating disorder) (American Psychiatric Association 1994)

Adapted from American Psychiatric Association Press. 1994. *Diagnostic and statistical manual of mental disorders*, 4th edition: DSM-IV. Washington, DC.

Female Athlete Triad

In 2007 the American College of Sports Medicine released an updated position stand on the female athlete triad (Nattiv et al. 2007). This term refers to the interrelationship among energy availability, menstrual function, and bone mineral density. Female athletes may be positioned all along a spectrum between health and disease, with those in the danger zone not exhibiting all of the clinical conditions at the same time. Low energy availability (with or without eating disorders), amenorrhea, and osteoporosis all pose significant health risks to physically active girls and women. Traditionally, body fat percent has been linked with the female athlete triad, whereas now, low energy availability (the amount of dietary energy remaining after training, metabolic processes, and activities of daily living are accounted for) seems to be the trigger. Some athletes reduce energy availability by increasing energy expenditure more than energy intake; others practice abnormal eating patterns using one or more of the inappropriate compensatory behaviors outlined earlier. Sustained low energy availability can impair both mental and physical health. All of the following are consequences of sustained low energy availability (Nattiv et al. 2007):

- Low self-esteem
- Depression
- Anxiety disorders
- Cardiovascular complications
- Endocrine complications
- Reproductive complications
- Skeletal complications
- Gastrointestinal complications
- Renal complications
- Central nervous complications

As the number of missed menstrual cycles accumulates secondary to sustained low energy intake, **bone mineral density (BMD)** declines; the loss of BMD may not be fully reversible, and the risk for stress fractures increases (Nattiv et al. 2007).

> ➤ bone mineral density (BMD)—The mineral content of bone; measured and used as a diagnostic criterion for osteopenia and osteoporosis.

It is important to be aware of disordered eating patterns and eating disorders among female athletes in order to prevent the downward spiral into the triad. The position stand (2007) makes several recommendations for screening and diagnosis of the triad:

1. Screening for the triad should occur at the preparticipation exam or the annual health screening exam. Athletes with one component of the triad should be assessed for the others.

2. Athletes with disordered eating should be referred to a mental health practitioner for evaluation, diagnosis, and recommendations for treatment.

3. To fully diagnose sustained low energy amenorrhea, other causes must be ruled out. A physical exam by a medical professional and the interpretation of laboratory results will help to rule out other causes of amenorrhea.

4. Finally, athletic administrators and the entire team of professionals working with female athletes should aim for triad prevention through education. Young female athletes often do not see that actions they are taking to enhance performance may cause future problems with bone density and fertility (Bonci et al. 2008; Michael and Pritchett 2002).

Professional Applications

Though the process of evaluation and athlete counseling is not likely to change dramatically in the upcoming years, the research on nutrition and supplementation for performance is always changing. In addition, the lists of banned substances change from year to year, as does the list of supplements certified as safe (through groups that test for banned substances). It is crucial that sport nutritionists stay current on all of this information so they can answer questions from athletes, coaches, and athletic training staff and be able to make specific, individualized recommendations to athletes. In the United States, many states require that the person providing medical nutrition therapy or individualized recommendations be a registered and licensed dietitian. However, those with sport nutrition certifications can provide general advice to athletes.

Sport nutrition is a field in a constant state of change; and it is vital that the sport nutritionist take a comprehensive look at an athlete's lifestyle, medical history, weight history, goals, injury report, lab work, body composition, and training program before helping the athlete develop a plan to achieve his goals. Along with a good base of knowledge of the latest sport science research and its application, it is crucial for the sport nutritionist to build a good rapport with each athlete, which will let the athlete know he can trust the sport nutritionist and therefore open up. Many clients may have a rational fear of opening up and talking about behavior they are ashamed of (such as binge eating or drinking, overeating, or disordered eating) and also fear that this personal information will be shared with others. Athletes must trust and be comfortable with sport nutritionists in order to talk about how they feel, exactly what they are eating and how much they are exercising, and what they think about their body. That trust may take some time to build and develops only through conversation.

This book includes many research findings that can be used to fine-tune a nutrition program but that also support some general recommendations that athletes need to be reminded of. The following are 10 general guidelines that will help athletes make wiser food choices:

1. Come back to earth. Choose the least processed forms of food most of the time.

2. Eat a rainbow often. Eat as many colorful fruits, vegetables, and whole grains as you can.

3. When it comes to protein, the less legs the better. Try to choose lean protein sources as often as possible.

4. Eat fats that give something back. Choose a variety of unsaturated fats and essential fatty acids in the diet.

5. Three for three. Eat mini meals consisting of carbohydrate, protein, and fat every 3 hours.

6. Eat breakfast every day. After you wake up, try to eat breakfast as soon as you can.

7. Hydrate. Be sure to meet your hydration needs.

8. Don't waste your workout. Consume a blend of carbohydrate and protein within 45 minutes of completing your training session or competition.

9. Supplement wisely. Check with your dietitian or doctor before starting a new supplement. Also, be aware of the rules and regulations of your sport's governing body when it comes to banned substances.

10. Get back in the kitchen. The more you can prepare your own food, the more control you will have over the nourishment of your own body.

SUMMARY POINTS

- The practice of sport nutrition is somewhere between science and art. Getting athletes to change the way they eat can positively affect performance, though bringing about behavior change is not always easy.

- Fitness professionals, though they may be knowledgeable about nutrition and performance, should make sure they have the appropriate credentials before providing nutrition information to athletes. Some laws restrict which professionals can provide nutrition counseling.

- When working on a nutrition plan, professionals should take care to keep medical information confidential.

- Always ask athletes' permission before sharing any information with their coach or other members of their team except in the case of a life-threatening condition or eating disorder.

- Building a good rapport with athletes is of utmost importance in helping them make changes.

- The steps in creating a nutrition plan include assessment, evaluation, intervention and education, and monitoring and evaluation.

- Using a systematic approach to assessment, evaluation of needs, and intervention and education and then building a deep relationship with the athlete during the monitoring phase not only sets up the nutrition program for success but also may help to change the way athletes view nutrition and the way they eat, well beyond their athletic careers.

- The sport nutritionist may be on the front line for detecting the female athlete triad of disordered eating, amenorrhea, and osteoporosis (or low bone density signaling a problem in young athletes).

References

Chapter 1

Antonio, J., and J.R. Stout. 2001. *Sports supplements.* Hagerstown, MD: Lippincott, Williams & Wilkins.

Applegate, E.A., and L.E. Grivetti. 1997. Search for the competitive edge: A history of dietary fads and supplements. *Journal of Nutrition* 127: 869S-873S.

Balsom, P.D., G.C. Gaitanos, K. Soderlund, and B. Ekblom. 1999. High-intensity exercise and muscle glycogen availability in humans. *Acta Physiologica Scandinavica* 165: 337-345.

Bell, A., K.D. Dorsch, D.R. McCreary, and R. Hovey. 2004. A look at nutritional supplement use in adolescents. *Journal of Adolescent Health* 34: 508-516.

Bigard, A.X., H. Sanchez, G. Claveyrolas, S. Martin, B. Thimonier, and M.J. Arnaud. 2001. Effects of dehydration and rehydration on EMG changes during fatiguing contractions. *Medicine and Science in Sports and Exercise* 33: 1694-1700.

Borsheim, E., K.D. Tipton, S.E. Wolf, and R.R. Wolfe. 2002. Essential amino acids and muscle protein recovery from resistance exercise. *American Journal of Physiology: Endocrinology and Metabolism* 283: E648-657.

Brooks, G.A. 1987. Amino acid and protein metabolism during exercise and recovery. *Medicine and Science in Sports and Exercise* 19: S150-156.

Campbell, B., R.B. Kreider, T. Ziegenfuss, P. La Bounty, M. Roberts, D. Burke, J. Landis, H. Lopez, and J. Antonio. 2007. International Society of Sports Nutrition position stand: Protein and exercise. *Journal of the International Society of Sports Nutrition* 4: 8.

Coggan, A.R., W.M. Kohrt, R.J. Spina, D.M. Bier, and J.O. Holloszy. 1990. Endurance training decreases plasma glucose turnover and oxidation during moderate-intensity exercise in men. *Journal of Applied Physiology* 68: 990-996.

Cupisti, A., C. D'Alessandro, S. Castrogiovanni, A. Barale, and E. Morelli. 2002. Nutrition knowledge and dietary composition in Italian adolescent female athletes and non-athletes. *International Journal of Sport Nutrition and Exercise Metabolism* 12: 207-219.

Currell, K., and A.E. Jeukendrup. 2008. Superior endurance performance with ingestion of multiple transportable carbohydrates. *Medicine and Science in Sports and Exercise* 40: 275-281.

Delamarche, P., J. Bittel, J.R. Lacour, and R. Flandrois. 1990. Thermoregulation at rest and during exercise in prepubertal boys. *European Journal of Applied Physiology and Occupational Physiology* 60: 436-440.

Drinkwater, B.L., I.C. Kupprat, J.E. Denton, J.L. Crist, and S.M. Horvath. 1977. Response of prepubertal girls and college women to work in the heat. *Journal of Applied Physiology* 43: 1046-1053.

Friedlander, A.L., G.A. Casazza, M.A. Horning, M.J. Huie, and G.A. Brooks. 1997. Training-induced alterations of glucose flux in men. *Journal of Applied Physiology* 82: 1360-1369.

Grandjean, A.C. 1997. Diets of elite athletes: Has the discipline of sports nutrition made an impact? *Journal of Nutrition* 127: 874S-877S.

Greenleaf, J.E., and B.L. Castle. 1971. Exercise temperature regulation in man during hypo-hydration and hyperhydration. *Journal of Applied Physiology* 30: 847-853.

Grivetti, L.E., and E.A. Applegate. 1997. From Olympia to Atlanta: A cultural-historical perspective on diet and athletic training. *Journal of Nutrition* 127: 860S-868S.

Hargreaves, M., and L. Spriet. 2006. *Exercise metabolism.* Champaign, IL: Human Kinetics.

Hoffman, J.R., A.D. Faigenbaum, N.A. Ratamess, R. Ross, J. Kang, and G. Tenenbaum. 2008. Nutritional supplementation and anabolic steroid use in adolescents. *Medicine and Science in Sports and Exercise* 40: 15-24.

Hurley, B.F., P.M. Nemeth, W.H. Martin 3rd, J.M. Hagberg, G.P. Dalsky, and J.O. Holloszy. 1986. Muscle triglyceride utilization during exercise: Effect of training. *Journal of Applied Physiology* 60: 562-567.

Jacobson, B.H., C. Sobonya, and J. Ransone. 2001. Nutrition practices and knowledge of college varsity athletes: A follow-up. *Journal of Strength and Conditioning Research* 15: 63-68.

Jeukendrup, A. 2003. Modulation of carbohydrate and fat utilization by diet, exercise and environment. *Biochemistry Society Transactions* 31(Pt 6): 1270-1273.

Jeukendrup, A.E., and L. Moseley. 2010. Multiple transportable carbohydrates enhance gastric emptying and fluid delivery. *Scandinavian Journal of Medicine and Science in Sports* 13: 452-457.

Kenney, W.L., and P. Chiu. 2001. Influence of age on thirst and fluid intake. *Medicine and Science in Sports and Exercise* 33: 1524-1532.

Lemon, P.W. 2000. Beyond the zone: Protein needs of active individuals. *Journal of the American College of Nutrition* 19: 513S-521S.

Lemon, P.W., and F.J. Nagle. 1981. Effects of exercise on protein and amino acid metabolism. *Medicine and Science in Sports and Exercise* 13: 141-149.

Lockwood, C.M., J.R. Moon, S.E. Tobkin, A.A. Walter, A.E. Smith, V.J. Dalbo, J.T. Cramer, and J.R. Stout. 2008. Minimal nutrition intervention with high-protein/low-carbohydrate and low-fat, nutrient-dense food supplement improves body composition and exercise benefits in overweight adults: A randomized controlled trial. *Nutrition and Metabolism* 5: 11.

Maughan, R.J., P.L. Greenhaff, J.B. Leiper, D. Ball, C.P. Lambert, and M. Gleeson. 1997. Diet composition and the performance of high-intensity exercise. *Journal of Sports Science and Medicine* 15: 265-275.

McArdle, W.D., F.I. Katch, and V.L. Katch. 2008. *Sports and exercise nutrition.* Philadelphia: Lippincott, Williams & Wilkins.

McNaughton, L.R. 1986. The influence of caffeine ingestion on incremental treadmill running. *British Journal of Sports Medicine* 20: 109-112.

Mittendorfer, B., and S. Klein. 2003. Physiological factors that regulate the use of endogenous fat and carbohydrate fuels during endurance exercise. *Nutrition Research Reviews* 16: 97-108.

Mougios, V. 2006. *Exercise biochemistry.* Champaign, IL: Human Kinetics.

Naitoh, M., and L.M. Burrell. 1998. Thirst in elderly subjects. *Journal of Health, Nutrition, and Aging* 2: 172-177.

Norton, L.E., and D.K. Layman. 2006. Leucine regulates translation initiation of protein synthesis in skeletal muscle after exercise. *Journal of Nutrition* 136: 533S-537S.

O'Dea, J.A. 2003. Consumption of nutritional supplements among adolescents: Usage and perceived benefits. *Health Education Research* 18: 98-107.

Phillips, S.M., S.A. Atkinson, M.A. Tarnopolsky, and J.D. MacDougall. 1993. Gender differences in leucine kinetics and nitrogen balance in endurance athletes. *Journal of Applied Physiology* 75: 2134-2141.

Raymond-Barker, P., A. Petroczi, and E. Quested. 2007. Assessment of nutritional knowledge in female athletes susceptible to the female athlete triad syndrome. *Journal of Occupational Medicine and Toxicology* 2: 10.

Robergs, R.A., D.R. Pearson, D.L. Costill, W.J. Fink, D.D. Pascoe, M.A. Benedict, C.P. Lambert, and J.J. Zachweija. 1991. Muscle glycogenolysis during differing intensities of weight-resistance exercise. *Journal of Applied Physiology* 70: 1700-1706.

Schaafsma, G. 2000. The protein digestibility-corrected amino acid score. *Journal of Nutrition* 130: 1865S-1867S.

Schoffstall, J.E., J.D. Branch, B.C. Leutholtz, and D.E. Swain. 2001. Effects of dehydration and rehydration on the one-repetition maximum bench press of weight-trained males. *Journal of Strength and Conditioning Research* 15: 102-108.

Shimomura, Y., Y. Yamamoto, G. Bajotto, J. Sato, T. Murakami, N. Shimomura, H. Kobayashi, and K. Mawatari. 2006. Nutraceutical effects of branched-chain amino acids on skeletal muscle. *Journal of Nutrition* 136: 529S-532S.

Stephens, F.B., M. Roig, G. Armstrong, and P.L. Greenhaff. 2008. Post-exercise ingestion of a unique, high molecular weight glucose polymer solution improves performance during a subsequent bout of cycling exercise. *Journal of Sports Science* 26: 149-154.

Tesch, P.A., L.L. Ploutz-Synder, L. Ystro, M.M. Castro, and G. Dudley. 1998. Skeletal muscle glycogen loss evoked by resistance exercise. *Journal of Strength and Conditioning Research* 12: 67.

Tipton, K.D., A.A. Ferrando, S.M. Phillips, D. Doyle Jr., and R.R. Wolfe. 1999. Postexercise net protein synthesis in human muscle from orally administered amino acids. *American Journal of Physiology* 276: E628-634.

U.S. Food and Drug Administration. 1994. Dietary Supplement Health and Education Act.

van Loon, L.J., A.E. Jeukendrup, W.H. Saris, and A.J. Wagenmakers. 1999. Effect of training status on fuel selection during submaximal exercise with glucose ingestion. *Journal of Applied Physiology* 87: 1413-1420.

Volek, J.S. 2004. Influence of nutrition on responses to resistance training. *Medicine and Science in Sports and Exercise* 36: 689-696.

Wagenmakers, A.J. 1998. Muscle amino acid metabolism at rest and during exercise: Role in human physiology and metabolism. *Exercise and Sport Sciences Reviews* 26: 287-314.

Walsh, R.M., T.D. Noakes, J.A. Hawley, and S.C. Dennis. 1994. Impaired high-intensity cycling performance time at low levels of dehydration. *International Journal of Sports Medicine* 15: 392-398.

Wexler, R.K. 2002. Evaluation and treatment of heat-related illness. *American Family Physician* 65: 2307.

Zinn, C., G. Schofield, and C. Wall. 2006. Evaluation of sports nutrition knowledge of New Zealand premier club rugby coaches. *International Journal of Sport Nutrition and Exercise Metabolism* 16: 214-225.

Chapter 2

Ahlborg, B.G., J. Bergström, J. Brohult, L.G. Ekelund, E. Hultman, and G. Maschino. 1967. Human muscle glycogen content and capacity for prolonged exercise after different diets. *Foersvarsmedicin* 3: 85-99.

Balsom, P.D., G.C. Gaitanis, K. Soderlund, and B. Ekblom. 1999. High-intensity exercise and muscle glycogen availability in humans. *Acta Physiologica Scandinavica* 165: 337-345.

Bergström, J., L. Hermansen, E. Hultman, and B. Saltin. 1967. Diet, muscle glycogen and physical performance. *Acta Physiologica Scandinavica* 71: 140-150.

Biolo, G., B.D. Williams, R.Y. Fleming, and R.R. Wolfe. 1999. Insulin action on muscle protein kinetics and amino acid transport after resistance exercise. *Diabetes* 48: 949-957.

Bosch, A.N., S.C. Dennis, and T.D. Noakes. 1994. Influence of carbohydrate ingestion on fuel substrate turnover and oxidation during prolonged exercise. *Journal of Applied Physiology* 76: 2364-2372.

Burke, L.M., G.R. Collier, and M. Hargreaves. 1998. Glycemic index: A new tool in sport nutrition. *International Journal of Sport Nutrition and Exercise Metabolism* 8: 401-415.

Casey, A., A.H. Short, S. Curtis, and P.L. Greenhaff. 1996. The effect of glycogen availability on power output and the metabolic response to repeated bouts of maximal, isokinetic exercise in man. *European Journal of Applied Physiology* 72: 249-255.

Coleman, E. 1994. Update on carbohydrate: Solid versus liquid. *International Journal of Sport Nutrition* 4: 80-88.

Conley, M.S., and M.H. Stone. 1996. Carbohydrate for resistance exercise and training. *Sports Medicine* 21: 7-17.

Costill, D. 1988. Carbohydrates for exercise: Dietary demands for optimal performance. *International Journal of Sports Medicine* 9: 1-18.

Coyle, E. 1995. Substrate utilization during exercise in active people. *American Journal of Clinical Nutrition* 61: 968S-979S.

Coyle, E.F., A.R. Coggan, M.K. Hemmert, and J.L. Ivy. 1986. Muscle glycogen utilization during prolonged strenuous exercise when fed carbohydrate. *Journal of Applied Physiology* 61: 165-172.

D'Adamo, P.D. 1990. Larch arabinogalactan. *Journal of Neuropathic Medicine* 6: 33-37.

Essen, B., and J. Henriksson. 1974. Glycogen content of individual muscle fibers in man. *Acta Physiologica Scandinavica* 90: 645-647.

Gollnick, P.D., J. Karlsson, K. Piehl, and B. Saltin. 1974. Selective glycogen depletion in skeletal muscle fibers of man following sustained contractions. *Journal of Physiology* 241: 59-67.

Haff, G.G., A.J. Koch, J.A. Potteiger, K.E. Kuphal, L.M. Magee, S.B. Green, and J.J. Jakicic. 2000. Carbohydrate supplementation attenuates muscle glycogen loss during acute bouts of resistance exercise. *International Journal of Sport Nutrition and Exercise Metabolism* 10: 326-339.

Haff, G.G., M.H. Stone, B.J. Warren, R. Keith, R.L. Johnson, D.C. Nieman, F. Williams JR, and K. Brett Kirksey. 1999. The effect of carbohydrate supplementation on multiple sessions and bouts of resistance exercise. *Journal of Strength and Conditioning Research* 13: 111-117.

Haff, G.G., M.J. Lehmkuhl, L.B. McCoy, and M.H. Stone. 2003. Carbohydrate and resistance training. *Journal of Strength and Conditioning Research* 17: 187-196.

Hargreaves, M. 2000. Carbohydrate replacement during exercise. In: *Nutrition in sport,* edited by R.J. Maughan. Oxford: Blackwell Science.

Hawley, J.A., E.J. Schabort, T.D. Noakes, and S.C. Dennis. 1997. Carbohydrate loading and exercise performance: An update. *Sports Medicine* 24: 73-81.

Hultman, E. 1967. Studies on muscle metabolism of glycogen and active phosphate in man with special reference to exercise and diet. *Scandinavian Journal of Clinical and Laboratory Investigation* 19: 1-63.

Ivy, J. 2001. Dietary strategies to promote glycogen synthesis after exercise. *Canadian Journal of Applied Physiology* 26: S236-S245.

Jeukendrup, A. 2004. Carbohydrate intake during exercise and performance. *Nutrition* 20: 669-677.

Jeukendrup, A.E., F. Brouns, A.J.M. Wagenmakers, and W.H.M. Saris. 1997. Carbohydrate-electrolyte feedings improve 1 h time trial cycling performance. *International Journal of Sports Medicine* 18(2): 125-129.

Jeukendrup, A., and R. Jentjens. 2000. Oxidation of carbohydrate feedings during prolonged exercise: Current thoughts, guidelines and directions for future research. *Sports Medicine* 29: 407-424.

Jeukendrup, A.E., A.J.M. Wagenmakers, J.H. Stegen, A.P. Gijsen, F. Brouns, and W.H. Saris. 1999. Carbohydrate ingestion can completely suppress endogenous glucose production during exercise. *American Journal of Physiology* 276: E672-E683.

Keizer, H., H. Kuipers, and G. van Kranenburg. 1987. Influence of liquid and solid meals on muscle glycogen resynthesis, plasma fuel hormone response, and maximal physical working capacity. *International Journal of Sports Medicine* 8: 99-104.

Kjaer, M. 1998. Hepatic glucose production during exercise. *Advances in Experimental Medicine and Biology* 441: 117-127.

Kulik, J.R., C.D. Touchberry, N. Kawamori, P.A. Blumert, A.J. Crum, and G.G. Haff. 2008. Supplemental carbohydrate ingestion does not improve performance of high-intensity resistance exercise. *Journal of Strength and Conditioning Research* 22: 1101-1107.

Leloir, L.F. 1971. Two decades of research on the biosynthesis of saccharides. *Science* 172: 1299-1303.

Liebman, B. 1998. Sugar: The sweetening of the American diet. *Nutrition Action Health Letter* 25: 1-8.

Lupton, J., and P. Trumbo. 2006. Dietary fiber. In: *Modern nutrition in health and disease,* edited by M. Shils. Philadelphia: Lippincott, Williams & Wilkins.

Marlett, J.A., M.I. McBurney, and J.L. Slavin. 2002. Position of the American Dietetic Association: Health implications of dietary fiber. *Journal of the American Dietetic Association* 102: 993-1000.

Maughan, R.J., P.L. Greenhaff, J.B. Leiper, D. Ball, C.P. Lambert, and M. Gleeson. 1997. Diet composition and the performance of high-intensity exercise. *Journal of Sports Science and Medicine* 15: 265-275.

McArdle, W.D., F.I. Katch, and V.L. Katch. 2009. *Sports and exercise nutrition.* Philadelphia: Lippincott, Williams & Wilkins.

Nardone, A., C. Romano, and M. Schieppati. 1989. Selective recruitment of high-threshold human motor units during voluntary isotonic lengthening of active muscles. *Journal of Physiology (London)* 409: 451-471.

National Academy of Sciences. 2002. *Dietary reference intakes for energy, carbohydrates, fiber, fat, protein and amino acids (macronutrients).* Washington, DC: National Academies Press.

Rauch, H.G., A. St Clair Gibson, E.V. Lambert, and T.D. Noakes. 2005. A signaling role for muscle glycogen in the regulation of pace during prolonged exercise. *British Journal of Sports Medicine* 39: 34-38.

Robergs, R.A., D.R. Pearson, D.L. Costill, W.J. Fink, D.D. Pascoe, M.A. Benedict, C.P. Lambert, and J.J. Zachweija. 1991. Muscle glycogenolysis during differing intensities of weight-resistance exercise. *International Journal of Sport Nutrition and Exercise Metabolism* 10 :326-339.

Rockwell, M.S., J.W. Rankin, and H. Dixon. 2003. Effects of muscle glycogen on performance of repeated sprints and mechanisms of fatigue. *International Journal of Sport Nutrition and Exercise Metabolism* 13: 1-14.

Roediger, W.E. 1989. Utilization of nutrients by isolated epithelial cells of the rat colon. *Gastroenternology* 83: 424-429.

Shulman, R., and D. Rothman. 2001. The "glycogen shunt" in exercising muscle: A role of glycogen in muscle energetics and fatigue. *Proceedings of the National Academy of Sciences* 98: 457-461.

Spriet, L.L. 1998. Regulation of fat/carbohydrate interaction in human skeletal muscle during exercise. *Advances in Experimental Medicine and Biology* 441: 249-261.

Tesch, P.A., E.B. Colliander, and P. Kaiser. 1986. Muscle metabolism during intense, heavy-resistance exercise. *European Journal of Applied Physiology* 4: 362-366.

Tesch, P.A., L.L. Ploutz-Snyder, L. Yström, M.J. Castro, and G.A. Dudley. 1998. Skeletal muscle glycogen loss evoked by resistance exercise. *Journal of Strength and Conditioning Research* 12: 67-73.

Tipton, K.D., B.B. Rasmussen, S.L. Miller, S.E. Wolf, S.K. Owens-Stovall, B.E. Petrini, and R.R. Wolfe. 2001. Timing of amino acid-carbohydrate ingestion alters anabolic response of muscle to resistance exercise. *American Journal of Physiology: Endocrinology and Metabolism* 281: E197-E206.

Tsintzas, K., and C. Williams. 1998. Human muscle glycogen metabolism during exercise: Effect of carbohydrate supplementation. *Sports Medicine* 25: 7-23.

Tsintzas, O.K., C. Williams, L. Boobis, and P. Greenhaff. 1995. Carbohydrate ingestion and glycogen utilization in different fiber types in man. *Journal of Physiology* 489: 243-250.

Van Hall, G. 2000. Lactate as fuel for mitochondrial respiration. *Acta Physiologica Scandinavica* 168: 643-656.

Chapter 3

Allred, C.D., K.F. Allred, Y.H. Ju, S.M. Virant, and W.G. Helferich. 2001. Soy diets containing varying amounts of genistein stimulate growth of estrogen-dependent (MCF-7) tumors in a dose-dependent manner. *Cancer Research* 61(13): 5045-5050.

Andersen, L.L., G. Tufekovic, M.K. Zebis, R.M. Crameri, G. Verlaan, M. Kjaer, C. Suetta, P. Magnusson, and P. Aagaard. 2005. The effect of resistance training combined with timed ingestion of protein on muscle fiber size and muscle strength. *Metabolism: Clinical and Experimental* 54(2): 151-156.

Antonio, J., and J.R. Stout, eds. 2001. *Sports supplements.* Philadelphia: Lippincott, Williams & Wilkins.

Badger, T.M., M.J. Ronis, and R. Hakkak. 2001. Developmental effects and health aspects of soy protein isolate, casein, and whey in male and female rats. *International Journal of Toxicology* 20(3): 165-174.

Baumrucker, C.R., M.H. Green, and J.W. Blum. 1994. Effects of dietary rhIGF-I in neonatal calves on the appearance of glucose, insulin, D-xylose, globulins and gamma-glutamyl transferase in blood. *Domestic Animal Endocrinology* 11(4): 393-403.

Beaufrere, B., M. Dangin, and Y. Boirie. 2000. The fast and slow protein concept. In: *Proteins, peptides and amino acids in enteral nutrition,* edited by P. Furst and V. Young, 121-133. Basel: Karger.

Berdanier, C.D. 2000. *Advanced nutrition: Micronutrients.* 2nd ed. Boca Raton, FL: CRC Press.

Bigard, A.X., P. Lavier, L. Ullmann, H. Legrand, P. Douce, and C.Y. Guezennec. 1996. Branched-chain amino acid supplementation during repeated prolonged skiing exercises at altitude. *International Journal of Sport Nutrition* 6(3): 295-306.

Bloomer, R.J., A.C. Fry, M.J. Falvo, and C.A. Moore. 2007. Protein carbonyls are acutely elevated following single set anaerobic exercise in resistance trained men. *Journal of Science and Medicine in Sport* 10(6): 411-417.

Bloomer, R.J., A.H. Goldfarb, L. Wideman, M.J. McKenzie, and L.A. Consitt. 2005. Effects of acute aerobic and anaerobic exercise on blood markers of oxidative stress. *Journal of Strength and Conditioning Research* 19(2): 276-285.

Boirie, Y., M. Dangin, P. Gachon, M.P. Vasson, J.L. Maubois, and B. Beaufrere. 1997. Slow and fast dietary proteins differently modulate postprandial protein accretion. *Proceedings of the National Academy of Sciences* 94(26) (Dec 23): 14930-14935.

Borsheim, E., A. Aarsland, and R.R. Wolfe. 2004. Effect of an amino acid, protein, and carbohydrate mixture on net muscle protein balance after resistance exercise. *International Journal of Sport Nutrition and Exercise Metabolism* 14(3): 255-271.

Borsheim, E., K.D. Tipton, S.E. Wolf, and R.R. Wolfe. 2002. Essential amino acids and muscle protein recovery from resistance exercise. *American Journal of Physiology: Endocrinology and Metabolism* 283(4): E648-E657.

Brown, E.C., R.A. DiSilvestro, A. Babaknia, and S.T. Devor. 2004. Soy versus whey protein bars: Effects on exercise training impact on lean body mass and antioxidant status. *Nutrition Journal* 8(3): 22.

Bucci, L., and L. Unlu. 2000. Proteins and amino acid supplements in exercise and sport. In: *Energy-yielding macronutrients and energy metabolism in sports nutrition,* edited by J. Driskell and I. Wolinsky. Boca Raton, FL: CRC Press.

Campbell, B., R.B. Kreider, T. Ziegenfuss, P. La Bounty, M. Roberts, D. Burke, J. Landis, H. Lopez, and J. Antonio. 2007. International society of sports nutrition position stand: Protein and exercise. *Journal of the International Society of Sports Nutrition* 4: 8.

Candow, D.G., N.C. Burke, T. Smith-Palmer, and D.G. Burke. 2006. Effect of whey and soy protein supplementation combined with resistance training in young adults. *International Journal of Sport Nutrition and Exercise Metabolism* 16: 233-244.

Candow, D.G., J.P. Little, P.D. Chilibeck, S. Abeysekara, G.A. Zello, M. Kazachkov, S.M. Cornish, and P.H. Yu. 2008. Low-dose creatine combined with protein during resistance training in older men. *Medicine and Science in Sports and Exercise* 40(9): 1645-1652.

Carli, G., M. Bonifazi, L. Lodi, C. Lupo, G. Martelli, and A. Viti. 1992. Changes in the exercise-induced hormone response to branched chain amino acid administration. *European Journal of Applied Physiology and Occupational Physiology* 64(3): 272-277.

Coombes, J.S., and L.R. McNaughton. 2000. Effects of branched-chain amino acid supplementation on serum creatine kinase and lactate dehydrogenase after prolonged exercise. *Journal of Sports Medicine and Physical Fitness* 40(3): 240-246.

Cribb, P.J., A.D. Williams, and A. Hayes. 2007. A creatine-protein-carbohydrate supplement enhances responses to resistance training. *Medicine and Science in Sports and Exercise* 39(11): 1960-1968.

De Feo, P., C. Di Loreto, P. Lucidi, G. Murdolo, N. Parlanti, A. De Cicco, F. Piccioni, and F. Santeusanio. 2003. Metabolic response to exercise. *Journal of Endocrinological Investigation* 26(9): 851-854.

Dewell, A., C.B. Hollenbeck, and B. Bruce. 2002. The effects of soy-derived phytoestrogens on serum lipids and lipoproteins in moderately hypercholesterolemic postmenopausal women. *Journal of Clinical Endocrinology and Metabolism* 87(1): 118-121.

Di Pasquale, M. 2000. Proteins and amino acids in exercise and sport. In: *Energy-yielding macronutrients and energy metabolism in exercise and sport,* edited by J. Driskell and I. Wolinsky. Boca Raton, FL: CRC Press.

Drăgan, I., V. Stroescu, I. Stoian, E. Georgescu, and R. Baloescu. 1992. Studies regarding the efficiency of Supro isolated soy protein in Olympic athletes. *Revue Roumaine de Physiologie* 29(3-4): 63-70.

Esmarck, B., J.L. Andersen, S. Olsen, E.A. Richter, M. Mizuno, and M. Kjaer. 2001. Timing of postexercise protein intake is important for muscle hypertrophy with resistance training in elderly humans. *Journal of Physiology* 535(Pt 1): 301-311.

FitzGerald, R.J., and H. Meisel. 2000. Milk protein-derived peptide inhibitors of angiotensin-I-converting enzyme. *British Journal of Nutrition* 84 Suppl 1: S33-S37.

Florisa, R., I. Recio, B. Berkhout, and S. Visser. 2003. Antibacterial and antiviral effects of milk proteins and derivatives thereof. *Current Pharmaceutical Design* 9(16): 1257-1275.

Friedman, J.E., and P.W. Lemon. 1989. Effect of chronic endurance exercise on retention of dietary protein. *International Journal of Sports Medicine* 10(2): 118-123.

Fruhbeck, G. 1998. Protein metabolism: Slow and fast dietary proteins. *Nature* 391: 843, 845.

Gattas, V.G. 1990. Protein-energy requirements of prepubertal school-age boys determined by using the nitrogen-balance response to a mixed-protein diet. *American Journal of Clinical Nutrition* 52(6): 1037-1042.

Gattas, V., G.A. Barrera, J.S. Riumallo, and R. Uauy. 1992. Protein-energy requirements of boys 12-14 y old determined by using the nitrogen-balance response to a mixed-protein diet. *American Journal of Clinical Nutrition* 56(3): 499-503.

Gleeson, M., G.I. Lancaster, and N.C. Bishop. 2001. Nutritional strategies to minimise exercise-induced immunosuppression in athletes. *Canadian Journal of Applied Physiology* 26 Suppl: S23-35.

Green, A.L., E. Hultman, I.A. Macdonald, D.A. Sewell, and P.L. Greenhaff. 1996. Carbohydrate ingestion augments skeletal muscle creatine accumulation during creatine supplementation in humans. *American Journal of Physiology* 271(5 Pt 1): E821-E826.

Hayes, A., and P.J. Cribb. 2008. Effect of whey protein isolate on strength, body composition and muscle hypertrophy during resistance training. *Current Opinion in Clinical Nutrition and Metabolic Care* 11(1): 40-44.

Hendler, S.S., and D. Rorvik, eds. 2001. *PDR for nutritional supplements.* 1st ed. Montvale, NJ: Thomson PDR.

Horton, B.S. 1995. Commercial utilization of minor milk components in the health and food industries. *Journal of Dairy Science* 78(11): 2584-2589.

Howarth, K.R., K.A. Burgomaster, S.M. Phillips, and M.J. Gibala. 2007. Exercise training increases branched-chain oxoacid dehydrogenase kinase content in human skeletal muscle. *American Journal of Physiology: Regulatory, Integrative and Comparative Physiology* 293(3): R1335-1341.

Hulmi, J.J., V. Kovanen, H. Selanne, W.J. Kraemer, K. Hakkinen, and A.A. Mero. 2009. Acute and long-term effects of resistance exercise with or without protein ingestion on muscle hypertrophy and gene expression. *Amino Acids* 37: 297-308.

Jenkins, D.J., C.W. Kendall, E. Vidgen, V. Vuksan, C.J. Jackson, L.S. Augustin, B. Lee, et al. 2000. Effect of soy-based breakfast cereal on blood lipids and oxidized low-density lipoprotein. *Metabolism: Clinical and Experimental* 49(11): 1496-1500.

Kalman, D., S. Feldman, M. Martinez, D.R. Krieger, and M.J. Tallon. 2007. Effect of protein source and resistance training on body composition and sex hormones. *Journal of the International Society of Sports Nutrition* 4: 4.

Kendrick, I.P., R.C. Harris, H.J. Kim, C.K. Kim, V.H. Dang, T.Q. Lam, T.T. Bui, M. Smith, and J.A. Wise. 2008. The effects of 10 weeks of resistance training combined with beta-alanine supplementation on whole body strength, force production, muscular endurance and body composition. *Amino Acids* 34(4): 547-554.

Kerksick, C., T. Harvey, J. Stout, B. Campbell, C. Wilborn, R. Kreider, D. Kalman, et al. 2008. International society of sports nutrition position stand: Nutrient timing. *Journal of the International Society of Sports Nutrition* 5: 17.

Kerksick, C.M., C.J. Rasmussen, S.L. Lancaster, B. Magu, P. Smith, C. Melton, M. Greenwood, A.L. Almada, C.P. Earnest, and R.B. Kreider. 2006. The effects of protein and amino acid supplementation on performance and training adaptations during ten weeks of resistance training. *Journal of Strength and Conditioning Research* 20(3): 643-653.

Kerksick, C.M., C. Rasmussen, S. Lancaster, M. Starks, P. Smith, C. Melton, M. Greenwood, A. Almada, and R. Kreider. 2007. Impact of differing protein sources and a creatine containing nutritional formula after 12 weeks of resistance training. *Nutrition* 23(9): 647-656.

Korhonen, H., and A. Pihlanto. 2003. Food-derived bioactive peptides—opportunities for designing future foods. *Current Pharmaceutical Design* 9(16): 1297-1308.

Kraemer, W.J., N.A. Ratamess, J.S. Volek, K. Hakkinen, M.R. Rubin, D.N. French, A.L. Gomez, et al. 2006. The effects of amino acid supplementation on hormonal responses to resistance training overreaching. *Metabolism: Clinical and Experimental* 55(3): 282-291.

Kreider, R.B., and S.M. Kleiner. 2000. Protein supplements for athletes: Need vs. convenience. *Your Patient and Fitness* 14(6): 12-18.

Kreider, R.B., B. Leutholtz, F.I. Katch, and V.L. Katch, eds. 2009. *Exercise and sport nutrition: Principles, promises, science, and recommendations*. Santa Barbara, CA: Fitness Technologies Press.

Kurzer, M.S. 2002. Hormonal effects of soy in premenopausal women and men. *Journal of Nutrition* 132(3): 570S-573S.

Lands, L.C., V.L. Grey, and A.A. Smountas. 1999. Effect of supplementation with a cysteine donor on muscular performance. *Journal of Applied Physiology* 87(4): 1381-1385.

Lemon, P. 2001. Protein requirements for strength athletes. In: *Sports supplements,* edited by J. Antonio and J.R. Stout, 301. Philadelphia: Lippincott, Williams & Wilkins.

Mero, A. 1999. Leucine supplementation and intensive training. *Sports Medicine* 27(6): 347-358.

Mero, A., H. Miikkulainen, J. Riski, R. Pakkanen, J. Aalto, and T. Takala. 1997. Effects of bovine colostrum supplementation on serum IGF-I, IgG, hormone, and saliva IgA during training. *Journal of Applied Physiology* 83(4): 1144-1151.

Messina, M. 1999. Soy, soy phytoestrogens (isoflavones), and breast cancer. *American Journal of Clinical Nutrition* 70(4): 574-575.

Messina, M., and V. Messina. 2000. Soyfoods, soybean isoflavones, and bone health: A brief overview. *Journal of Renal Nutrition* 10(2): 63-68.

Nelson, A.G., D.A. Arnall, J. Kokkonen, R. Day, and J. Evans. 2001. Muscle glycogen supercompensation is enhanced by prior creatine supplementation. *Medicine and Science in Sports and Exercise* 33(7): 1096-1100.

Nicholls, J., B.L. Lasley, S.T. Nakajima, K.D. Setchell, and B.O. Schneeman. 2002. Effects of soy consumption on gonadotropin secretion and acute pituitary responses to gonadotropin-releasing hormone in women. *Journal of Nutrition* 132(4): 708-714.

Pelligrini, A. 2003. Antimicrobial peptides from food proteins. *Current Pharmaceutical Design* 9(16): 1225-1238.

Pino, A.M., L.E. Valladares, M.A. Palma, A.M. Mancilla, M. Yanez, and C. Albala. 2000. Dietary isoflavones affect sex hormone-binding globulin levels in postmenopausal women. *Journal of Clinical Endocrinology and Metabolism* 85(8): 2797-2800.

Potter, S.M. 1995. Overview of proposed mechanisms for the hypocholesterolemic effect of soy. *Journal of Nutrition* 125(3 Suppl): 606S-611S.

Puntis, J.W., P.A. Ball, M.A. Preece, A. Green, G.A. Brown, and I.W. Booth. 1989. Egg and breast milk based nitrogen sources compared. *Archives of Disease in Childhood* 64(10): 1472-1477.

Rowlands, D.S., K. Rossler, R.M. Thorp, D.F. Graham, B.W. Timmons, S.R. Stannard, and M.A. Tarnopolsky. 2008. Effect of dietary protein content during recovery from high-intensity cycling on subsequent performance and markers of stress, inflammation, and muscle damage in well-trained men. *Applied Physiology, Nutrition, and Metabolism* 33(1): 39-51.

Roy, B.D. 2008. Milk: The new sports drink? A review. *Journal of the International Society of Sports Nutrition* 5: 15.

Shirreffs, S.M., P. Watson, and R.J. Maughan. 2007. Milk as an effective post-exercise rehydration drink. *British Journal of Nutrition* 98: 173-180.

Solerte, S.B., C. Gazzaruso, R. Bonacasa, M. Rondanelli, M. Zamboni, C. Basso, E. Locatelli, N. Schifino, A. Giustina, and M. Fioravanti. 2008. Nutritional supplements with oral amino acid mixtures increases whole-body lean mass and insulin sensitivity in elderly subjects with sarcopenia. *American Journal of Cardiology* 101(11A): 69E-77E.

Takatsuka, N., C. Nagata, Y. Kurisu, S. Inaba, N. Kawakami, and H. Shimizu. 2000. Hypocholesterolemic effect of soymilk supplementation with usual diet in premenopausal normolipidemic japanese women. *Preventive Medicine* 31(4): 308-314.

Tang, J.E., J.J. Manolakos, G.W. Kujbida, P.J. Lysecki, D.R. Moore, and S.M. Phillips. 2007. Minimal whey protein with carbohydrate stimulates muscle protein synthesis following resistance exercise in trained young men. *Applied Physiology, Nutrition, and Metabolism* 32(6): 1132-1138.

Tarnopolsky, M.A., J.D. MacDougall, and S.A. Atkinson. 1988. Influence of protein intake and training status on nitrogen balance and lean body mass. *Journal of Applied Physiology* 64(1): 187-193.

Tikkanen, M.J., and H. Adlercreutz. 2000. Dietary soy-derived isoflavone phytoestrogens: Could they have a role in coronary heart disease prevention? *Biochemical Pharmacology* 60(1): 1-5.

Tipton, K.D., T.A. Elliott, M.G. Cree, A.A. Aarsland, A.P. Sanford, and R.R. Wolfe. 2007. Stimulation of net muscle protein synthesis by whey protein ingestion before and after exercise. *American Journal of Physiology: Endocrinology and Metabolism* 292(1): E71-E76.

Tipton, K.D., T.A. Elliott, M.G. Cree, S.E. Wolf, A.P. Sanford, and R.R. Wolfe. 2004. Ingestion of casein and whey proteins result in muscle anabolism after resistance exercise. *Medicine and Science in Sports and Exercise* 36(12): 2073-2081.

Tipton, K.D., and A.A. Ferrando. 2008. Improving muscle mass: Response of muscle metabolism to exercise, nutrition and anabolic agents. *Essays in Biochemistry* 44: 85-98.

Tipton, K.D., A.A. Ferrando, S.M. Phillips, D. Doyle Jr., and R.R. Wolfe. 1999. Postexercise net protein synthesis in human muscle from orally administered amino acids. *American Journal of Physiology* 276(4 Pt 1): E628-E634.

Tipton, K.D., B.B. Rasmussen, S.L. Miller, S.E. Wolf, S.K. Owens-Stovall, B.E. Petrini, and R.R. Wolfe. 2001. Timing of amino acid-carbohydrate ingestion alters anabolic response of muscle to resistance exercise. *American Journal of Physiology: Endocrinology and Metabolism* 281(2): E197-E206.

Toba, Y., Y. Takada, Y. Matsuoka, Y. Morita, M. Motouri, T. Hirai, T. Suguri, et al. 2001. Milk basic protein promotes bone formation and suppresses bone resorption in healthy adult men. *Bioscience, Biotechnology, and Biochemistry* 65(6): 1353-1357.

Tomas, F.M., S.E. Knowles, P.C. Owens, C.S. Chandler, G.L. Francis, L.C. Read, and F.J. Ballard. 1992. Insulin-like growth factor-I (IGF-I) and especially IGF-I variants are anabolic in dexamethasone-treated rats. *Biochemical Journal* 282(Pt 1): 91-97.

Wagenmakers, A.J. 1998. Muscle amino acid metabolism at rest and during exercise: Role in human physiology and metabolism. *Exercise and Sport Sciences Reviews* 26: 287-314.

Watson, P., T.D. Love, R.J. Maughan, and S.M. Shirreffs. 2008. A comparison of the effects of milk and a carbohydrate-electrolyte drink on the restoration of fluid balance and exercise capacity in a hot, humid environment. *European Journal of Applied Physiology* 104(4): 633-642.

Williams, M.H. 2002. *Nutrition for health, fitness, and sport.* 6th ed. New York: McGraw-Hill.

Willoughby, D.S., J.R. Stout, and C.D. Wilborn. 2007. Effects of resistance training and protein plus amino acid supplementation on muscle anabolism, mass, and strength. *Amino Acids* 32(4): 467-477.

Wong, C.W., A.H. Liu, G.O. Regester, G.L. Francis, and D.L. Watson. 1997. Influence of whey and purified whey proteins on neutrophil functions in sheep. *Journal of Dairy Research* 64(2): 281-288.

Zawadzki, K.M., B.B. Yaspelkis 3rd, and J.L. Ivy. 1992. Carbohydrate-protein complex increases the rate of muscle glycogen storage after exercise. *Journal of Applied Physiology* 72(5): 1854-1859.

Chapter 4

Ahrén, B., A. Mari, C.L. Fyfe, F. Tsofliou, A.A. Sneddon, K.W. Wahle, M.S. Winzell, G. Pacini, and L.M. Williams. 2009. Effects of conjugated linoleic acid plus n-3 polyunsaturated fatty acids on insulin secretion and estimated insulin sensitivity in men. *European Journal of Clinical Nutrition* 63(6): 778-786.

Andersson, A., A. Sjodin, A. Hedman, R. Olsson, and B. Vessby. 2000. Fatty acid profile of skeletal muscle phospholipids in trained and untrained young men. *American Journal of Physiology: Endocrinology and Metabolism* 279(4): E744-E751.

Aoyama, T., N. Nosaka, and M. Kasai. 2007. Research on the nutritional characteristics of medium-chain fatty acids. *Journal of Medical Investigation* 54(3-4): 385-388.

Archer, S., D. Green, M. Chamberlain, A. Dyer, and K. Liu. 1998. Association of dietary fish and n-3 fatty acid intake with hemostatic factors in the coronary artery risk development in young adults (CARDIA) study. *Arteriosclerosis, Thrombosis, and Vascular Biology* 18: 1119-1123.

Arterburn, L.M., E.B. Hall, and H. Oken. 2006. Distribution, interconversion, and dose response of n-3 fatty acids in humans. *American Journal of Clinical Nutrition* 83(6 Suppl): 1467S-1476S.

Bastard, J.P., M. Maachi, C. Lagathu, M.J. Kim, M. Caron, H. Vidal, J. Capeau, and B. Feve. 2006. Recent advances in the relationship between obesity, inflammation, and insulin resistance. *European Cytokine Network* 17(1): 4-12.

Boudreau, M.D., P.S. Chanmugam, S.B. Hart, S.H. Lee, and D.H. Hwang. 1991. Lack of dose response by dietary n-3 fatty acids at a constant ratio of n-3 to n-6 fatty acids in suppressing eicosanoid biosynthesis from arachidonic acid. *American Journal of Clinical Nutrition* 54(1): 111-117.

Breslow, J. 2006. n-3 fatty acids and cardiovascular disease. *American Journal of Clinical Nutrition* 83(6 Suppl): 1477S-1482S.

Brooks, G.A. 1997. Importance of the "crossover" concept in exercise metabolism. *Clinical and Experimental Pharmacology and Physiology* 24(11): 889-895.

Browning, L. 2003. n-3 Polyunsaturated fatty acids, inflammation and obesity-related disease. *Proceedings of the Nutrition Society* 62(2): 447-453.

Calabrese, C., S. Myer, S. Munson, P. Turet, and T.C. Birdsall. 1999. A cross-over study of the effect of a single oral feeding of medium chain triglyceride oil vs. canola oil on post-ingestion plasma triglyceride levels in healthy men. *Alternative Medicine Review* 4(1): 23-28.

Calder, P. 2006. n-3 polyunsaturated fatty acids, inflammation, and inflammatory diseases. *American Journal of Clinical Nutrition* 83(6 Suppl): 1505S-1519S.

Cannon, J.G., M.A. Fiatarone, M. Meydani, J. Gong, L. Scott, J.B. Blumberg, and W.J. Evans. 1995. Aging and dietary modulation of elastase and interleukin-1 beta secretion. *American Journal of Physiology* 268(1 Pt 2): R208-213.

Childs, C.E., M. Romeu-Nadal, G.C. Burdge, and P.C. Calder. 2008. Gender differences in the n-3 fatty acid content of tissues. *Proceedings of the Nutrition Society* 67(1): 19-27.

Curtis, C.L., C.E. Hughes, C.R. Flannery, C.B. Little, J.L. Harwood, and B. Caterson. 2000. n-3 fatty acids specifically modulate catabolic factors involved in articular cartilage degradation. *Journal of Biological Chemistry* 275(2): 721-724.

Delarue, J., O. Matzinger, C. Binnert, P. Schneiter, R. Chiolero, and L. Tappy. 2003. Fish oil prevents the adrenal activation elicited by mental stress in healthy men. *Diabetes and Metabolism* 29(3): 289-295.

Dorgan, J.F., J.T. Judd, C. Longcope, C. Brown, A. Schatzkin, B.A. Clevidence, W.S. Campbell, P.P. Nair, C. Franz, L. Kahle, and P.R. Taylor. 1996. Effects of dietary fat and fiber on plasma and urine androgens and estrogens in men: A controlled feeding study. *American Journal of Clinical Nutrition* 64(6): 850-855.

Ehringer, W., D. Belcher, S.R. Wassall, and W. Stillwell. 1990. A comparison of the effects of linolenic (18:3 omega 3) and docosahexaenoic (22:6 omega 3) acids on phospholipid bilayers. *Chemistry of Physics and Lipids* 54(2): 79-88.

Endres, S., R. Ghorbani, V. Kelley, K. Georgilis, G.J. Lonnemann, J. van der Meer, J. Cannon, T. Rogers, M. Klempner, and P. Weber. 1989. The effect of dietary supplementation with n-3 polyunsaturated fatty acids on the synthesis of interleukin-1 and tumor necrosis factor by mononuclear cells. *New England Journal of Medicine* 320(5): 265-271.

Fernandes, G., R. Lawrence, and D. Sun. 2003. Protective role of n-3 lipids and soy protein in osteoporosis. *Prostaglandins, Leukotrienes and Essential Fatty Acids* 68(6): 361-372.

Fleming, J., M.J. Sharman, N.G. Avery, D.M. Love, A.L. Gomez, T.P. Scheett, W.J. Kraemer, and J.S. Volek. 2003. Endurance capacity and high-intensity exercise performance responses to a high fat diet. *International Journal of Sport Nutrition and Exercise Metabolism* 13(4): 466-478.

Flickinger, B.D., and N. Matsuo. 2003. Nutritional characteristics of DAG oil. *Lipids* 38(2): 129-132.

Hamalainen, E.K., H. Adlercreutz, P. Puska, and P. Pietinen. 1983. Decrease of serum total and free testosterone during a low-fat high-fibre diet. *Journal of Steroid Biochemistry* 18(3): 369-370.

Hargreaves, M., J. Hawley, and A. Jeukendrup. 2004. Pre-exercise carbohydrate and fat ingestion: Effects on metabolism and performance. *Journal of Sports Science and Medicine* 22: 31-38.

Hawley, J.A., S.C. Dennis, F.H. Lindsay, and T.D. Noakes. 1995. Nutritional practices of athletes: Are they sub-optimal? *Journal of Sports Science and Medicine* 13: S75-S81.

Helge, J.W., B.J. Wu, M. Willer, J.R. Daugaard, L.H. Storlien, and B. Kiens. 2001. Training affects muscle phospholipid fatty acid composition in humans. *Journal of Applied Physiology* 90(2): 670-677.

Hoffman, D.R., R.C. Theuer, Y.S. Castañeda, D.H. Wheaton, R.G. Bosworth, A.R. O'Connor, S.E. Morale, L.E. Wiedemann, and E.E. Birch. 2004. Maturation of visual acuity is accelerated in breast-fed term infants fed baby food containing DHA-enriched egg yolk. *Journal of Nutrition* 134(9): 2307-2313.

Horowitz, J.F., R. Mora-Rodriguez, L.O. Byerley, and E.F. Coyle. 2000. Preexercise medium-chain triglyceride ingestion does not alter muscle glycogen use during exercise. *Journal of Applied Physiology* 88(1): 219-225.

Horvath, P.J., C.K. Eagen, N.M. Fisher, J.J. Leddy, and D.R. Pendergast. 2000. The effects of varying dietary fat on performance and metabolism in trained male and female runners. *Journal of the American College of Nutrition* 19(1): 52-60.

Innis, S. 2008. Dietary omega 3 fatty acids and the developing brain. *Brain Research* 1237: 35-43.

Institute of Medicine. 2002. *Dietary reference intakes for energy, carbohydrate, fiber, fat, fatty acids, cholesterol, protein, and amino acids,* 335-432. Washington, DC: National Academies Press.

Institute of Medicine. 2005. *Dietary reference intakes for energy, carbohydrate, fiber, fat, fatty acids, cholesterol, protein, and amino acids.* Washington, DC: National Academies Press.

Jeukendrup, A.E., J.J. Thielen, A.J. Wagenmakers, F. Brouns, and W.H. Saris. 1998. Effect of medium-chain triacylglycerol and carbohydrate ingestion during exercise on substrate utilization and subsequent cycling performance. *American Journal of Clinical Nutrition* 67(3): 397-404.

Kapoor, R., and Y.S. Huang. 2006. Gamma linolenic acid: An antiinflammatory omega-6 fatty acid. *Current Pharmaceutical Biotechnology* 7(6): 531-534.

Klein, S., E.F. Coyle, and R.R. Wolfe. 1994. Fat metabolism during low-intensity exercise in endurance-trained and untrained men. *American Journal of Physiology* 267(6) Pt 1: E934-940.

Kremer, J., W. Jubiz, A. Michalek, R. Rynes, L. Bartholomew, J. Bigaouette, M. Timchalk, D. Beeler, and L. Lininger. 1987. Fish-oil fatty acid supplementation in active rheumatoid arthritis: A double-blinded, controlled, crossover study. *Annals of Internal Medicine* 106: 497-503.

Lenn, J., T. Uhl, C. Mattacola, G. Boissonneault, J. Yates, W. Ibrahim, and G. Bruckner. 2002. The effects of fish oil and isoflavones on delayed onset muscle soreness. *Medicine and Science in Sports and Exercise* 34(10): 1605-1613.

Lindgren, B.F., E. Ruokonen, K. Magnusson-Borg, and J. Takala. 2001. Nitrogen sparing effect of structured triglycerides containing both medium-and long-chain fatty acids in critically ill patients; a double blind randomized controlled trial. *Clinical Nutrition* 20(1): 43-48.

Logan, A. 2003. Neurobehavioral aspects of omega-3 fatty acids: Possible mechanisms and therapeutic value in major depression. *Alternative Medicine Review* 8(4): 410-425.

Lowery, L. 1999. Effects of conjugated linoleic acid on body composition and strength in novice male bodybuilders. In: *International Conference on Weight Lifting and Strength Training conference book,* edited by K. Hakkinen, 241-242. Lahti, Finland: Gummerus.

Lowery, L. 2004. Dietary fat and sports nutrition: A primer. *Journal of Sports Science and Medicine* 3: 106-117.

Mann, N.J., L.G. Johnson, G.E. Warrick, and A.J. Sinclair. 1995. The arachidonic acid content of the Australian diet is lower than previously estimated. *Journal of Nutrition* 125(10): 2528-2535.

Mathews, E.M., and D.R. Wagner. 2008. Prevalence of overweight and obesity in collegiate American football players, by position. *Journal of American College Health* 57(1): 33-38.

McDonald, B. 2004. The Canadian experience: Why Canada decided against an upper limit for cholesterol. *Journal of the American College of Nutrition* 23(6 Suppl): 616S-620S.

Mensink, R.P. 2005. Effects of stearic acid on plasma lipid and lipoproteins in humans. *Lipids* 40(12): 1201-1205.

Meyer, B.J., N.J. Mann, J.L. Lewis, G.C. Milligan, A.J. Sinclair, and P.R. Howe. 2003. Dietary intakes and food sources of omega-6 and omega-3 polyunsaturated fatty acids. *Lipids* 38(4): 391-398.

Mickleborough, T.D., R.L. Murray, A.A. Ionescu, and M.R. Lindley. 2003. Fish oil supplementation reduces severity of exercise-induced bronchoconstriction in elite athletes. *American Journal of Respiratory and Critical Care Medicine* 168(10): 1181-1189.

Morcos, N.C., and K. Camilo. 2001. Acute and chronic toxicity study of fish oil and garlic combination. *International Journal for Vitamin and Nutrition Research* 71(5): 306-312.

Muskiet, F.A., M.R. Fokkema, A. Schaafsma, E.R. Boersma, and M.A. Crawford. 2004. Is docosahexaenoic acid (DHA) essential? Lessons from DHA status regulation, our ancient diet, epidemiology and randomized controlled trials. *Journal of Nutrition* 134(1): 183-186.

Pariza, M., Y. Park, and M. Cook. 2001. The biologically active isomers of conjugated linoleic acid. *Progress in Lipid Research* 40: 283-298.

Park, Y., K.J. Albright, W. Liu, J.M. Storkson, M.E. Cook, and M.W. Pariza. 1997. Effect of conjugated linoleic acid on body composition in mice. *Lipids* 32(8): 853-858.

Perez-Jimenez, F., J. Lopez-Miranda, and P. Mata. 2002. Protective effect of dietary mono-unsaturated fat on arteriosclerosis: Beyond cholesterol. *Atherosclerosis* 163(2): 385-398.

Phillips, T., A.C. Childs, D.M. Dreon, S. Phinney, and C. Leeuwenburgh. 2003. A dietary supplement attenuates IL-6 and CRP after eccentric exercise in untrained males. *Medicine and Science in Sports and Exercise* 35(12): 2032-2037.

Piper, S.N., K.D. Röhm, J. Boldt, B. Odermatt, W.H. Maleck, and S.W. Suttner. 2008. Hepatocellular integrity in patients requiring parenteral nutrition: Comparison of structured MCT/LCT vs. a standard MCT/LCT emulsion and a LCT emulsion. *European Journal of Anaesthesiology* 25(7): 557-565.

Raatz, S.K., D. Bibus, W. Thomas, and P. Kris-Etherton. 2001. Total fat intake modifies plasma fatty acid composition in humans. *Journal of Nutrition* 131(2): 231-234.

Rasmussen, O.W., C.H. Thomsen, K.W. Hansen, M. Vesterlund, E. Winther, and K. Hermansen. 1995. Favourable effect of olive oil in patients with non-insulin-dependent diabetes. The effect on blood pressure, blood glucose and lipid levels of a high-fat diet rich in mono-unsaturated fat compared with a carbohydrate-rich diet. *Ugeskr Laeger* 157(8): 1028-1032.

Reed, M.J., R.W. Cheng, M. Simmonds, W. Richmond, and V.H. James. 1987. Dietary lipids: An additional regulator of plasma levels of sex hormone binding globulin. *Journal of Clinical Endocrinology and Metabolism* 64(5): 1083-1085.

Richter, W. 2003. Long-chain omega-3 fatty acids from fish reduce sudden cardiac death in patients with coronary heart disease. *European Journal of Medical Research* 8(8): 332-336.

Riechman, S.E., R.D. Andrews, D.A. Maclean, and S. Sheather. 2007. Statins and dietary and serum cholesterol are associated with increased lean mass following resistance training. *Journals of Gerontology: Biological Sciences and Medical Sciences* 62(10): 1164-1171.

Sidossis, L.S., A. Gastaldelli, S. Klein, and R.R. Wolfe. 1997. Regulation of plasma fatty acid oxidation during low- and high-intensity exercise. *American Journal of Physiology* 272(6) Pt 1: E1065-1070.

Simopoulos, A. 2002. The importance of the ratio of omega-6/omega-3 essential fatty acids. *Biomedicine and Pharmacotherapy* 56(8): 365-379.

Simopoulos, A. 2007. Omega-3 fatty acids and athletics. *Current Sports Medicine Reports* 6(4): 230-236.

Stepto, N. 2002. Effect of short term fat adaptation on high intensity training. *Medicine and Science in Sports and Exercise* 34: 449-455.

Su, H.M., L. Bernardo, M. Mirmiran, X.H. Ma, P.W. Nathanielsz, and J.T. Brenna. 1999. Dietary 18:3n-3 and 22:6n-3 as sources of 22:6n-3 accretion in neonatal baboon brain and associated organs. *Lipids* 34 Suppl: S347-S350.

Su, K.P., S.Y. Huang, C.C. Chiu, and W.W. Shen. 2003. Omega-3 fatty acids in major depressive disorder. A preliminary double-blind, placebo-controlled trial. *European Neuropsychopharmacology* 13(4): 267-271.

Takeuchi, H., S. Sekine, K. Kojima, and T. Aoyama. 2008. The application of medium-chain fatty acids: Edible oil with a suppressing effect on body fat accumulation. *Asia Pacific Journal of Clinical Nutrition* 17 Suppl 1: 320-323.

Terpstra, A.H. 2004. Effect of conjugated linoleic acid on body composition and plasma lipids in humans: An overview of the literature. *American Journal of Clinical Nutrition* 79(3): 352-361.

Thomsen, C., O.W. Rasmussen, K.W. Hansen, M. Vesterlund, and K. Hermansen. 1995. Comparison of the effects on the diurnal blood pressure, glucose, and lipid levels of a diet rich in monounsaturated fatty acids with a diet rich in polyunsaturated fatty acids in type 2 diabetic subjects. *Diabetic Medicine* 12(7): 600-606.

U.S. Department of Health and Human Services and U.S. Department of Agriculture. 2005. *Dietary guidelines for Americans.* Washington, DC: U.S. Government Printing Office.

van Loon, L.J., R. Koopman, R. Manders, W. van der Weegen, G.P. van Kranenburg, and H.A. Keizer. 2004. Intramyocellular lipid content in type 2 diabetes patients compared with overweight sedentary men and highly trained endurance athletes. *American Journal of Physiology: Endocrinology and Metabolism* 287(3): E558-E565.

Van Zant, R.S., J.M. Conway, and J.L. Seale. 2002. A moderate carbohydrate and fat diet does not impair strength performance in moderately trained males. *Journal of Sports Medicine and Physical Fitness* 42(1): 31-37.

Venkatraman, J.T., X. Feng, and D. Pendergast. 2001. Effects of dietary fat and endurance exercise on plasma cortisol, prostaglandin E2, interferon-gamma and lipid peroxides in runners. *Journal of the American College of Nutrition* 20(5) (Oct): 529-536.

Venkatraman, J.T., J. Leddy, and D. Pendergast. 2000. Dietary fats and immune status in athletes: Clinical implications. *Medicine and Science in Sports and Exercise* 32(7 Suppl): S389-S395.

Vistisen, B., L. Nybo, X. Xu, C.E. Høy, and B. Kiens. 2003. Minor amounts of plasma medium-chain fatty acids and no improved time trial performance after consuming lipids. *Journal of Applied Physiology* 95(6): 2434-2443.

Vogt, M., A. Puntschart, H. Howald, B. Mueller, C. Mannhart, L. Gfeller-Tuescher, P. Mullis, and H. Hoppeler. 2003. Effects of dietary fat on muscle substrates, metabolism, and performance in athletes. *Medicine and Science in Sports and Exercise* 35(6) (Jun): 952-960.

Wang, Y.W., and P.J. Jones. 2004. Conjugated linoleic acid and obesity control: Efficacy and mechanisms. *International Journal of Obesity and Related Metabolic Disorders* 28(8): 941-955.

Weisinger, H.S., A.J. Vingrys, and A.J. Sinclair. 1996. The effect of docosahexaenoic acid on the electroretinogram of the guinea pig. *Lipids* 31(1): 65-70.

Whigham, L.D., A.C. Watras, and D.A. Schoeller. 2007. Efficacy of conjugated linoleic acid for reducing fat mass: A meta-analysis in humans. *American Journal of Clinical Nutrition* 85(5): 1203-1211.

Williams, M. 2005. *Nutrition for health, fitness and sport.* New York: McGraw-Hill.

Zderic, T.W., C.J. Davidson, S. Schenk, L.O. Byerley, and E.F. Coyle. 2004. High-fat diet elevates resting intramuscular triglyceride concentration and whole body lipolysis during exercise. *American Journal of Physiology: Endocrinology and Metabolism* 286(2): E217-E225.

Chapter 5

Armstrong, L.E., C.M. Maresh, J.W. Castellani, M.F. Bergeson, R.W. Kenefick, K.E. LaGasse, and D. Riebe. 1994. Urinary indices of hydration status. *International Journal of Sport Nutrition* 4(3): 265-279.

Ballauff, A., M. Kersting, and F. Manz. 1988. Do children have an adequate intake? Water balance studies carried out at home. *Annals of Nutrition and Metabolism* 32: 332-339.

Bar-Or, O. 1980. Climate and the exercising child. *International Journal of Sports Medicine* 1: 53-65.

Bar-Or, O. 1989. Temperature regulation during exercise in children and adolescents. In: *Perspectives in exercise science and sports medicine: Youth, exercise and sport,* edited by C.V. Gisolfi and D.R. Lamb. Carmel, IN: Benchmark Press.

Bar-Or, O. 1996. Thermoregulation in females from a life span perspective. In: *Perspectives in exercise science and sports medicine: Exercise and the female. A life span approach,* edited by O. Bar-Or, D.R. Lamb, and P.M. Clarkson. Carmel, IN: Cooper Publishing Group.

Bar-Or, O., S. Barr, M. Bergeron, R. Carey, P. Clarkson, L. Houtkooper, A. Rivera-Brown, T. Rowland, and S. Steen. 1997. Youth in sport: Nutritional needs. *Gatorade Sport Science Institute Sports Science Exchange Roundtable* 8(4).

Bar-Or, O., C.J.R. Blimkie, J.A. Hay, J.D. MacDougall, D.S. Ward, and W.M. Wilson. 1992. Voluntary dehydration and heat tolerance in patients with cystic fibrosis. *Lancet* 339: 696-699.

Beetham, R. 2000. Biochemical investigation of suspected rhabdomyolysis. *Annals of Clinical Biochemistry* 37: 581-587.

Bergeron, M.F., D.B. McKeag, D.J. Casa, P.M. Clarkson, R.W. Dick, E.R. Elchner, C.A. Horswill, A.C. Luke, F. Mueller, T.A. Munce, W.O. Roberts, and T.W. Rowland. 2005. Youth football: Heat stress and injury risk. *Medicine and Science in Sports and Exercise* 37: 1421-1430.

Burrell, L.M., J.M. Palmer, and P.H. Baylis. 1992. Atrial natriuretic peptide inhibits fluid intake in hyperosmolar subjects. *Clinical Science* 83: 35-39.

Campbell, W.W., and R.A. Geik. 2004. Nutritional considerations for the older adult. *Nutrition* 20: 603-608.

Cheuvront, S.N., R. Carter III, S.J. Montain, and M.N. Sawka. 2004. Daily body mass variability and stability in active men undergoing exercise-heat stress. *International Journal of Sport Nutrition and Exercise Metabolism* 14: 532-540.

Crowe, M.J., M.L. Forsling, B.J. Rolls, P.A. Phillips, J.G.G. Ledingham, and R.F. Smith. 1987. Altered water secretion in healthy elderly men. *Age and Aging* 16: 285-293.

Dunford, M. 2006. *Sports nutrition: A practice manual for professionals.* Chicago: American Dietetic Association.

Dunford, M., and J.A. Doyle. 2008. *Nutrition for sport and exercise.* Belmont, CA: Thompson Higher Education.

Epstein, M., and N.K. Hollenberg. 1976. Age as a determinant of renal sodium concentration. *Journal of Laboratory and Clinical Medicine* 87: 411-417.

Falk, B., O. Bar-Or, and J.D. MacDougall. 1992. Thermoregulatory responses of pre-mid- and late-pubertal boys. *Medicine and Science in Sports and Exercise* 24: 688-694.

Godek, S.F., A.R. Bartolozzi, R. Burkholder, E. Sugarman, and C. Peduzzi. 2008. Sweat rates and fluid turnover in professional football players: A comparison of National Football League lineman and backs. *Journal of Athletic Training* 43(2): 184-189.

Greiwe, J.S., K.S. Staffey, D.R. Melrose, M.D. Narve, and R.G. Knowlton. 1998. Effects of dehydration on isometric muscular strength and endurance. *Medicine and Science in Sports and Exercise* 30: 284-288.

Hayes, L.D., and C.I. Morse. 2010. The effects of progressive dehydration on strength and power: Is there a dose response? *European Journal of Applied Physiology* 108: 701-707.

Hew-Butler, T., C. Almond, J.C. Ayus, J. Dugas, W. Meeuwisse, T. Noakes, S. Reid, A. Siegel, D. Speedy, K. Stuempfle, J. Verbalis, and L. Weschler. 2005. Consensus statement of the 1st International Exercise-Associated Hyponatremia Consensus Development Conference, Cape Town, South Africa. *Clinical Journal of Sports Medicine* 15(4): 206-211.

Institute of Medicine. 1994. *Fluid replacement and heat stress.* Washington, DC: Committee on Military Nutrition Research, Food and Nutrition Board, Institute of Medicine.

Institute of Medicine. 2005. *Dietary reference intakes for water, sodium, chloride, potassium and sulfate,* 73-185. Washington, DC: National Academies Press.

Jeukendrup, A.E., R. Jentjens, and L. Moseley. 2005. Nutritional considerations in triathlon. *Sports Medicine* 35: 163-181.

Judelson, D.A., C.M. Maresh, J.M. Anderson, D.J. Casa, W.J. Kraemer, and J.S. Volek. 2007a. Hydration and muscular performance: Does fluid balance affect strength, power and high-intensity endurance? *Sports Medicine* 37: 907-921.

Judelson, D.A., C.M. Maresh, M.J. Farrell, L.M. Yamamoto, L.E. Armstrong, W.J. Kraemer, J.S. Volek, B.A. Spiering, D.J. Casa, and J.M. Anderson. 2007b. Effect of hydration state on strength, power, and resistance exercise performance. *Medicine and Science in Sports and Exercise* 39: 1817-1824.

Judelson, D.A., C.M. Maresh, L.M. Yamamoto, M.F. Farrell, L.E. Armstrong, W.J. Kraemer, J.S. Volek, B.A. Spiering, D.J. Casa, and J.M. Anderson. 2008. Effect of hydration state on resistance exercise-induced endocrine markers of anabolism, catabolism and metabolism. *Journal of Applied Physiology* 105: 816-824.

Kenney, W.L., and P. Chiu. 2001. Influence of age on thirst and fluid intake. *Medicine and Science in Sports and Exercise* 33(9): 1524-1532.

Kenney, W.L., and S.R. Fowler. 1988. Methylcholine-activated eccrine sweat gland density and output as a function of age. *Journal of Applied Physiology* 65: 1082-1086.

Kenney, W.L., C.G. Tankersley, D.L. Newswanger, D.E. Hyde, S.M. Puhl, and S.L. Turner. 1990. Age and hypohydration independently influence the peripheral vascular system response to heat stress. *Journal of Applied Physiology* 68: 1902-1908.

Kiningham, R.B., and D.W. Gorenflo. 2001. Weight loss methods of high school wrestlers. *Medicine and Science in Sports and Exercise* 33(5): 810-813.

Kirchengast, S., and M. Gartner. 2002. Changes in fat distribution (WHR) and body weight across the menstrual cycle. *Collegium Antropologicum* 26 Suppl: 47-57.

Knochel, J.P. 1992. Hypophosphatemia and rhabdomyolysis. *American Journal of Medicine* 92: 455-457.

Laursen, P.B., R. Suriano, M.J. Quod, H. Lee, C.R. Abbiss, K. Nosaka, D.T. Martin, and D. Bishop. 2006. Core temperature and hydration status during an Ironman triathlon. *British Journal of Sports Medicine* 40: 320-325.

Maughan, R., and S.M. Shirreffs. 2008. Development of individual hydration strategies for athletes. *International Journal of Sport Nutrition and Exercise Metabolism* 18: 457-472.

McArdle, W.D., F.I. Katch, and V.L. Katch. 2006. Factors affecting physiological function: The environment and special aids to performance. In: *Essentials of exercise physiology.* Baltimore: McGraw-Hill.

Meyer, F., O. Bar-Or, J.D. MacDougall, and J.F. Heigenhauser. 1992. Sweat electrolyte loss during exercise in the heat: Effects of gender and maturation. *Medicine and Science in Sports and Exercise* 24: 776-781.

Montain, S. 2008. Strategies to prevent hyponatremia during prolonged exercise. *Current Sports Medicine Reports* 7(4): S28-S35.

Noonan, B., G. Mack, and N. Stachenfeld. 2007. The effects of hockey protective equipment on high-intensity intermittent exercise. *Medicine and Science in Sports and Exercise* 39(8): 1327-1335.

Olsson, K., and B. Saltin. 2008. Variation in total body water with muscle glycogen changes in man. *Acta Physiologica Scandinavica* 80: 11-18.

Petrie, H.J., E.A. Stover, and C.A. Horswill. 2004. Nutritional concerns for the child and adolescent competitor. *Nutrition* 20: 620-631.

Phillips, P.A., M. Bretherton, C.I. Johnston, and L. Gray. 1993a. Reduced osmotic thirst in healthy elderly men. *American Journal of Physiology* 261: R166-R171.

Phillips, P.A., M. Bretherton, J. Risvanis, D. Casley, C. Johnston, and L. Gray. 1993b. Effects of drinking on thirst and vasopressin in dehydrated elderly men. *American Journal of Physiology* 264: R877-R881.

Ray, M.L., M.W. Bryan, T.M. Ruden, S.M. Baier, R.L. Sharp, and D.S. King. 1998. Effect of sodium in a rehydration beverage when consumed as a fluid or meal. *Journal of Applied Physiology* 85: 1329-1336.

Reaburn, P. 2000. Nutrition and the ageing athlete. In: *Clinical sports nutrition,* edited by L. Burke and V. Deakin. Melbourne: McGraw-Hill.

Rehrer, N.J., F. Brouns, E.J. Beckers, F. ten Hoor, and W.H. Saris. 1990. Gastric emptying with repeated drinking during running and bicycling. *International Journal of Sports Medicine* 11(3): 238-243.

Rolls, B.J., and P.A. Phillips. 1990. Aging and disturbances of thirst and fluid balance. *Nutrition Reviews* 48(3): 137-144.

Rosenbloom, C.A., and A. Dunaway. 2007. Nutrition recommendations for masters athletes. *Clinical Sports Medicine* 26: 91-100.

Rosenfeld, D., D. Livne, O. Nevo, L. Dayan, V. Milloul, S. Lavi, and G. Jacob. 2008. Hormonal and volume dysregulation in women with premenstrual syndrome. *Hypertension* 51(4): 1225-1230.

Sawka, M.N., L.M. Burke, E.R. Eichner, R.J. Maughan, S.J. Montain, and N.S. Stachenfeld. 2007. Exercise and fluid replacement position stand. *Medicine and Science in Sports and Exercise* 39(2): 377-389.

Sawka, M.N., and K.B. Pandolf. 1990. Effects of body water loss in physiological function and exercise performance. In: *Perspectives in exercise science and sports medicine: Fluid homeostasis during exercise,* edited by D.R. Lamb and C.V. Gisolfi. Indianapolis: Benchmark Press.

Sawka, M.N., C.B. Wenger, and K.B. Pandolf. 1996. Thermoregulatory responses to acute exercise-heat stress and heat acclimation. In: *Handbook of physiology, section 4: Environmental physiology,* edited by C.M. Blatteis and M.J. Fregly. New York: Oxford University Press for the American Physiological Society.

Seckl, J.R., T.D.M. Williams, and S.L. Lightman. 1986. Oral hypertonic saline causes transient fall of vasopressin in humans. *American Journal of Physiology* 251: R214-R217.

Seifert, J., J. Harmon, and P. DeClercq. 2006. Protein added to a sports drink improves fluid retention. *International Journal of Sport Nutrition and Exercise Metabolism* 16(4): 420-429.

Speedy, D.B., T.D. Noakes, and C. Schneider. 2001. Exercise-associated hyponatremia: A review. *Emergency Medicine Journal* 13: 17-27.

Tarnopolsky, M.A. 2008. Nutritional consideration in the aging athlete. *Clinical Journal of Sports Medicine* 18(6): 531-538.

Thompson, C.J., J. Burd, and P.H. Baylis. 1987. Acute suppression of plasma vasopressin and thirst after drinking in hypernatremic humans. *American Journal of Physiology* 240: R1138-R1142.

Unnithan, V.B., and S. Goulopoulou. 2004. Nutrition for the pediatric athlete. *Current Sports Medicine Reports* 3: 206-211.

Yamamoto, L.M., D.A. Judelson, M.F. Farrell, E.C. Lee, L.E. Armstrong, D.J. Casa, W.J. Kraemer, J.S. Volek, and C.M. Maresh. 2008. Effects of hydration state and resistance exercise on markers of muscle damage. *Journal of Strength and Conditioning Research* 22(5): 1387-1393.

Chapter 6

Aguilo, A., P. Tauler, A. Sureda, N. Cases, J. Tur, and A. Pons. 2007. Antioxidant diet supplementation enhances aerobic performance in amateur sportsmen. *Journal of Sports Sciences* 25(11): 1203-1210.

Beals, K.A., and M.M. Manore. 1998. Nutritional status of female athletes with subclinical eating disorders. *Journal of the American Dietetic Association* 98(4): 419-425.

Belko, A.Z., M.P. Meredith, H.J. Kalkwarf, E. Obarzanek, S. Weinberg, R. Roach, G. McKeon, and D.A. Roe. 1985. Effects of exercise on riboflavin requirements: Biological validation in weight reducing women. *American Journal of Clinical Nutrition* 41(2): 270-277.

Belko, A.Z., E. Obarzanek, R. Roach, M. Rotter, G. Urban, S. Weinberg, and D.A. Roe. 1984. Effects of aerobic exercise and weight loss on riboflavin requirements of moderately obese, marginally deficient young women. *American Journal of Clinical Nutrition* 40(3): 553-561.

Benson, J., D.M. Gillen, K. Bourdet, and A.R. Loosli. 1985. Inadequate nutrition and chronic calorie restriction in adolescent ballerinas. *Physician and SportsMedicine* 13: 79-90.

Beshgetoor, D., and J.F. Nichols. 2003. Dietary intake and supplement use in female master cyclists and runners. *International Journal of Sport Nutrition and Exercise Metabolism* 13(2): 166-172.

Bischoff-Ferrari, H.A., T. Dietrich, E.J. Orav, F.B. Hu, Y. Zhang, E.W. Karlson, and B. Dawson-Hughes. 2004. Higher 25-hydroxyvitamin D concentrations are associated with better lower-extremity function in both active and inactive persons aged > or =60 y. *American Journal of Clinical Nutrition* 80(3): 752-758.

Bredle, D.L., J.M. Stager, W.F. Brechue, and M.O. Farber. 1988. Phosphate supplementation, cardiovascular function, and exercise performance in humans. *Journal of Applied Physiology* 65(4): 1821-1826.

Brilla, L.R., and T.F. Haley. 1992. Effect of magnesium supplementation on strength training in humans. *Journal of the American College of Nutrition* 11(3): 326-329.

Brownlie, T. 4th, V. Utermohlen, P.S. Hinton, and J.D. Haas. 2004. Tissue iron deficiency without anemia impairs adaptation in endurance capacity after aerobic training in previously untrained women. *American Journal of Clinical Nutrition* 79(3): 437-443.

Brun, J.F., C. Dieu-Cambrezy, A. Charpiat, C. Fons, C. Fedou, J.P. Micallef, M. Fussellier, L. Bardet, and A. Orsetti. 1995. Serum zinc in highly trained adolescent gymnasts. *Biological Trace Element Research* 47(1-3): 273-278.

Brutsaert, T.D., S. Hernandez-Cordero, J. Rivera, T. Viola, G. Hughes, and J.D. Haas. 2003. Iron supplementation improves progressive fatigue resistance during dynamic knee extensor exercise in iron-depleted, nonanemic women. *American Journal of Clinical Nutrition* 77(2): 441-448.

Cannell, J.J., B.W. Hollis, M.B. Sorenson, T.N. Taft, and J.J. Anderson. 2009. Athletic performance and vitamin D. *Medicine and Science in Sports and Exercise* 41(5): 1102-1110.

Cannell, J.J., B.W. Hollis, M. Zasloff, and R.P. Heaney. 2008. Diagnosis and treatment of vitamin D deficiency. *Expert Opinion on Pharmacotherapy* 9(1): 107-118.

Ciocoiu, M., M. Badescu, and I. Paduraru. 2007. Protecting antioxidative effects of vitamins E and C in experimental physical stress. *Journal of Physiology and Biochemistry* 63(3): 187-194.

Cohen, J.L., L. Potosnak, O. Frank, and H. Baker. 1985. A nutritional and hematological assessment of elite ballet dancers. *Physician and SportsMedicine* 13: 43-54.

Cook, J.D., M.B. Reddy, J. Burri, M.A. Juillerat, and R.F. Hurrell. 1997. The influence of different cereal grains on iron absorption from infant cereal foods. *American Journal of Clinical Nutrition* 65(4): 964-969.

Deuster, P.A., and J.A. Cooper. 2006. Choline. In: *Sports nutrition,* edited by J.A. Driskell and I. Wolinsky. Boca Raton, FL: CRC Press.

Deuster, P.A., E. Dolev, S.B. Kyle, R.A. Anderson, and E.B. Schoomaker. 1987. Magnesium homeostasis during high-intensity anaerobic exercise in men. *Journal of Applied Physiology* 62(2): 545-550.

Deuster, P.A., S.B. Kyle, P.B. Moser, R.A. Vigersky, A. Singh, and E.B. Schoomaker. 1986. Nutritional survey of highly trained women runners. *American Journal of Clinical Nutrition* 44(6): 954-962.

Doyle, M.R., M.J. Webster, and L.D. Erdmann. 1997. Allithiamine ingestion does not enhance isokinetic parameters of muscle performance. *International Journal of Sport Nutrition* 7(1): 39-47.

Dressendorfer, R.H., and R. Sockolov. 1980. Hypozincemia in runners. *Physician and Sports-Medicine* 8: 97-100.

Economos, C.D., S.S. Bortz, and M.E. Nelson. 1993. Nutritional practices of elite athletes. Practical recommendations. *Sports Medicine (Auckland, NZ)* 16(6): 381-399.

Edgerton, V.R., Y. Ohira, J. Hettiarachchi, B. Senewiratne, G.W. Gardner, and R.J. Barnard. 1981. Elevation of hemoglobin and work tolerance in iron-deficient subjects. *Journal of Nutritional Science and Vitaminology* 27(2): 77-86.

Evans, G.W. 1989. The effect of chromium picolinate on insulin-controlled parameters in humans. *International Journal of Bioscience and Medical Research* 11: 163-180.

Faber, M., and A.J. Benade. 1991. Mineral and vitamin intake in field athletes (discus-, hammer-, javelin-throwers and shotputters). *International Journal of Sports Medicine* 12(3): 324-327.

Filaire, E., and G. Lac. 2002. Nutritional status and body composition of juvenile elite female gymnasts. *Journal of Sports Medicine and Physical Fitness* 42(1): 65-70.

Fletcher, R.H., and K.M. Fairfield. 2002. Vitamins for chronic disease prevention in adults. Clinical applications. *Journal of the American Medical Association* 287: 3127-3129.

Fogelholm, G.M., J.J. Himberg, K. Alopaeus, C.G. Gref, J.T. Laakso, J.J. Lehto, and H. Mussalo-Rauhamaa. 1992. Dietary and biochemical indices of nutritional status in male athletes and controls. *Journal of the American College of Nutrition* 11(2): 181-191.

Fogelholm, M., I. Ruokonen, J.T. Laakso, T. Vuorimaa, and J.J. Himberg. 1993. Lack of association between indices of vitamin B1, B2, and B6 status and exercise-induced blood lactate in young adults. *International Journal of Sport Nutrition* 3(2): 165-176.

Gaeini, A.A., N. Rahnama, and M.R. Hamedinia. 2006. Effects of vitamin E supplementation on oxidative stress at rest and after exercise to exhaustion in athletic students. *Journal of Sports Medicine and Physical Fitness* 46(3): 458-461.

Galbo, H., J.J. Holst, N.J. Christensen, and J. Hilsted. 1976. Glucagon and plasma catecholamines during beta-receptor blockade in exercising man. *Journal of Applied Physiology* 40(6): 855-863.

Gardner, G.W., V.R. Edgerton, B. Senewiratne, R.J. Barnard, and Y. Ohira. 1977. Physical work capacity and metabolic stress in subjects with iron deficiency anemia. *American Journal of Clinical Nutrition* 30(6): 910-917.

Golf, S.W., D. Bohmer, and P.E. Nowacki. 1993. Is magnesium a limiting factor in competitive exercise? A summary of relevant scientific data. In: *Magnesium,* edited by S. Golf, D. Dralle, and L. Vecchiet, 209-220. London: John Libbey.

Guilland, J.C., T. Penaranda, C. Gallet, V. Boggio, F. Fuchs, and J. Klepping. 1989. Vitamin status of young athletes including the effects of supplementation. *Medicine and Science in Sports and Exercise* 21(4): 441-449.

Haas, J.D., and T. Brownlie 4th. 2001. Iron deficiency and reduced work capacity: A critical review of the research to determine a causal relationship. *Journal of Nutrition* 131(2S-2): 676S, 688S; discussion 688S-690S.

Hallberg, L., M. Brune, M. Erlandsson, A.S. Sandberg, and L. Rossander-Hulten. 1991. Calcium: Effect of different amounts on nonheme- and heme-iron absorption in humans. *American Journal of Clinical Nutrition* 53(1): 112-119.

Hallberg, L., L. Hulten, and E. Gramatkovski. 1997. Iron absorption from the whole diet in men: How effective is the regulation of iron absorption? *American Journal of Clinical Nutrition* 66(2): 347-356.

Haymes, E.M. 2006. Iron. In: *Sports nutrition,* edited by J.A. Driskell and I. Wolinsky, 203-216. Boca Raton, FL: CRC Press.

Heath, E.M. 2006. Niacin. In: *Sports nutrition,* edited by J.A. Driskell and I. Wolinsky, 69-80. Boca Raton, FL: CRC Press.

Herrmann, M., R. Obeid, J. Scharhag, W. Kindermann, and W. Herrmann. 2005. Altered vitamin B12 status in recreational endurance athletes. *International Journal of Sport Nutrition and Exercise Metabolism* 15(4): 433-441.

Hickson, J.F. Jr., J. Schrader, and L.C. Trischler. 1986. Dietary intakes of female basketball and gymnastics athletes. *Journal of the American Dietetic Association* 86(2): 251-253.

Hinton, P.S., C. Giordano, T. Brownlie, and J.D. Haas. 2000. Iron supplementation improves endurance after training in iron-depleted, nonanemic women. *Journal of Applied Physiology* 88(3): 1103-1111.

Holick, M.F. 2007. Vitamin D deficiency. *New England Journal of Medicine* 357(3): 266-281.

Hoogendijk, W.J., P. Lips, M.G. Dik, D.J. Deeg, A.T. Beekman, and B.W. Penninx. 2008. Depression is associated with decreased 25-hydroxyvitamin D and increased parathyroid hormone levels in older adults. *Archives of General Psychiatry* 65(5): 508-512.

Institute of Medicine, Food and Nutrition Board. 1997. *Dietary reference intakes for calcium, phosphorus, magnesium, vitamin D, and fluoride.* Washington, DC: National Academies Press.

Institute of Medicine, Food and Nutrition Board. 1998. *Dietary references intakes for thiamin, riboflavin, niacin, vitamin B12, folate, pantothenic acid, biotin, and choline.* Washington, DC: National Academy Press.

Institute of Medicine, Food and Nutrition Board. 2000. *Dietary reference intakes for vitamin C, vitamin E, selenium, and carotenoids.* Washington, DC: National Academy Press.

Institute of Medicine, Food and Nutrition Board. 2001. *Dietary reference intakes for vitamin A, vitamin K, arsenic, boron, chromium, copper, iodine, iron, manganese, molybdenum, nickel, silicon, vanadium, and zinc.* Washington, DC: National Academy Press.

Institute of Medicine, Food and Nutrition Board. 2003. *Dietary reference intakes: Applications in dietary planning.* Washington, DC: National Academy Press.

Institute of Medicine, Food and Nutrition Board. 2005. *Dietary reference intakes for water, potassium, chloride, and sodium.* Washington, DC: National Academy Press.

Isaacson, A., and A. Sandow. 1963. Effects of zinc on responses of skeletal muscle. *Journal of General Physiology* 46: 655-677.

Johnston, C.S., P.D. Swan, and C. Corte. 1999. Substrate utilization and work efficiency during submaximal exercise in vitamin C depleted-repleted adults. *International Journal for Vitamin and Nutrition Research* 69(1): 41-44.

Keith, R.E. 2006. Ascorbic acid. In: *Sports nutrition,* edited by J.A. Driskell and I. Wolinsky, 29-46. Boca Raton, FL: CRC Press.

Keith, R.E., and L.A. Alt. 1991. Riboflavin status of female athletes consuming normal diets. *Nutrition Research* 11: 727-734.

Keith, R.E., K.A. O'Keeffe, L.A. Alt, and K.L. Young. 1989. Dietary status of trained female cyclists. *Journal of the American Dietetic Association* 89(11): 1620-1623.

Keys, A., A.F. Henschel, O. Michelsen, and J.M. Brozek. 1943. The performance of normal young men on controlled thiamin intakes. *Journal of Nutrition* 26: 399-415.

Khaled, S., J.F. Brun, J.P. Micallel, L. Bardet, G. Cassanas, J.F. Monnier, and A. Orsetti. 1997. Serum zinc and blood rheology in sportsmen (football players). *Clinical Hemorheology and Microcirculation* 17(1): 47-58.

Kirchner, E.M., R.D. Lewis, and P.J. O'Connor. 1995. Bone mineral density and dietary intake of female college gymnasts. *Medicine and Science in Sports and Exercise* 27(4): 543-549.

Kreider, R.B., G.W. Miller, M.H. Williams, C.T. Somma, and T.A. Nasser. 1990. Effects of phosphate loading on oxygen uptake, ventilatory anaerobic threshold, and run performance. *Medicine and Science in Sports and Exercise* 22(2): 250-256.

Krotkiewski, M., M. Gudmundsson, P. Backstrom, and K. Mandroukas. 1982. Zinc and muscle strength and endurance. *Acta Physiologica Scandinavica* 116(3): 309-311.

Lawrence, J.D., R.C. Bower, W.P. Riehl, and J.L. Smith. 1975. Effects of alpha-tocopherol acetate on the swimming endurance of trained swimmers. *American Journal of Clinical Nutrition* 28(3): 205-208.

Leklem, J.E. 1990. Vitamin B-6: A status report. *Journal of Nutrition* 120(Suppl 11): 1503-1507.

Lemmel, G. 1938. Vitamin C deficiency and general capacity for work. *Munchener Medizinische Wochenschrift* 85: 1381.

Loosli, A.R., and J. Benson. 1990. Nutritional intake in adolescent athletes. *Pediatric Clinics of North America* 37(5): 1143-1152.

Loosli, A.R., J. Benson, D.M. Gillen, and K. Bourdet. 1986. Nutritional habits and knowledge in competitive adolescent female gymnasts. *Physician and SportsMedicine* 14: 118-121.

Lukaski, H. 1999. Chromium as a supplement. *Annual Review of Nutrition* 19: 279-302.

Lukaski, H. 2004. Vitamin and mineral status: Effects on physical performance. *Nutrition* 20(7-8): 632-644.

Lukaski, H.C. 2005. Low dietary zinc decreases erythrocyte carbonic anhydrase activities and impairs cardiorespiratory function in men during exercise. *American Journal of Clinical Nutrition* 81(5): 1045-1051.

Lukaski, H.C. 2006. Zinc. In: *Sports nutrition,* edited by J.A. Driskell and I. Wolinsky, 217-234. Boca Raton, FL: CRC Press.

Lukaski, H.C. 2007. Effects of chromium(III) as a nutritional supplement. In: *The nutritional biochemistry of chromium(III),* edited by J.B. Vincent, 71-84. New York: Elsevier.

Lukaski, H.C., C.B. Hall, and W.A. Siders. 1991. Altered metabolic response of iron-deficient women during graded, maximal exercise. *European Journal of Applied Physiology and Occupational Physiology* 63(2): 140-145.

Lukaski, H.C., B.S. Hoverson, S.K. Gallagher, and W.W. Bolonchuk. 1990. Physical training and copper, iron, and zinc status of swimmers. *American Journal of Clinical Nutrition* 51(6): 1093-1099.

Lukaski, H.C., and F.H. Nielsen. 2002. Dietary magnesium depletion affects metabolic responses during submaximal exercise in postmenopausal women. *Journal of Nutrition* 132(5): 930-935.

Magkos, F., and M. Yannakoulia. 2003. Methodology of dietary assessment in athletes: Concepts and pitfalls. *Current Opinion in Clinical Nutrition and Metabolic Care* 6(5): 539-549.

Manore, M.M. 2000. Effect of physical activity on thiamine, riboflavin, and vitamin B-6 requirements. *American Journal of Clinical Nutrition* 72(2 Suppl): 598S-606S.

Marzani, B., M. Balage, A. Vénien, T. Astruc, I. Papet, D. Dardevet, and L. Mosoni. 2008. Antioxidant supplementation restores defective leucine stimulation of protein synthesis in skeletal muscle from old rats. *Journal of Nutrition* 138(11): 2205-2211.

Matter, M., T. Stittfall, J. Graves, K. Myburgh, B. Adams, P. Jacobs, and T.D. Noakes. 1987. The effect of iron and folate therapy on maximal exercise performance in female marathon runners with iron and folate deficiency. *Clinical Science* 72(4): 415-422.

McClung, J.P., L.J. Marchitelli, K.E. Friedl, and A.J. Young. 2006. Prevalence of iron deficiency and iron deficiency anemia among three populations of female military personnel in the US army. *Journal of the American College of Nutrition* 25(1): 64-69.

Monsen, E.R. 1988. Iron nutrition and absorption: Dietary factors which impact iron bioavailability. *Journal of the American Dietetic Association* 88(7): 786-790.

Montoye, H.J., P.J. Spata, V. Pinckney, and L. Barron. 1955. Effects of vitamin B12 supplementation on physical fitness and growth of young boys. *Journal of Applied Physiology* 7(6): 589-592.

Murray, R., W.P. Bartoli, D.E. Eddy, and M.K. Horn. 1995. Physiological and performance responses to nicotinic-acid ingestion during exercise. *Medicine and Science in Sports and Exercise* 27(7): 1057-1062.

Niekamp, R.A., and J.T. Baer. 1995. In-season dietary adequacy of trained male cross-country runners. *International Journal of Sport Nutrition* 5(1): 45-55.

Nielsen, F.H., and H.C. Lukaski. 2006. Update on the relationship between magnesium and exercise. *Magnesium Research* 19(3): 180-189.

Pernow, B., and B. Saltin. 1971. Availability of substrates and capacity for prolonged heavy exercise in man. *Journal of Applied Physiology* 31(3): 416-422.

Peters, A.J., R.H. Dressendorfer, J. Rimar, and C.L. Keen. 1986. Diet of endurance runners competing in a 20-day road race. *Physician and SportsMedicine* 14: 63-70.

Pfeifer, M., B. Begerow, and H.W. Minne. 2002. Vitamin D and muscle function. *Osteoporosis International* 13(3): 187-194.

Plotnikoff, G.A., and J.M. Quigley. 2003. Prevalence of severe hypovitaminosis D in patients with persistent, nonspecific musculoskeletal pain. *Mayo Clinic Proceedings* 78(12): 1463-1470.

Read, M.H., and S.L. McGuffin. 1983. The effect of B-complex supplementation on endurance performance. *Journal of Sports Medicine and Physical Fitness* 23(2): 178-184.

Richardson, J.H., and P.D. Drake. 1979. The effects of zinc on fatigue of striated muscle. *Journal of Sports Medicine and Physical Fitness* 19(2): 133-134.

Rodriguez, N.R., N.M. DiMarco, and S. Langley. 2009. Position of the American Dietetic Association, Dietitians of Canada, and the American College of Sports Medicine: Nutrition and athletic performance. *Journal of the American Dietetic Association* 109(3): 509-527.

Rokitzki, L., E. Logemann, G. Huber, E. Keck, and J. Keul. 1994. Alpha-tocopherol supplementation in racing cyclists during extreme endurance training. *International Journal of Sport Nutrition* 4(3) (Sep): 253-264.

Rowland, T.W., M.B. Deisroth, G.M. Green, and J.F. Kelleher. 1988. The effect of iron therapy on the exercise capacity of nonanemic iron-deficient adolescent runners. *American Journal of Diseases of Children* 142(2): 165-169.

Schoene, R.B., P. Escourrou, H.T. Robertson, K.L. Nilson, J.R. Parsons, and N.J. Smith. 1983. Iron repletion decreases maximal exercise lactate concentrations in female athletes with minimal iron-deficiency anemia. *Journal of Laboratory and Clinical Medicine* 102(2): 306-312.

Sharman, I.M., M.G. Down, and N.G. Norgan. 1976. The effects of vitamin E on physiological function and athletic performance of trained swimmers. *Journal of Sports Medicine and Physical Fitness* 16(3): 215-225.

Sharman, I.M., M.G. Down, and R.N. Sen. 1971. The effects of vitamin E and training on physiological function and athletic performance in adolescent swimmers. *British Journal of Nutrition* 26(2): 265-276.

Shephard, R.J., R. Campbell, P. Pimm, D. Stuart, and G.R. Wright. 1974. Vitamin E, exercise, and the recovery from physical activity. *European Journal of Applied Physiology and Occupational Physiology* 33(2): 119-126.

Short, S.H., and W.R. Short. 1983. Four-year study of university athletes' dietary intake. *Journal of the American Dietetic Association* 82(6): 632-645.

Siegenberg, D., R.D. Baynes, T.H. Bothwell, B.J. Macfarlane, R.D. Lamparelli, N.G. Car, P. MacPhail, U. Schmidt, A. Tal, and F. Mayet. 1991. Ascorbic acid prevents the dose-dependent inhibitory effects of polyphenols and phytates on nonheme-iron absorption. *American Journal of Clinical Nutrition* 53(2): 537-541.

Simon-Schnass, I., and H. Pabst. 1988. Influence of vitamin E on physical performance. *International Journal for Vitamin and Nutrition Research* 58(1): 49-54.

Singh, A., P.A. Deuster, and P.B. Moser. 1990. Zinc and copper status in women by physical activity and menstrual status. *Journal of Sports Medicine and Physical Fitness* 30(1): 29-36.

Singh, A., F.M. Moses, and P.A. Deuster. 1992. Chronic multivitamin-mineral supplementation does not enhance physical performance. *Medicine and Science in Sports and Exercise* 24: 726-732.

Soric, M., M. Misigoj-Durakovic, and Z. Pedisic. 2008. Dietary intake and body composition of prepubescent female aesthetic athletes. *International Journal of Sport Nutrition and Exercise Metabolism* 18(3): 343-354.

South, P.K., and D.D. Mille. 1998. Iron binding by tannic acid: Effects of selected ligands. *Food Chemistry* 63(2): 167-172.

Speich, M., A. Pineau, and F. Ballereau. 2001. Minerals, trace elements and related biological variables in athletes and during physical activity. *Clinical Chimica Acta* 312: 1-11.

Stacewicz-Sapuntzakis, M., and G. Borthakur. 2006. Vitamin A. In: *Sports nutrition,* edited by J.A. Driskell and I. Wolinsky, 163-174. Boca Raton, FL: CRC Press.

Steen, S.N., K. Mayer, K.D. Brownell, and T.A. Wadden. 1995. Dietary intake of female collegiate heavyweight rowers. *International Journal of Sport Nutrition* 5(3): 225-231.

Steen, S.N., and S. McKinney. 1986. Nutritional assessment of college wrestlers. *Physician and SportsMedicine* 14: 101-116.

Stofan, J.R., J.J. Zachwieja, C.A. Horswill, R. Murray, S.A. Anderson, and E.R. Eichner. 2005. Sweat and sodium losses in NCAA football players: A precursor to heat cramps? *International Journal of Sport Nutrition and Exercise Metabolism* 15(6): 641-652.

Suboticanec, K., A. Stavljenic, W. Schalch, and R. Buzina. 1990. Effects of pyridoxine and riboflavin supplementation on physical fitness in young adolescents. *International Journal for Vitamin and Nutrition Research* 60(1): 81-88.

Telford, R.D., E.A. Catchpole, V. Deakin, A.G. Hahn, and A.W. Plank. 1992. The effect of 7 to 8 months of vitamin/mineral supplementation on athletic performance. *International Journal of Sport Nutrition* 2(2): 135-153.

Tin-May-Than, Ma-Win-May, Khin-Sann-Aung, and M. Mya-Tu. 1978. The effect of vitamin B12 on physical performance capacity. *British Journal of Nutrition* 40(2): 269-273.

van der Beek, E.J., W. van Dokkum, J. Schrijver, A. Wesstra, C. Kistemaker, and R.J. Hermus. 1990. Controlled vitamin C restriction and physical performance in volunteers. *Journal of the American College of Nutrition* 9(4): 332-339.

van der Beek, E.J., W. van Dokkum, M. Wedel, J. Schrijver, and H. van den Berg. 1994. Thiamin, riboflavin and vitamin B6: Impact of restricted intake on physical performance in man. *Journal of the American College of Nutrition* 13(6): 629-640.

Van Loan, M.D., B. Sutherland, N.M. Lowe, J.R. Turnlund, and J.C. King. 1999. The effects of zinc depletion on peak force and total work of knee and shoulder extensor and flexor muscles. *International Journal of Sport Nutrition* 9(2): 125-135.

Vincent, J.B. 2003. The potential value and toxicity of chromium picolinate as a nutritional supplement, weight loss agent and muscle development agent. *Sports Medicine* 33(3): 213-30.

Virk, R.S., N.J. Dunton, J.C. Young, and J.E. Leklem. 1999. Effect of vitamin B-6 supplementation on fuels, catecholamines, and amino acids during exercise in men. *Medicine and Science in Sports and Exercise* 31(3): 400-408.

Volek, J.S., R. Silvestre, J.P. Kirwan, M.J. Sharman, D.A. Judelson, B.A. Spiering, J.L. Vingren, C.M. Maresh, J.L. Vanheest, and W.J. Kraemer. 2006. Effects of chromium supplementation on glycogen synthesis after high-intensity exercise. *Medicine and Science in Sports and Exercise* 38(12): 2102-2109.

Volpe, S.L. 2007. Micronutrient requirements for athletes. *Clinics in Sports Medicine* 26(1): 119-130.

Wald, G., L. Brougha, and R. Johnson. 1942. Experimental human vitamin A deficiency and ability to perform muscular exercise. *American Journal of Physiology* 137: 551-554.

Watt, T., T.T. Romet, I. McFarlane, D. McGuey, C. Allen, and R.C. Goode. 1974. Letter: Vitamin E and oxygen consumption. *Lancet* 2(7876): 354-355.

Webster, M.J. 1998. Physiological and performance responses to supplementation with thiamin and pantothenic acid derivatives. *European Journal of Applied Physiology and Occupational Physiology* 77(6): 486-491.

Weight, L.M., K.H. Myburgh, and T.D. Noakes. 1998. Vitamin and mineral supplementation: Effect on the running performance of trained athletes. *American Journal of Clinical Nutrition* 47: 192-195.

Welch, P.K., K.A. Zager, J. Endres, and S.W. Poon. 1987. Nutrition education, body composition and dietary intake of female college athletes. *Physician and SportsMedicine* 15: 63-74.

Williams, M.H. 2004. Dietary supplements and sports performance: Introduction and vitamins. *Journal of the International Society of Sports Nutrition* 1(2): 1-6.

Williams, M.H. 2005. Dietary supplements and sports performance: Minerals. *Journal of the International Society of Sports Nutrition* 2(1): 43-49.

Wood, B., A. Gijsbers, A. Goode, S. Davis, J. Mulholland, and K. Breen. 1980. A study of partial thiamin restriction in human volunteers. *American Journal of Clinical Nutrition* 33(4): 848-861.

Woolf, K., and M.M. Manore. 2006. B-vitamins and exercise: Does exercise alter requirements? *International Journal of Sport Nutrition and Exercise Metabolism* 16(5): 453-484.

Ziegler, P.J., J.A. Nelson, and S.S. Jonnalagadda. 1999. Nutritional and physiological status of U.S. national figure skaters. *International Journal of Sport Nutrition* 9(4): 345-360.

Chapter 7

Armstrong, L.E. 2002. Caffeine, body fluid-electrolyte balance, and exercise performance. *International Journal of Sport Nutrition and Exercise Metabolism* 12: 189-206.

Balsom, P.D., K. Soderlund, and B. Ekblom. 1994. Creatine in humans with special reference to creatine supplementation. *Sports Medicine* 18(4): 268-280.

Besset, A., A. Bonardet, G. Rondouin, B. Descomps, and P. Passouant. 1982. Increase in sleep related GH and Prl secretion after chronic arginine aspartate administration in man. *Acta Endocrinologica (Copenhagen)* 99: 18-23.

Biolo, G., S.P. Maggi, B.D. Williams, K.D. Tipton, and R.R. Wolfe. 1995. Increased rates of muscle protein turnover and amino acid transport after resistance exercise in humans. *American Journal of Physiology* 268(3 Pt 1): E514-E20.

Biolo, G., K.D. Tipton, S. Klein, and R.R. Wolfe. 1997. An abundant supply of amino acids enhances the metabolic effect of exercise on muscle protein. *American Journal of Physiology* 273(1 Pt 1): E122-E129.

Boirie, Y., M. Dangin, P. Gachon, M.P. Vasson, J.L. Maubois, and B. Beaufrere. 1997. Slow and fast dietary proteins differently modulate postprandial protein accretion. *Proceedings of the National Academy of Sciences* 94(26): 14930-14935.

Branch, J.D. 2003. Effect of creatine supplementation on body composition and performance: A meta-analysis. *International Journal of Sport Nutrition and Exercise Metabolism* 13(2): 198-226.

Brose, A., G. Parise, and M.A. Tarnopolsky. 2003. Creatine supplementation enhances isometric strength and body composition improvements following strength exercise training in older adults. *Journals of Gerontology: Series A, Biological Sciences and Medical Sciences* 58(1): B11-B19.

Brown, G.A., M.D. Vukovich, E.R. Martini, M.L. Kohut, W.D. Franke, D.A. Jackson, and D.S. King. 2000. Endocrine responses to chronic androstenedione intake in 30- to 56-year-old men. *Journal of Clinical Endocrinology and Metabolism* 85: 4074-4080.

Brown, G.A., M.D. Vukovich, R.L. Sharp, T.A. Reifenrath, K.A. Parsons, and D.S. King. 1999. Effect of oral DHEA on serum testosterone and adaptations to resistance training in young men. *Journal of Applied Physiology* 87: 2274-2283.

Buford, T.W., R.B. Kreider, J.R. Stout, M. Greenwood, B. Campbell, M. Spano, T. Ziegenfuss, H. Lopez, J. Landis, and J. Antonio. 2007. International society of sports nutrition position stand: Creatine supplementation and exercise. *Journal of the International Society of Sports Nutrition* 4: 6.

Campbell, B., R.B. Kreider, T. Ziegenfuss, P. La Bounty, M. Roberts, D. Burke, J. Landis, H. Lopez, and J. Antonio. 2007. International society of sports nutrition position stand: Protein and exercise. *Journal of the International Society of Sports Nutrition* 4: 8.

Campbell, B., M. Roberts, C. Kerksick, C. Wilborn, B. Marcello, L. Taylor, E. Nassar, B. Leutholtz, R. Bowden, C. Rasmussen, M. Greenwood, and R. Kreider. 2006. Pharmacokinetics, safety, and effects on exercise performance of l-arginine alpha-ketoglutarate in trained adult men. *Nutrition* 22: 872-881.

Candow, D.G., P.D. Chilibeck, D.G. Burke, K.S. Davison, and T. Smith-Palmer. 2001. Effect of glutamine supplementation combined with resistance training in young adults. *European Journal of Applied Physiology* 86: 142-149.

Castell, L.M., and E.A. Newsholme. 1997. The effects of oral glutamine supplementation on athletes after prolonged, exhaustive exercise. *Nutrition* 13(7-8): 738-742.

Chrusch, M.J., P.D. Chilibeck, K.E. Chad, K.S. Davison, and D.G. Burke. 2001. Creatine supplementation combined with resistance training in older men. *Medicine and Science in Sports and Exercise* 33(12): 2111-2117.

Clarkson, P.M. 1993. Nutritional ergogenic aids: Caffeine. *International Journal of Sport Nutrition* 3: 103-111.

Costill, D.L., G.P. Dalsky, and W.J. Fink. 1978. Effects of caffeine ingestion on metabolism and exercise performance. *Medicine and Science in Sports* 10: 155-158.

Cribb, P.J., A.D. Williams, M.F. Carey, and A. Hayes. 2006. The effect of whey isolate and resistance training on strength, body composition, and plasma glutamine. *International Journal of Sport Nutrition and Exercise Metabolism* 16(5): 494-509.

Dangin, M., Y. Boirie, C. Garcia-Rodenas, P. Gachon, J. Fauquant, P. Callier, O. Ballevre, and B. Beaufrere. 2001. The digestion rate of protein is an independent regulating factor of postprandial protein retention. *American Journal of Physiology: Endocrinology and Metabolism* 280(2): E340-348.

Demling, R.H., and L. DeSanti. 2000. Effect of a hypocaloric diet, increased protein intake and resistance training on lean mass gains and fat mass loss in overweight police officers. *Annals of Nutrition and Metabolism* 44(1): 21-29.

Driskell, J., and I. Wolinsky. 2000. *Energy-yielding macronutrients and energy metabolism in sports nutrition.* Boca Raton, FL: CRC Press.

Dunnett, M., and R.C. Harris. 1999. Influence of oral beta-alanine and L-histidine supplementation on the carnosine content of the gluteus medius. *Equine Veterinary Journal Supplement* 30: 499-504.

Earnest, C.P., P.G. Snell, R. Rodriguez, A.L. Almada, and T.L. Mitchell. 1995. The effect of creatine monohydrate ingestion on anaerobic power indices, muscular strength and body composition. *Acta Physiologica Scandinavica* 153(2): 207-209.

Eckerson, J.M., J.R. Stout, G.A. Moore, N.J. Stone, K. Nishimura, and K. Tamura. 2004. Effect of two and five days of creatine loading on anaerobic working capacity in women. *Journal of Strength and Conditioning Research* 18: 168.

Elam, R.P., D.H. Hardin, R.A. Sutton, and L. Hagen. 1989. Effects of arginine and ornithine on strength, lean body mass and urinary hydroxyproline in adult males. *Journal of Sports Medicine and Physical Fitness* 29: 52-56.

Esmarck, B., J.L. Andersen, S. Olsen, E.A. Richter, M. Mizuno, and M. Kjaer. 2001. Timing of postexercise protein intake is important for muscle hypertrophy with resistance training in elderly humans. *Journal of Physiology* 535(Pt 1): 301-311.

Falkoll, P., R. Sharp, S. Baier, D. Levenhagen, C. Carr, and S. Nissen. 2004. Effect of beta-hydroxy-beta-methylbutyrate, arginine, and lysine supplementation on strength, functionality, body composition, and protein metabolism in elderly women. *Nutrition* 20(5): 445-451.

Forslund, A.H., A.E. El-Khoury, R.M. Olsson, A.M. Sjodin, L. Hambraeus, and V.R. Young. 1999. Effect of protein intake and physical activity on 24-h pattern and rate of macronutrient utilization. *American Journal of Physiology* 276(5 Pt 1): E964-E976.

Friedman, J.E., and P.W. Lemon. 1989. Effect of chronic endurance exercise on retention of dietary protein. *International Journal of Sports Medicine* 10(2): 118-123.

Gallagher, P.M., J.A. Carrithers, M.P. Godard, K.E. Schulze, and S.W. Trappe. 2000a. Beta-hydroxy-beta-methylbutyrate ingestion, part I: Effects on strength and fat free mass. *Medicine and Science in Sports and Exercise* 32(12): 2109-2115.

Gallagher, P.M., J.A. Carrithers, M.P. Godard, K.E. Schulze, and S.W. Trappe. 2000b. Beta-hydroxy-beta-methylbutyrate ingestion, part II: Effects on hematology, hepatic and renal function. *Medicine and Science in Sports and Exercise* 32(12): 2116-2119.

Graham, T.E., and L.L. Spriet. 1991. Performance and metabolic responses to a high caffeine dose during prolonged exercise. *Journal of Applied Physiology* 71: 2292-2298.

Greenwood, M., J. Farris, R. Kreider, L. Greenwood, and A. Byars. 2000. Creatine supplementation patterns and perceived effects in select division I collegiate athletes. *Clinical Journal of Sport Medicine* 10(3): 191-194.

Greenwood, M., D.S. Kalman, and J. Antonio, eds. 2008. *Nutritional supplements in sports and exercise.* New York: Humana Press.

Greenwood, M., R.B. Kreider, C. Melton, C. Rasmussen, S. Lancaster, E. Cantler, P. Milnor, and A. Almada. 2003. Creatine supplementation during college football training does not increase the incidence of cramping or injury. *Molecular and Cellular Biochemistry* 244: 83-88.

Harris, R.C., C.A. Hill, H.J. Kim, L. Boobis, C. Sale, D.B. Harris, and J.A. Wise. 2005. Beta-alanine supplementation for 10 weeks significantly increased muscle carnosine levels. *FASEB Journal* 19: A1125.

Harris, R.C., M.J. Tallon, M. Dunnett, L. Boobis, J. Coakley, H.J. Kim, J.L. Fallowfield, C.A. Hill, C. Sale, and J.A. Wise. 2006. The absorption of orally supplied β-alanine and its effect on muscle carnosine synthesis in human vastus lateralis. *Amino Acids* 30(3): 279-289.

Heymsfield, S.B., C. Arteaga, C. McManus, J. Smith, and S. Moffitt. 1983. Measurement of muscle mass in humans: Validity of the 24-hour urinary creatinine method. *American Journal of Clinical Nutrition* 37(3): 478-494.

Hirvonen, J., S. Rehunen, H. Rusko, and M. Harkonen. 1987. Breakdown of high-energy phosphate compounds and lactate accumulation during short supramaximal exercise. *European Journal of Applied Physiology and Occupational Physiology* 56(3): 253-259.

Hoffman, J.R., J. Cooper, M. Wendell, J. Im, and J. Kang. 2004. Effects of b-hydroxy-b-methylbutyrate on power performance and indices of muscle damage and stress during high intensity training. *Journal of Strength and Conditioning Research* 18(94): 745-752.

Hoffman, J.R., N.A. Ratamess, A.D. Faigenbaum, R. Ross, J. Kang, J.R. Stout, and J.A. Wise. 2008a. Short duration beta-alanine supplementation increases training volume and reduces subject feelings of fatigue in college football players. *Nutrition Research* 28(1): 31-35.

Hoffman, J., N. Ratamess, J. Kang, G. Mangine, A. Faigenbaum, and J. Stout. 2006. Effect of creatine and beta-alanine supplementation on performance and endocrine responses in strength/power athletes. *International Journal of Sport Nutrition and Exercise Metabolism* 16(4): 430-446.

Hoffman, J., N.A. Ratamess, R. Ross, J. Kang, J. Magrelli, K. Neese, A.D. Faigenbaum, and J.A. Wise. 2008b. Beta-alanine and the hormonal response to exercise. *International Journal of Sports Medicine* 29(12): 952-958.

Hoffman, J.R., and J.R. Stout. 2008. Performance enhancing supplements. In: *Essentials of strength training and conditioning,* edited by T.R. Baechle and R.W. Earle. Champaign, IL: Human Kinetics.

Jones, A.M., T. Atter, and K.P. Georg. 1999. Oral creatine supplementation improves multiple sprint performance in elite ice-hockey players. *Journal of Sports Medicine and Physical Fitness* 39(3): 189-196.

Joyner, M.J. 2000. Over-the-counter supplements and strength training. *Exercise and Sport Sciences Reviews* 28: 2-3.

Kendrick, I.P., R.C. Harris, H.J. Kim, C.K. Kim, V.H. Dang, T.Q. Lam, T.T. Bui, M. Smith, and J.A. Wise. 2008. The effects of 10 weeks of resistance training combined with beta-alanine supplementation on whole body strength, force production, muscular endurance and body composition. *Amino Acids* 34(4): 547-554.

Kerksick, C.M., C.J. Rasmussen, S.L. Lancaster, B. Magu, P. Smith, C. Melton, M. Greenwood, A.L. Almada, C.P. Earnest, and R.B. Kreider. 2006. The effects of protein and amino acid supplementation on performance and training adaptations during ten weeks of resistance training. *Journal of Strength and Conditioning Research* 20(3): 643-653.

King, D.S., R.L. Sharp, M.D. Vukovich, G.A. Brown, T.A. Reifenrath, N.L. Uhl, K.A. Parsons, et al. 1999. Effect of oral androstenedione on serum testosterone and adaptations to resistance training in young men: A randomized controlled trial. *Journal of the American Medical Association* 281: 2020-2028.

Kirksey, K.B., M.H. Stone, B.J. Warren, R.L. Johnson, M. Stone, G.G. Haff, F.E. Williams, and C. Proulx. 1999. The effects of 6 weeks of creatine monohydrate supplementation on performance measures and body composition in collegiate track and field athletes. *Journal of Strength and Conditioning Research* 13: 148.

Knitter, A.E., L. Panton, J.A. Rathmacher, A. Petersen, and R. Sharp. 2000. Effects of beta-hydroxy-beta-methylbutyrate on muscle damage after a prolonged run. *Journal of Applied Physiology* 89(4): 1340-1344.

Kreider, R.B. 2003a. Effects of creatine supplementation on performance and training adaptations. *Molecular and Cellular Biochemistry* 244(1-2): 89-94.

Kreider, R.B. 2003b. Species-specific responses to creatine supplementation. *American Journal of Physiology: Regulatory, Integrative and Comparative Physiology* 285(4): R725-R726.

Kreider, R.B., M. Ferreira, M. Wilson, and A.L. Almada. 1999. Effects of calcium beta-hydroxy-beta-methylbutyrate (HMB) supplementation during resistance-training on markers of catabolism, body composition and strength. *International Journal of Sports Medicine* 20(8): 503-9.

Kreider, R.B., M. Ferreira, M. Wilson, P. Grindstaff, S. Plisk, J. Reinardy, E. Cantler, and A.L. Almada. 1998. Effects of creatine supplementation on body composition, strength, and sprint performance. *Medicine and Science in Sports and Exercise* 30(1): 73-82.

Kreider, R.B., R. Klesges, K. Harmon, P. Grindstaff, L. Ramsey, D. Bullen, L. Wood, Y. Li, and A. Almada. 1996. Effects of ingesting supplements designed to promote lean tissue accretion on body composition during resistance training. *International Journal of Sport Nutrition* 6(3): 234-246.

Kreider, R.B., B.C. Leutholtz, and M. Greenwood. 2004. Creatine. In: *Nutritional ergogenic aids,* edited by I. Wolinsky and J. Driskel, 81-104. Boca Raton, FL: CRC Press.

Kreider, R.B., C. Melton, C.J. Rasmussen, M. Greenwood, S. Lancaster, E.C. Cantler, P. Milnor, and A.L. Almada. 2003. Long-term creatine supplementation does not significantly affect clinical markers of health in athletes. *Molecular and Cellular Biochemistry* 244: 95-104.

Lamont, L.S., D.G. Patel, and S.C. Kalhan. 1990. Leucine kinetics in endurance-trained humans. *Journal of Applied Physiology* 69(1): 1-6.

Lemon, P.W. 1991. Protein and amino acid needs of the strength athlete. *International Journal of Sport Nutrition* 1(2): 127-145.

Lemon, P.W. 1998. Effects of exercise on dietary protein requirements. *International Journal of Sport Nutrition* 8(4): 426-447.

Lemon, P.W., M.A. Tarnopolsky, J.D. MacDougall, and S.A. Atkinson. 1992. Protein requirements and muscle mass/strength changes during intensive training in novice bodybuilders. *Journal of Applied Physiology* 73(2): 767-775.

Meredith, C.N., M.J. Zackin, W.R. Frontera, and W.J. Evans. 1989. Dietary protein requirements and body protein metabolism in endurance-trained men. *Journal of Applied Physiology* 66(6): 2850-2856.

Mero, A.A., K.L. Keskinen, M.T. Malvela, and J.M. Sallinen. 2004. Combined creatine and sodium bicarbonate supplementation enhances interval swimming. *Journal of Strength and Conditioning Research* 18(2): 306-310.

Mujika, I., S. Padilla, J. Ibanez, M. Izquierdo, and E. Gorostiaga. 2000. Creatine supplementation and sprint performance in soccer players. *Medicine and Science in Sports and Exercise* 32(2): 518-525.

Nissen, S., T.D. Faidley, D.R. Zimmerman, R. Izard, and C.T. Fisher. 1994. Colostral milk fat percentage and pig performance are enhanced by feeding the leucine metabolite beta-hydroxy-beta-methyl butyrate to sows. *Journal of Animal Science* 72(9): 2331-2337.

Nissen, S., R. Sharp, M. Ray, J.A. Rathmacher, D. Rice, J.C. Fuller Jr., A.S. Connelly, and N. Abumrad. 1996. Effect of leucine metabolite beta-hydroxy-beta-methylbutyrate on muscle metabolism during resistance-exercise training. *Journal of Applied Physiology* 81(5): 2095-2104.

Noonan, D., K. Berg, R.W. Latin, J.C. Wagner, and K. Reimers. 1998. Effects of varying dosages of oral creatine relative to fat free body mass on strength and body composition. *Journal of Strength and Conditioning Research* 12: 104.

O'Connor, D.M., and M.J. Crowe. 2003. Effects of beta-hydroxy-beta-methylbuterate and creatine monohydrate supplementation on the aerobic and anaerobic capacity of highly trained athletes. *Journal of Sports Medicine and Physical Fitness* 43: 64-68.

Ostojic, S.M. 2004. Creatine supplementation in young soccer players. *International Journal of Sport Nutrition and Exercise Metabolism* 14(1): 95-103.

Peeters, B., C. Lantz, and J. Mayhew. 1999. Effects of oral creatine monohydrate and creatine phosphate supplementation on maximal strength indices, body composition, and blood pressure. *Journal of Strength and Conditioning Research* 13: 3.

Peterson, A.L., M.A. Qureshi, P.R. Ferket, and J.C. Fuller Jr. 1999a. Enhancement of cellular and humoral immunity in young broilers by the dietary supplementation of beta-hydroxy-beta-methylbutyrate. *Immunopharmacology and Immunotoxicology* 21(2): 307-330.

Peterson, A.L., M.A. Qureshi, P.R. Ferket, and J.C. Fuller Jr. 1999b. In vitro exposure with beta-hydroxy-beta-methylbutyrate enhances chicken macrophage growth and function. *Veterinary Immunology and Immunopathology* 67(1): 67-78.

Phillips, S.M., S.A. Atkinson, M.A. Tarnopolsky, and J.D. MacDougall. 1993. Gender differences in leucine kinetics and nitrogen balance in endurance athletes. *Journal of Applied Physiology* 75(5): 2134-2141.

Phillips, S.M., K.D. Tipton, A. Aarsland, S.E. Wolf, and R.R. Wolfe. 1997. Mixed muscle protein synthesis and breakdown after resistance exercise in humans. *American Journal of Physiology* 273(1 Pt 1): E99-E107.

Phillips, S., K. Tipton, A. Ferrando, and R. Wolfe. 1999. Resistance training reduces the acute exercise-induced increase in muscle protein turnover. *American Journal of Physiology* 276(1 Pt 1): E118-E124.

Preen, D., B. Dawson, C. Goodman, S. Lawrence, J. Beilby, and S. Ching. 2001. Effect of creatine loading on long-term sprint exercise performance and metabolism. *Medicine and Science in Sports and Exercise* 33(5): 814-821.

Rasmussen, B.B., E. Volpi, D.C. Gore, and R.R. Wolfe. 2000. Androstenedione does not stimulate muscle protein anabolism in young healthy men. *Journal of Clinical Endocrinology and Metabolism* 85: 55-59.

Rennie, M.J., H. Wackerhage, E.E. Spangenburg, and F.W. Booth. 2004. Control of the size of the human muscle mass. *Annual Review of Physiology* 66: 799-828.

Rohle, D., C. Wilborn, L. Taylor, C. Mulligan, R. Kreider, and D. Willoughby. 2007. Effects of eight weeks of an alleged aromatase inhibiting nutritional supplement 6-OXO (androst-4-ene-3,6,17-trione) on serum hormone profiles and clinical safety markers in resistance-trained, eugonadal males. *Journal of the International Society of Sports Nutrition* 19(4): 13.

Skare, O.C., Skadberg, and A.R. Wisnes. 2001. Creatine supplementation improves sprint performance in male sprinters. *Scandinavian Journal of Medicine and Science in Sports* 11(2): 96-102.

Slater, G., D. Jenkins, P. Logan, H. Lee, M. Vukovich, J.A. Rathmacher, and A.G. Hahn. 2001. Beta-hydroxy-beta-methylbutyrate (HMB) supplementation does not affect changes in strength or body composition during resistance training in trained men. *International Journal of Sport Nutrition and Exercise Metabolism* 11(3): 384-396.

Stone, M.H., K. Sanborn, L.L. Smith, H.S. O'Bryant, T. Hoke, A.C. Utter, R L. Johnson, R. Boros, J. Hruby, K.C. Pierce, M.E. Stone, and B. Garner. 1999. Effects of in-season (5 weeks) creatine and pyruvate supplementation on anaerobic performance and body composition in american football players. *International Journal of Sport Nutrition* 9(2): 146-165.

Stout, J.R., J.T. Cramer, M. Mielke, J. O'Kroy, D.J. Torok, and R.F. Zoeller. 2006. Effects of twenty-eight days of beta-alanine and creatine monohydrate supplementation on the physical working capacity at neuromuscular fatigue threshold. *Journal of Strength and Conditioning Research* 20(4): 928-931.

Stout, J., J. Eckerson, K. Ebersole, G. Moore, S. Perry, T. Housh, A. Bull, J. Cramer, and A. Batheja. 2000. Effect of creatine loading on neuromuscular fatigue threshold. *Journal of Applied Physiology* 88(1): 109-112.

Stout, J.R., J. Eckerson, and D. Noonan. 1999. Effects of 8 weeks of creatine supplementation on exercise performance and fat-free weight in football players during training. *Nutrition Research* 19: 217.

Stout, J.R., B.S. Graves, A.E. Smith, M.J. Hartman, J.T. Cramer, T.W. Beck, and R.C. Harris. 2008. The effect of beta-alanine supplementation on neuromuscular fatigue in elderly (55-92 years): A double-blind randomized study. *Journal of the International Society of Sports Nutrition* 5: 21.

Tarnopolsky, M. 2004. Protein requirements for endurance athletes. *Nutrition* 20(7-8): 662-668.

Tarnopolsky, M.A., S.A. Atkinson, J.D. MacDougall, A. Chesley, S. Phillips, and H.P. Schwarcz. 1992. Evaluation of protein requirements for trained strength athletes. *Journal of Applied Physiology* 73(5): 1986-1995.

Tarnopolsky, M.A., and D.P. MacLennan. 2000. Creatine monohydrate supplementation enhances high-intensity exercise performance in males and females. *International Journal of Sport Nutrition and Exercise Metabolism* 10(4): 452-463.

Theodorou, A.S., C.B. Cooke, R.F. King, C. Hood, T. Denison, B.G. Wainwright, and K. Havenetidis. 1999. The effect of longer-term creatine supplementation on elite swimming performance after an acute creatine loading. *Journal of Sports Sciences* 17(11): 853-859.

Tipton, K.D., T.A. Elliot, M.G. Cree, S.E. Wolf, A.P. Sanford, and R.R. Wolf. 2004. Ingestion of casein and whey proteins result in muscle anabolism after resistance exercise. *Medicine and Science in Sports and Exercise* 36(12): 2073-2081.

Tipton, K.D., A.A. Ferrando, S.M. Phillips, D. Doyle Jr., and R.R. Wolfe. 1999. Postexercise net protein synthesis in human muscle from orally administered amino acids. *American Journal of Physiology* 276(4 Pt 1): E628-E634.

Vandenberghe, K., M. Goris, P. Van Hecke, M. Van Leemputte, L. Vangerven, and P. Hespel. 1997. Long-term creatine intake is beneficial to muscle performance during resistance training. *Journal of Applied Physiology* 83(6): 2055-2063.

Van Koevering, M.T., H.G. Dolezal, D.R. Gill, F.N. Owens, C.A. Strasia, D.S. Buchanan, R. Lake, and S. Nissen. 1994. Effects of beta-hydroxy-beta-methyl butyrate on performance and carcass quality of feedlot steers. *Journal of Animal Science* 72(8): 1927-1935.

van Loon, L.J., A.M. Oosterlaar, F. Hartgens, M.K. Hesselink, R.J. Snow, and A.J. Wagenmakers. 2003. Effects of creatine loading and prolonged creatine supplementation on body composition, fuel selection, sprint and endurance performance in humans. *Clinical Science* 104(2): 153-162.

van Someren, K.A., A.J. Edwards, and G. Howatson. 2003. The effects of HMB supplementation on indices of exercise induced muscle damage in man. *Medicine and Science in Sports and Exercise* 35(5): 270.

van Someren, K.A., A.J. Edwards, and G. Howatson. 2005. Supplementation with beta-hydroxy-beta-methylbutyrate (HMB) and alpha-ketoisocaproic acid (KIC) reduces signs and symptoms of exercise-induced muscle damage in man. *International Journal of Sport Nutrition and Exercise Metabolism* 15(4): 413-424.

Volek, J.S., N.D. Duncan, S.A. Mazzetti, R.S. Staron, M. Putukian, A.L. Gomez, D.R. Pearson, W.J. Fink, and W.J. Kraemer. 1999. Performance and muscle fiber adaptations to creatine supplementation and heavy resistance training. *Medicine and Science in Sports and Exercise* 3(8): 1147-1156.

Volek, J.S., W.J. Kraemer, J.A. Bush, M. Boetes, T. Incledon, K.L. Clark, and J.M. Lynch. 1997. Creatine supplementation enhances muscular performance during high-intensity resistance exercise. *Journal of the American Dietetic Association* 97(7): 765-770.

Vukovich, M.D., N.B. Stubbs, and R.M. Bohlken. 2001. Body composition in 70-year-old adults responds to dietary beta-hydroxy-beta-methylbutyrate similarly to that of young adults. *Journal of Nutrition* 131(7): 2049-2052.

Wagenmakers, A.J. 1999. Tracers to investigate protein and amino acid metabolism in human subjects. *Proceedings of the Nutrition Society* 58(4): 987-1000.

Welbourne, T.C. 1995. Increased plasma bicarbonate and growth hormone after an oral glutamine load. *American Journal of Clinical Nutrition* 61: 1058-1061.

Willoughby, D.S., and J. Rosene. 2001. Effects of oral creatine and resistance training on myosin heavy chain expression. *Medicine and Science in Sports and Exercise* 33(10): 1674-1681.

Willoughby, D.S., J.R. Stout, and C.D. Wilborn. 2007. Effects of resistance training and protein plus amino acid supplementation on muscle anabolism, mass, and strength. *Amino Acids* 32(4): 467-477.

Willoughby, D.S., C. Wilborn, L. Taylor, and B. Campbell. 2007. Eight weeks of aromatase inhibition using the nutritional supplement Novedex XT: Effects in young, eugonadal men. *International Journal of Sport Nutrition and Exercise Metabolism* 17: 92-108.

Wiroth, J.B., S. Bermon, S. Andrei, E. Dalloz, X. Hebuterne, and C. Dolisi. 2001. Effects of oral creatine supplementation on maximal pedalling performance in older adults. *European Journal of Applied Physiology* 84(6): 533-539.

Zoeller, R.F., J.R. Stout, J.A. O'kroy, D.J. Torok, and M. Mielke. 2007. Effects of 28 days of beta-alanine and creatine monohydrate supplementation on aerobic power, ventilatory and lactate thresholds, and time to exhaustion. *Amino Acids* 33(3): 505-510.

Chapter 8

Acheson, K.J., Y. Schutz, T. Bessard, K. Anantharaman, J.P. Flatt, and E. Jéquier. 1988. Glycogen storage capacity and de novo lipogenesis during massive carbohydrate overfeeding in man. *American Journal of Clinical Nutrition* 48(2): 240-247.

American College of Sports Medicine, American Dietetic Association, and Dietitians of Canada. 2000. Joint position statement: Nutrition and athletic performance. *Medicine and Science in Sports and Exercise* 32(12): 2130-2145.

Aulin, K.P., K. Soderlund, and F. Hultman. 2000. Muscle glycogen resynthesis rate in humans after supplementation of drinks containing carbohydrates with low and high molecular masses. *European Journal of Applied Physiology* 81: 346-351.

Baker, L.B., T.A. Munce, and W.L. Kenney. 2005. Sex differences in voluntary fluid intake by older adults during exercise. *Medicine and Science in Sports and Exercise* 37: 789-796.

Banister, E.W., M.E. Allen, I.B. Mekjavic, A.K. Singh, B. Legge, and B.J.C. Mutch. 1983. The time course of ammonia and lactate accumulation in blood during bicycle exercise. *European Journal of Applied Physiology* 51: 195-202.

Barr, S.I. 1999. Effects of dehydration on exercise performance. *Canadian Journal of Applied Physiology* 24(2): 164-172.

Bassit, R.A., L.A. Sawada, R.F.P. Bacarau, F. Navarro, and L.F.B.P. Costa Rosa. 2000. The effect of BCAA supplementation upon the immune response of triathletes. *Medicine and Science in Sports and Exercise* 32: 1214-1219.

Bell, D.G., and T.M. McLellan. 2003. Effect of repeated caffeine ingestion on repeated exhaustive exercise aerobic endurance. *Medicine and Science in Sports and Exercise* 35(8): 1348-1354.

Berardi, J.M., T.B. Price, E.E. Noreen, and P.W. Lemon. 2006. Postexercise muscle glycogen recovery enhanced with a carbohydrate-protein supplement. *Medicine and Science in Sports and Exercise* 38(60): 1106-1113.

Bernadot, D. 2006. *Advanced sports nutrition.* Champaign, IL: Human Kinetics.

Betts, J.A., C. Williams, L. Boobis, and K. Tsintzas. 2008. Increased carbohydrate oxidation after ingesting carbohydrate with added protein. *Medicine and Science in Sports and Exercise* 40(5): 903-912.

Blomstrand, E., E. Celsing, and E.A. Newsholme. 1988. Changes in plasma concentrations of aromatic and branched-chain amino acids during sustained exercise in man and their possible role in fatigue. *Acta Physiologica Scandinavica* 133(1): 115-121.

Blomstrand, E., P. Hassmen, S. Ek, B. Ekblom, and E.A. Newsholme. 1997. Influence of ingesting a solution of branched-chain amino acids on perceived exertion during exercise. *Acta Physiologica Scandinavica* 159(1): 41-49.

Blomstrand, E., P. Hassmen, B. Ekblom, and E.A. Newsholme. 1991. Administration of branched-chain amino acids during sustained exercise; effect on performance and on plasma concentration of some amino acids. *European Journal of Applied Physiology* 63: 83-88.

Brouns, F. 1991. Heat-sweat-dehydration-rehydration: A praxis oriented approach. *Journal of Sports Science* 9: 143-152.

Butterfield, G.E., and D.H. Calloway. 1984. Physical activity improves protein utilization in young men. *British Journal of Nutrition* 51: 171-184.

Carli, G., M. Bonifazi, L. Lodi, C. Lupo, G. Martelli, and A. Viti. 1992. Changes in the exercise-induced hormone response to branched chain amino acid administration. *European Journal of Applied Physiology and Occupational Physiology* 64: 272-277.

Castell, L.M. 2003. Glutamine supplementation in vitro and vivo, in exercise and in immunodepression. *Sports Medicine* 33: 323-345.

Coggan, A.R., and E.F. Coyle. 1991. Carbohydrate ingestion during prolonged exercise: Effects on metabolism and performance. *Exercise and Sport Sciences Reviews* 19: 1-40.

Coombes, J.S., and L.R. McNaughton. 2000. Effects of branched-chain amino acid supplementation on serum creatine kinase and lactate dehydrogenase after prolonged exercise. *Journal of Sports Medicine and Physical Fitness* 40: 240-246.

Cureton, K.J., G.L. Warren, M.L. Millard-Stafford, J.E. Wingo, J. Trilk, and M. Buyckx. 2007. Caffeinated sports drink: Ergogenic effects and possible mechanisms. *International Journal of Sport Nutrition and Exercise Metabolism* 17: 35-55.

Currell, K., and A.E. Jeukendrup. 2008. Superior aerobic endurance performance with ingestion of multiple transportable carbohydrates. *Medicine and Science in Sports and Exercise* 40(2): 275-281.

Demura, S., T. Yamada, and N. Terasawa. 2007. Effect of coffee ingestion on physiological responses and ratings of perceived exertion during submaximal aerobic endurance exercise. *Perceptual and Motor Skills* 105(3 Pt 2): 1109-1116.

Doherty, M., and P.M. Smith. 2004. Effects of caffeine ingestion on exercise testing: A meta-analysis. *International Journal of Sport Nutrition and Exercise Metabolism* 14(6): 626-646.

Dulloo, A.G., C.A. Geissler, T. Horton, A. Collins, and D.S. Miller. 1989. Normal caffeine consumption: Influence on thermogenesis and daily energy expenditure in lean and postobese human volunteers. *American Journal of Clinical Nutrition* 49(1): 44-50.

Dunford, M. 2006. *Sports nutrition: A practice manual for professionals.* 4th ed. American Dietetic Association. Chicago, IL.

Fredholm, B., K. Battig, J. Holmen, A. Nehlig, and E.E. Zvartau. 1999. Actions of caffeine in the brain with special reference to factors that contribute to its widespread use. *Pharmacological Reviews* 51(1): 83-133.

Fujisawa, T., J. Riby, and N. Kretchmer. 1991. Intestinal absorption of fructose in the rat. *Gastroenterology* 101: 360-367.

Gleeson, M. 2005. Interrelationship between physical activity and branched-chain amino acids. *Journal of Nutrition* 135: 1591S-1595S.

Goodpaster, B.H., D.L. Costill, W.J. Fink, T.A. Trappe, A.C. Jozi, R.D. Starling, and S.W. Trappe. 1996. The effects of pre-exercise starch ingestion on aerobic endurance performance. *International Journal of Sports Medicine* 17(5): 366-372.

Graham, T.E. 2001. Caffeine and exercise: Metabolism, aerobic endurance and performance. *Sports Medicine* 31: 785-807.

Graham, T.E., and L.L. Spriet. 1996. Caffeine and exercise performance. *Gatorade Sports Science Exchange* 9(1): 1-5.

Green, M.S., B.T. Corona, J.A. Doyle, and C.P. Ingalls. 2008. Carbohydrate-protein drinks do not enhance recovery from exercise-induced muscle injury. *International Journal of Sport Nutrition and Exercise Metabolism* 18: 1-18.

Greer, B.K., J.L. Woodard, J.P. White, E.M. Arguello, and E.M. Haymes. 2007. Branched-chain amino acid supplementation and indicators of muscle damage after aerobic endurance exercise. *International Journal of Sport Nutrition and Exercise Metabolism* 17: 595-607.

Halton, T.L., and F.B. Hu. 2004. The effects of high protein diets on thermogenesis, satiety and weight loss: A critical review. *Journal of the American College of Nutrition* 23(5): 373-385.

Hargreaves, M. 2004. Muscle glycogen and metabolic regulation. *Proceedings of the Nutrition Society* 63(2): 217-220.

Hassmen, P., E. Blomstrand, B. Ekblom, and E.A. Newsholme. 1994. Branched-chain amino acid supplementation during 30-km competitive run: Mood and cognitive performance. *Nutrition* 10(5): 405-410.

Hawley, J.A., and T. Reilly. 1997. Fatigue revisited. *Journal of Sports Science* 15: 245-246.

Hoffman, J.R., J. Kang, N.A. Ratamess, P.F. Jennings, G.T. Mangine, and A.D. Faigenbaum. 2007. Effect of nutritionally enriched coffee consumption on aerobic and anaerobic exercise performance. *Journal of Strength and Conditioning Research* 21(2): 456-459.

Jentjens, R.L., J. Achten, and A.E. Jeukendrup. 2004. High oxidation rates from combined carbohydrates ingested during exercise. *Medicine and Science in Sports and Exercise* 36: 1551-1558.

Jeukendrup, A., and M. Gleeson. 2004. *Sports nutrition: An introduction to energy production and performance.* Champaign, IL: Human Kinetics.

Johannsen, N.M., and R.L. Sharp. 2007. Effect of preexercise ingestion of modified cornstarch on substrate oxidation during aerobic endurance exercise. *International Journal of Sport Nutrition Exercise Metabolism* 17(3): 232-243.

Jozsi, A.C., T.A. Trappe, R.D. Starling, B.H. Goodpaster, S.W. Trappe, W.J. Fink, and D.L. Costill. 1996. The influence of starch structure on glycogen resynthesis and subsequent cycling performance. *International Journal of Sports Medicine* 17(5): 373-378.

Kiens, B., A.B. Raben, A.K. Valeur, and E.A. Richter. 1990. Benefit of dietary simple carbohydrates on the early post-exercise muscle glycogen repletion in male athletes. *Medicine ad Science in Sports and Exercise* 22: S88.

Koopman, R., D.L.E. Pannemans, A.E. Jeukendrup, A.P. Gijsen, J.M.G. Senden, D. Halliday, W.H. Saris, L.J. van Loon, and A.J. Wagenmakers. 2004. Combined ingestion of protein and carbohydrate improves protein balance during ultra-aerobic endurance exercise. *American Journal of Physiology, Endocrinology and Metabolism* 287: E712-E720.

Lamont, L.S., A.J. McCullough, and S.C. Kalhan. 1999. Comparison of leucine kinetics in aerobic endurance-trained and sedentary humans. *Journal of Applied Physiology* 86: 320-325.

Latner, J.D., and M. Schwartz. 1999. The effects of a high-carbohydrate, high-protein or balanced lunch upon later food intake and hunger ratings. *Appetite* 33(1): 119-128.

Leiper, J.B., K.P. Aulin, and K. Soderlund. 2000. Improved gastric emptying rate in humans of a unique glucose polymer with gel-forming properties. *Scandinavian Journal of Gastroenterology* 35: 1143-1149.

Lemon, P.W.R. 1998. Effects of exercise on dietary protein requirements. *International Journal of Sport Nutrition* 8: 426-447.

Lemon, P.W., and D.N. Proctor. 1991. Protein intake and athletic performance. *Sports Medicine* 12: 313-325.

Luden, N.D., M.J. Saunders, and M.K. Todd. 2007. Postexercise carbohydrate-protein-antioxidant ingestion decreases plasma creatine kinase and muscle soreness. *International Journal of Sport Nutrition and Exercise Metabolism* 17: 109-123.

Maughan, R.J. 1991. Fluid and electrolyte loss and replacement in exercise. *Journal of Sports Science* 9: 117-142.

Maughan, R.J., and R. Murray. 2001. Gastric emptying and intestinal absorption of fluids, carbohydrates, and electrolytes. In: *Sports drinks: Basic science and practical aspects.* New York: CRC Press.

McLellan, T.M., G.D. Bell, and G.H. Kamimori. 2004. Caffeine improves physical performance during 24 h of active wakefulness. *Aviation, Space, and Environmental Medicine* 75(8): 666-672.

Millard-Stafford, M.L., K.J. Cureton, J.E. Wingo, J. Trilk, G.J. Warren, and M. Buyckx. 2007. Hydration during exercise in warm, humid conditions: Effect of a caffeinated sports drink. *International Journal of Sport Nutrition and Exercise Metabolism* 17: 163-177.

Morgan, R.M., M.J. Patterson, and M.A. Nimmo. 2004. Acute effects of dehydration on sweat composition in men during prolonged exercise in the heat. *Acta Physiologica Scandinavica* 182(1): 37-43.

Murray, R., and W.L. Kenney. 2008. Sodium balance and exercise. *Current Sports Medicine Reports* 7(4): S1-S2.

Murray, R., G.L. Paul, J.G. Seifert, D.E. Eddy, and G.A. Halaby. 1989. The effects of glucose, fructose, and sucrose ingestion during exercise. *Medicine and Science in Sports and Exercise* 21: 275-282.

National Collegiate Athletic Association. 2009-10 NCAA banned drugs. June 10, 2009. Accessed August 25, 2010.

Noakes, T.D. 1993. Fluid replacement during exercise. In: *Exercise and sport sciences reviews* 21, edited by J.O. Holloszy. Baltimore: Williams & Wilkins.

Ohtani, M., M. Sugita, and K. Maryuma. 2006. Amino acid mixture improves training efficiency in athletes. *Journal of Nutrition* 136: 538S-543S.

Otukonyong, E.E., and D.D. Oyebola. 1994. Electrolyte loss during exercise in apparently healthy Nigerians. *Central African Journal of Medicine* 40(3): 74-77.

Paddon-Jones, D., M. Sheffield-Moore, X.J. Zhang, E. Volpi, S.E. Wolf, A. Aarsland, A.A. Ferrando, and R.R. Wolfe. 2004. Amino acid ingestion improves protein synthesis in the young and elderly. *American Journal of Physiology: Endocrinology and Metabolism* 286: E321-E328.

Paik, I.Y., M.H. Jeong, H.E. Jin, Y.I. Kim, A.R. Suh, S.Y. Cho, H.T. Roh, C.H. Jin, and S.H. Suh. 2009. Fluid replacement following dehydration reduces oxidative stress during recovery. *Biochemical and Biophysical Research Communications.* [e-pub ahead of print]

Pederson, D.L., S.J. Lessard, V.G. Coffey, E.G. Churchley, A.M. Wootton, T. Ng, M.J. Watt, and J.A. Hawley. 2008. High rates of muscle glycogen resynthesis after exhaustive exercise when carbohydrate is coingested with caffeine. *Journal of Applied Physiology* 105(1): 7-13.

Rehrer, N.J. 2001. Fluid and electrolyte balance in ultra-aerobic endurance sport. *Sports Medicine* 31(10): 701-715.

Requena, B., M. Zabala, P. Padial, and B. Feriche. 2005. Sodium bicarbonate and sodium citrate: Ergogenic aids? *Journal of Strength and Conditioning Research* 19(1): 213-224.

Roberts, M., C. Lockwood, V.J. Dalbo, P. Tucker, A. Frye, R. Polk, J. Volek, and C. Kerksick. 2009. Ingestion of a high molecular weight modified waxy maize starch alters metabolic responses to prolonged exercise in trained cyclists. FASEB abstract.

Rowlands, D.S., R.M. Thorp, K. Rossler, D.F. Graham, and M.J. Rockell. 2007. Effect of protein-rich feeding on recovery after intense exercise. *International Journal of Sport Nutrition and Exercise Metabolism* 17: 521-543.

Sanders, B., T.D. Noakes, and S.C. Dennis. 1999. Water and electrolyte shifts with partial fluid replacement during exercise. *European Journal of Applied Physiology* 80: 318-323.

Sawka, M.N., L.M. Burke, R.E. Eichner, R.J. Maughan, S.J. Montain, and N.S. Stachenfeld. 2007. American College of Sports Medicine position stand: Exercise and fluid replacement. *Medicine and Science Sports and Exercise* 39: 377-390.

Seifert, J., J. Harmon, and P. DeClercq. 2006. Protein added to a sports drink improves fluid retention. *International Journal of Sport Nutrition and Exercise Metabolism* 16(4): 420-429.

Shirreffs, S.M., L.E. Armstrong, and S.N. Cheuvront. 2004. Fluid and electrolyte needs for preparation and recovery from training and competition. *Journal of Sports Science* 22: 57-63.

Shirreffs, S.M., L.F. Aragon-Vargas, M. Keil, T.D. Love, and S. Phillips. 2007. Rehydration after exercise in the heat: A comparison of 4 commonly used drinks. *International Journal of Sport Nutrition and Exercise Metabolism* 17: 244-258.

Shirreffs, S.M., and R.J. Maughan. 1998. Volume repletion after exercise-induced volume depletion in humans: Replacement of water and sodium losses. *American Journal of Physiology* 274: F868-F875.

Smith, A., A. Kendrick, A. Maben, and J. Salmon. 1994. Effects of breakfast and caffeine on cognitive performance, mood and cardiovascular functioning. *Appetite* 22(1): 39-55.

Struder, H.K., W. Hollman, P. Platen, R. Wöstmann, A. Ferrauti, and K. Weber. 1997. Effect of exercise intensity on free tryptophan to branched-chain amino acids ratio and plasma prolactin during aerobic endurance exercise. *Canadian Journal of Applied Physiology* 22(3): 280-291.

Tipton, K.D., and R.R. Wolfe. 1998. Exercise-induced changes in protein metabolism. *Acta Physiologica Scandinavica* 162: 377-387.

Tipton, K.D., and R.R. Wolfe. 2004. Protein and amino acids for athletes. *Journal of Sports Science* 22: 65-79.

Turinsky, J., and C.L. Long. 1990. Free amino acids in muscle: Effect of muscle fiber population and denervation. *American Journal of Physiology* 258: E485-E491.

U.S. Anti-Doping Agency. n.d. DRO drug reference online. www.usada.org/dro/search/search.aspx.

Van Hall, G., J.S. Raaymakers, W.H. Saris, and A.J. Wagenmakers. 1995. Ingestion of branched-chain amino acids and tryptophan during sustained exercise in man: Failure to affect performance. *Journal of Physiology* 486(Pt 3): 789-94.

Van Hall, G., S.M. Shirreffs, and J.A. Calbet. 2000. Muscle glycogen resynthesis during recovery from cycle exercise: No effect of additional protein ingestion. *Journal of Applied Physiology* 88(5): 1631-1636.

Van Nieuwenhoven, M.A., R.B. Brummer, and F. Brouns. 2000. Gastrointestinal function during exercise: Comparison of water, sports drink, and sports drink with caffeine. *Journal of Applied Physiology* 89: 1079-1085.

Vist, G.E., and R.J. Maughan. 1994. Gastric emptying of ingested solutions in man: Effect of beverage glucose concentration. *Medicine and Science in Sports and Exercise* 10: 1269-1273.

Wolfe, R.R., M.H. Wolfe, E.R. Nadel, and J.H. Shaw. 1984. Isotopic determination of amino acid-urea interactions in exercise in humans. *Journal of Applied Physiology* 56: 221-229.

Yeo, S.E., R.L. Jentjens, G.A. Wallis, and A.E. Jeukendrup. 2005. Caffeine increases exogenous carbohydrate oxidation during exercise. *Journal of Applied Physiology* 99: 844-850.

Zawadzki, K.M., B.B. Yaspelkis 3rd, and J.L. Ivy. 1992. Carbohydrate-protein complex increases the rate of muscle glycogen storage after exercise. *Journal of Applied Physiology* 72(5): 1854-1859.

Chapter 9

American College of Sports Medicine, American Dietetic Association, and Dietitians of Canada. 2000. Joint position statement: Nutrition and athletic performance. *Medicine and Science in Sports and Exercise* 32(12): 2130-2145.

Baty, J.J., H. Hwang, Z. Ding, J.R. Bernard, B. Wang, B. Kwon, and J.L. Ivy. 2007. The effect of a carbohydrate and protein supplement on resistance exercise performance, hormonal response, and muscle damage. *Journal of Strength and Conditioning Research* 21(2): 321-329.

Beelen, M., R. Koopman, A.P. Gijsen, H. Vandereyt, A.K. Kies, H. Kuipers, W.H. Saris, and L.J. Van Loon. 2008. Protein coingestion stimulates muscle protein synthesis during resistance-type exercise. *American Journal of Physiology: Endocrinology and Metabolism* 295(1): E70-77.

Berardi, J.M., E.E. Noreen, and P.W. Lemon. 2008. Recovery from a cycling time trial is enhanced with carbohydrate-protein supplementation vs. isoenergetic carbohydrate supplementation. *Journal of the International Society of Sports Nutrition* 5: 24.

Berardi, J.M., T.B. Price, E.E. Noreen, and P.W. Lemon. 2006. Postexercise muscle glycogen recovery enhanced with a carbohydrate-protein supplement. *Medicine and Science in Sports and Exercise* 38(6): 1106-1113.

Bergstrom, J., L. Hermansen, E. Hultman, and B. Saltin. 1967. Diet, muscle glycogen and physical performance. *Acta Physiologica Scandinavica* 71(2): 140-150.

Bergstrom, J., and E. Hultman. 1966. Muscle glycogen synthesis after exercise: An enhancing factor localized to the muscle cells in man. *Nature* 210(5033): 309-310.

Biolo, G., K.D. Tipton, S. Klein, and R.R. Wolfe. 1997. An abundant supply of amino acids enhances the metabolic effect of exercise on muscle protein. *American Journal of Physiology* 273(1 Pt 1): E122-129.

Bird, S.P., K.M. Tarpenning, and F.E. Marino. 2006a. Effects of liquid carbohydrate/essential amino acid ingestion on acute hormonal response during a single bout of resistance exercise in untrained men. *Nutrition* 22(4): 367-375.

Bird, S.P., K.M. Tarpenning, and F.E. Marino. 2006b. Independent and combined effects of liquid carbohydrate/essential amino acid ingestion on hormonal and muscular adaptations following resistance training in untrained men. *European Journal of Applied Physiology* 97(2): 225-238.

Bird, S.P., K.M. Tarpenning, and F.E. Marino. 2006c. Liquid carbohydrate/essential amino acid ingestion during a short-term bout of resistance exercise suppresses myofibrillar protein degradation. *Metabolism: Clinical and Experimental* 55(5): 570-577.

Boirie, Y., M. Dangin, P. Gachon, M.P. Vasson, J.L. Maubois, and B. Beaufrere. 1997. Slow and fast dietary proteins differently modulate postprandial protein accretion. *Proceedings of the National Academy of Sciences* 94(26): 14930-14935.

Borsheim, E., M.G. Cree, K.D. Tipton, T.A. Elliott, A. Aarsland, and R.R. Wolfe. 2004. Effect of carbohydrate intake on net muscle protein synthesis during recovery from resistance exercise. *Journal of Applied Physiology* 96(2): 674-678.

Borsheim, E., K.D. Tipton, S.E. Wolf, and R.R. Wolfe. 2002. Essential amino acids and muscle protein recovery from resistance exercise. *American Journal of Physiology: Endocrinology and Metabolism* 283(4): E648-657.

Bosch, A.N., S.C. Dennis, and T.D. Noakes. 1993. Influence of carbohydrate loading on fuel substrate turnover and oxidation during prolonged exercise. *Journal of Applied Physiology* 74(4): 1921-1927.

Bucci, L., and U. Lm. 2000. Proteins and amino acid supplements in exercise and sport. In: *Energy-yield macronutrients and energy metabolism in sports nutrition,* edited by J. Driskell and I. Wolinsky, 191-212. Boca Raton, FL: CRC Press.

Buford, T.W., R.B. Kreider, J.R. Stout, M. Greenwood, B. Campbell, M. Spano, T. Ziegenfuss, H. Lopez, J. Landis, and J. Antonio. 2007. International society of sports nutrition position stand: Creatine supplementation and exercise. *Journal of the International Society of Sports Nutrition* 4: 6.

Burke, L.M. 2001. Nutritional needs for exercise in the heat. *Comparative Biochemistry and Physiology* 128: 735-748.

Burke, L.M., B. Kiens, and J.L. Ivy. 2004. Carbohydrates and fat for training and recovery. *Journal of Sports Science* 22: 15-30.

Bussau, V.A., T.J. Fairchild, A. Rao, P. Steele, and P.A. Fournier. 2002. Carbohydrate loading in human muscle: An improved 1 day protocol. *European Journal of Applied Physiology* 87(3): 290-295.

Candow, D.G., N.C. Burke, T. Smith-Palmer, and D.G. Burke. 2006. Effect of whey and soy protein supplementation combined with resistance training in young adults. *International Journal of Sport Nutrition and Exercise Metabolism* 16(3): 233-244.

Coburn, J.W., D.J. Housh, T.J. Housh, M.H. Malek, T.W. Beck, J.T. Cramer, G.O. Johnson, and P.E. Donlin. 2006. Effects of leucine and whey protein supplementation during eight weeks of unilateral resistance training. *Journal of Strength and Conditioning Research* 20(2): 284-291.

Conlee, R.K., R.M. Lawler, and P.E. Ross. 1987. Effects of glucose or fructose feeding on glycogen repletion in muscle and liver after exercise or fasting. *Annals of Nutrition and Metabolism* 31: 126-132.

Coyle, E.F., A.R. Coggan, M.K. Hemmert, and J.E. Ivy. 1986. Muscle glycogen utilization during prolonged strenuous exercise when fed carbohydrate. *Journal of Applied Physiology* 61(1): 165-172.

Coyle, E.F., A.R. Coggan, M.K. Hemmert, R.C. Lowe, and T.J. Walters. 1985. Substrate usage during prolonged exercise following a preexercise meal. *Journal of Applied Physiology* 59(2): 429-433.

Cribb, P.J., and A. Hayes. 2006. Effects of supplement timing and resistance exercise on skeletal muscle hypertrophy. *Medicine and Science in Sports and Exercise* (11): 1918-1925.

Cribb, P.J., A.D. Williams, and A. Hayes. 2007. A creatine-protein-carbohydrate supplement enhances responses to resistance training. *Medicine and Science in Sports and Exercise* 39(11): 1960-1968.

Cribb, P.J., A.D. Williams, C.G. Stathis, M.F. Carey, and A. Hayes. 2007. Effects of whey isolate, creatine, and resistance training on muscle hypertrophy. *Medicine and Science in Sports and Exercise* 39(2): 298-307.

Currell, K., and A.E. Jeukendrup. 2008. Superior endurance performance with ingestion of multiple transportable carbohydrates. *Medicine and Science in Sports and Exercise* 40(2): 275-281.

Dangin, M., Y. Boirie, C. Garcia-Rodenas, P. Gachon, J. Fauquant, P. Callier, O. Ballevre, and B. Beaufrere. 2001. The digestion rate of protein is an independent regulating factor of postprandial protein retention. *American Journal of Physiology: Endocrinology and Metabolism* 280(2): E340-348.

Dennis, S.C., T.D. Noakes, and J.A. Hawley. 1997. Nutritional strategies to minimize fatigue during prolonged exercise: Fluid, electrolyte and energy replacement. *Journal of Sports Science* 15(3): 305-313.

Earnest, C.P., S.L. Lancaster, C.J. Rasmussen, C.M. Kerksick, A. Lucia, M.C. Greenwood, A.L. Almada, P.A. Cowan, and R.B. Kreider. 2004. Low vs. high glycemic index carbohydrate gel ingestion during simulated 64-km cycling time trial performance. *Journal of Strength and Conditioning Research* 18(3): 466-472.

Erickson, M.A., R.J. Schwarzkopf, and R.D. Mckenzie. 1987. Effects of caffeine, fructose, and glucose ingestion on muscle glycogen utilization during exercise. *Medicine and Science in Sports and Exercise* 19(6): 579-583.

Febbraio, M.A., A. Chiu, D.J. Angus, M.J. Arkinstall, and J.A. Hawley. 2000a. Effects of carbohydrate ingestion before and during exercise on glucose kinetics and performance. *Journal of Applied Physiology* 89(6): 2220-2226.

Febbraio, M.A., J. Keenan, D.J. Angus, S.E. Campbell, and A.P. Garnham. 2000b. Preexercise carbohydrate ingestion, glucose kinetics, and muscle glycogen use: Effect of the glycemic index. *Journal of Applied Physiology* 89(5): 1845-1851.

Febbraio, M.A., and K.L. Stewart. 1996. CHO feeding before prolonged exercise: Effect of glycemic index on muscle glycogenolysis and exercise performance. *Journal of Applied Physiology* 81(3): 1115-1120.

Fielding, R.A., D.L. Costill, W.J. Fink, D.S. King, M. Hargreaves, and J.E. Kovaleski. 1985. Effect of carbohydrate feeding frequencies and dosage on muscle glycogen use during exercise. *Medicine and Science in Sports and Exercise* 17(4): 472-476.

Foster, C., D.L. Costill, and W.J. Fink. 1979. Effects of preexercise feedings on endurance performance. *Medicine and Science in Sports and Exercise* 11: 1-5.

Gleeson, M., D.C. Nieman, and B.K. Pedersen. 2004. Exercise, nutrition and immune function. *Journal of Sports Science* 22: 115-125.

Goforth, H.W., D. Laurent, W.K. Prusaczyk, K.E. Schneider, K.F. Petersen, and G.I. Shulman. 2003. Effects of depletion exercise and light training on muscle glycogen supercompensation in men. *American Journal of Physiology: Endocrinology and Metabolism* 285: 1304-1311.

Haff, G.G., A.J. Koch, J.A. Potteiger, K.E. Kuphal, L.M. Magee, S.B. Green, and J.J. Jakicic. 2000. Carbohydrate supplementation attenuates muscle glycogen loss during acute bouts of resistance exercise. *International Journal of Sport Nutrition and Exercise Metabolism* 10(3): 326-339.

Hargreaves, M., D.L. Costill, A. Coggan, W.J. Fink, and I. Nishibata. 1984. Effect of carbohydrate feedings on muscle glycogen utilization and exercise performance. *Medicine and Science in Sports and Exercise* 16(3): 219-222.

Hartman, J.W., J.E. Tang, S.B. Wilkinson, M.A. Tarnopolsky, R.L. Lawrence, A.V. Fullerton, and S.M. Phillips. 2007. Consumption of fat-free fluid milk after resistance exercise promotes greater lean mass accretion than does consumption of soy or carbohydrate in young, novice, male weightlifters. *American Journal of Clinical Nutrition* 86: 373-81.

Hawley, J.A., A.N. Bosch, S.M. Weltan, S.C. Dennis, and T.D. Noakes. 1994. Glucose kinetics during prolonged exercise in euglycaemic and hyperglycaemic subjects. *Pflugers Archives* 426(5): 378-386.

Hawley, J.A., and L.M. Burke. 1997. Effect of meal frequency and timing on physical performance. *British Journal of Nutrition* 77(Suppl 1): S91-S103.

Hawley, J.A., E.J. Schabort, T.D. Noakes, and S.C. Dennis. 1997. Carbohydrate-loading and exercise performance. An update. *Sports Medicine* 24(2): 73-81.

Hoffman, J.R., N.A. Ratamess, C.P. Tranchina, S.L. Rashti, J. Kang, and A.D. Faigenbaum. 2009. Effect of protein-supplement timing on strength, power, and body-composition changes in resistance-trained men. *International Journal of Sport Nutrition and Exercise Metabolism* 19(2): 172-185.

Ivy, J.L. 1998. Glycogen resynthesis after exercise: Effect of carbohydrate intake. *International Journal of Sports Medicine* 19 Suppl 2: S142-145.

Ivy, J.L., H.W. Goforth Jr., B.M. Damon, T.R. Mccauley, E.C. Parsons, and T.B. Price. 2002. Early postexercise muscle glycogen recovery is enhanced with a carbohydrate-protein supplement. *Journal of Applied Physiology* 93(4): 1337-1344.

Ivy, J.L., P.T. Res, R.C. Sprague, and M.O. Widzer. 2003. Effect of a carbohydrate-protein supplement on endurance performance during exercise of varying intensity. *International Journal of Sport Nutrition and Exercise Metabolism* 13(3): 382-395.

Jentjens, R., J. Achten, and A.E. Jeukendrup. 2004. High rates of exogenous carbohydrate oxidation from multiple transportable carbohydrates ingested during prolonged exercise. *Medicine and Science in Sports and Exercise* 36(9): 1551-1558.

Jentjens, R., and A.E. Jeukendrup. 2003. Determinants of post-exercise glycogen synthesis during short-term recovery. *Sports Medicine* 33: 117-144.

Jentjens, R., and A.E. Jeukendrup. 2005. High exogenous carbohydrate oxidation rates from a mixture of glucose and fructose ingested during prolonged cycling exercise. *British Journal of Nutrition* 93(4): 485-492.

Jentjens, R.L., L. Moseley, R.H. Waring, L.K. Harding, and A.E. Jeukendrup. 2004. Oxidation of combined ingestion of glucose and fructose during exercise. *Journal of Applied Physiology* 96(4): 1277-1284.

Jentjens, R., C. Shaw, T. Birtles, R.H. Waring, L.K. Harding, and A.E. Jeukendrup. 2005. Oxidation of combined ingestion of glucose and sucrose during exercise. *Metabolism: Clinical and Experimental* 54: 610-618.

Jentjens, R., M.C. Venables, and A.E. Jeukendrup. 2004. Oxidation of exogenous glucose, sucrose, and maltose during prolonged cycling exercise. *Journal of Applied Physiology* 96: 1285-1291.

Jentjens, R.L.P.G., L. Van Loon, C.H. Mann, A.J.M. Wagenmakers, and A.E. Jeukendrup. 2001. Addition of protein and amino acids to carbohydrates does not enhance postexercise muscle glycogen synthesis. *Journal of Applied Physiology* 91: 839-846.

Jeukendrup, A.E. 2004. Carbohydrate intake during exercise and performance. *Nutrition* 20(7-8): 669-677.

Jeukendrup, A.E., and R. Jentjens. 2000. Oxidation of carbohydrate feedings during prolonged exercise: Current thoughts, guidelines and directions for future research. *Sports Medicine* 29(6): 407-424.

Jeukendrup, A.E., R.L. Jentjens, and L. Moseley. 2005. Nutritional considerations in triathlon. *Sports Medicine* 35(2): 163-181.

Karlsson, J., and B. Saltin. 1971. Diet, muscle glycogen, and endurance performance. *Journal of Applied Physiology* 31(2): 203-206.

Kavouras, S.A., J.P. Troup, and J.R. Berning. 2004. The influence of low versus high carbohydrate diet on a 45-min strenuous cycling exercise. *International Journal of Sport Nutrition and Exercise Metabolism* 14(1): 62-72.

Keizer, H., H. Kuipers, and G. Van Kranenburg. 1987. Influence of liquid and solid meals on muscle glycogen resynthesis, plasma fuel hormone response, and maximal physical working capacity. *International Journal of Sports Medicine* 8: 99-104.

Kerksick, C., T. Harvey, J. Stout, B. Campbell, C. Wilborn, R. Kreider, D. Kalman, T. Ziegenfuss, H. Lopez, J. Landis, J. Ivy, and J. Antonio. 2008. International society of sports nutrition position stand: Nutrient timing. *Journal of the International Society of Sports Nutrition* 5(1): 17.

Kerksick, C.M., C.J. Rasmussen, S.L. Lancaster, B. Magu, P. Smith, C. Melton, M. Greenwood, A.L. Almada, C.P. Earnest, and R.B. Kreider. 2006. The effects of protein and amino acid supplementation on performance and training adaptations during ten weeks of resistance training. *Journal of Strength and Conditioning Research* 20(3): 643-653.

Kerksick, C.M., C. Rasmussen, S. Lancaster, M. Starks, P. Smith, C. Melton, M. Greenwood, A. Almada, and R. Kreider. 2007. Impact of differing protein sources and a creatine containing nutritional formula after 12 weeks of resistance training. *Nutrition* 23(9): 647-656.

Koopman, R., D.L. Pannemans, A.E. Jeukendrup, A.P. Gijsen, J.M. Senden, D. Halliday, W.H. Saris, L.J. Van Loon, and A.J. Wagenmakers. 2004. Combined ingestion of protein and carbohydrate improves protein balance during ultra-endurance exercise. *American Journal of Physiology: Endocrinology and Metabolism* 287(4): E712-720.

Kraemer, W.J., D.L. Hatfield, B.A. Spiering, J.L. Vingren, M.S. Fragala, J.Y. Ho, J.S. Volek, J.M. Anderson, and C.M. Maresh. 2007. Effects of a multi-nutrient supplement on exercise performance and hormonal responses to resistance exercise. *European Journal of Applied Physiology* 101(5): 637-646.

Kreider, R.B. 2003. Effects of creatine supplementation on performance and training adaptations. *Molecular and Cellular Biochemistry* 244(1-2): 89-94.

Levenhagen, D.K., J.D. Gresham, M.G. Carlson, D.J. Maron, M.J. Borel, and P.J. Flakoll. 2001. Postexercise nutrient intake timing in humans is critical to recovery of leg glucose and protein homeostasis. *American Journal of Physiology: Endocrinology and Metabolism* 280(6): E982-993.

McConell, G., R.J. Snow, J. Proietto, and M. Hargreaves. 1999. Muscle metabolism during prolonged exercise in humans: Influence of carbohydrate availability. *Journal of Applied Physiology* 87(3): 1083-1086.

Miller, S.L., K.D. Tipton, D.L. Chinkes, S.E. Wolf, and R.R. Wolfe. 2003. Independent and combined effects of amino acids and glucose after resistance exercise. *Medicine and Science in Sports and Exercise* 35(3): 449-455.

Neufer, P.D., D.L. Costill, M.G. Flynn, J.P. Kirwan, J.B. Mitchell, and J. Houmard. 1987. Improvements in exercise performance: Effects of carbohydrate feedings and diet. *Journal of Applied Physiology* 62(3): 983-988.

Nicholas, C.W., P.A. Green, and R.D. Hawkins. 1997. Carbohydrate intake and recovery of intermittent running capacity. *International Journal of Sport Nutrition* 7: 251-260.

Nicholas, C.W., C. Williams, H.K. Lakomy, G. Phillips, and A. Nowitz. 1995. Influence of ingesting a carbohydrate-electrolyte solution on endurance capacity during intermittent, high-intensity shuttle running. *Journal of Sports Sciences* 13(4): 283-290.

Patterson, S.D., and S.C. Gray. 2007. Carbohydrate-gel supplementation and endurance performance during intermittent high-intensity shuttle running. *International Journal of Sport Nutrition and Exercise Metabolism* 17(5): 445-455.

Phillips, S.M., K.D. Tipton, A.A. Ferrando, and R.R. Wolfe. 1999. Resistance training reduces the acute exercise-induced increase in muscle protein turnover. *American Journal of Physiology* 276: E118-E124.

Pitkanen, H.T., T. Nykanen, J. Knuutinen, K. Lahti, O. Keinanen, M. Alen, P.V. Komi, and A.A. Mero. 2003. Free amino acid pool and muscle protein balance after resistance exercise. *Medicine and Science in Sports and Exercise* 35(5): 784-792.

Rasmussen, B.B., K.D. Tipton, S.L. Miller, S.E. Wolf, and R.R. Wolfe. 2000. An oral essential amino acid-carbohydrate supplement enhances muscle protein anabolism after resistance exercise. *Journal of Applied Physiology* 88(2): 386-392.

Reed, M.J., J.T. Brozinick, M.C. Lee, and J.L. Ivy. 1989. Muscle glycogen storage postexercise: Effect of mode of carbohydrate administration. *Journal of Applied Physiology* 66(2): 720-726.

Saunders, M.J., M.D. Kane, and M.K. Todd. 2004. Effects of a carbohydrate-protein beverage on cycling endurance and muscle damage. *Medicine and Science in Sports and Exercise* 36(7): 1233-1238.

Saunders, M.J., N.D. Luden, and J.E. Herrick. 2007. Consumption of an oral carbohydrate-protein gel improves cycling endurance and prevents postexercise muscle damage. *Journal of Strength and Conditioning Research* 21(3): 678-684.

Sherman, W.M., G. Brodowicz, D.A. Wright, W.K. Allen, J. Simonsen, and A. Dernbach. 1989. Effects of 4 h preexercise carbohydrate feedings on cycling performance. *Medicine and Science in Sports and Exercise* 21(5): 598-604.

Sherman, W.M., D.L. Costill, W.J. Fink, F.C. Hagerman, L.E. Armstrong, and T.F. Murray. 1983. Effect of a 42.2-km footrace and subsequent rest or exercise on muscle glycogen and enzymes. *Journal of Applied Physiology* 55: 1219-1224.

Sherman, W.M., D.L. Costill, W.J. Fink, and J.M. Miller. 1981. Effect of exercise-diet manipulation on muscle glycogen and its subsequent utilization during performance. *International Journal of Sports Medicine* 2(2): 114-118.

Tarnopolsky, M.A., M. Bosman, J.R. Macdonald, D. Vandeputte, J. Martin, and B.D. Roy. 1997. Postexercise protein-carbohydrate and carbohydrate supplements increase muscle glycogen in men and women. *Journal of Applied Physiology* 83(6): 1877-1883.

Tarnopolsky, M.A., M. Gibala, A.E. Jeukendrup, and S.M. Phillips. 2005. Nutritional needs of elite endurance athletes. Part I: Carbohydrate and fluid requirements. *European Journal of Sport Science* 5(1): 3-14.

Tarnopolsky, M.A., G. Parise, N.J. Yardley, C.S. Ballantyne, S. Olatinji, and S.M. Phillips. 2001. Creatine-dextrose and protein-dextrose induce similar strength gains during training. *Medicine and Science in Sports and Exercise* 33(12): 2044-2052.

Tipton, K.D., T.A. Elliott, M.G. Cree, A. Aarsland, A.P. Sanford, and R.R. Wolfe. 2007. Stimulation of net muscle protein synthesis by whey protein ingestion before and after exercise. *American Journal of Physiology: Endocrinology and Metabolism* 292: E71-E76.

Tipton, K.D., T.A. Elliott, M.G. Cree, S.E. Wolf, A.P. Sanford, and R.R. Wolfe. 2004. Ingestion of casein and whey proteins results in muscle anabolism after resistance exercise. *Medicine and Science in Sports and Exercise* 36(12): 2073-2081.

Tipton, K.D., A.A. Ferrando, S.M. Phillips, D.J. Doyle, and R.R. Wolfe. 1999a. Postexercise net protein synthesis in human muscle from orally administered amino acids. *American Journal of Physiology* 276(4 Pt 1): E628-634.

Tipton, K.D., B.E. Gurkin, S. Matin, and R.R. Wolfe. 1999b. Nonessential amino acids are not necessary to stimulate net muscle protein synthesis in healthy volunteers. *Journal of Nutritional Biochemistry* 10: 89-95.

Tipton, K.D., B.B. Rasmussen, S.L. Miller, S.E. Wolf, S.K. Owens-Stovall, B.E. Petrini, and R.R. Wolfe. 2001. Timing of amino acid-carbohydrate ingestion alters anabolic response of muscle to resistance exercise. *American Journal of Physiology: Endocrinology and Metabolism* 281(2): E197-206.

Tipton, K.D., and R.R. Wolfe. 2001. Exercise, protein metabolism, and muscle growth. *International Journal of Sport Nutrition and Exercise Metabolism* 11(1): 109-132.

Van Loon, L.J., W.H. Saris, M. Kruijshoop, and A.J. Wagenmakers. 2000. Maximizing postexercise muscle glycogen synthesis: Carbohydrate supplementation and the application of amino acid or protein hydrolysate mixtures. *American Journal of Clinical Nutrition* 72(1): 106-111.

Wallis, G.A., D.S. Rowlands, C. Shaw, R. Jentjens, and A.E. Jeukendrup. 2005. Oxidation of combined ingestion of maltodextrins and fructose during exercise. *Medicine and Science in Sports and Exercise* 37(3): 426-432.

White, J.P., J.M. Wilson, K.G. Austin, B.K. Greer, N. St John, and L.B. Panton. 2008. Effect of carbohydrate-protein supplement timing on acute exercise-induced muscle damage. *Journal of the International Society of Sports Nutrition* 5: 5.

Widrick, J.J., D.L. Costill, W.J. Fink, M.S. Hickey, G.K. Mcconell, and H. Tanaka. 1993. Carbohydrate feedings and exercise performance: Effect of initial muscle glycogen concentration. *Journal of Applied Physiology* 74(6): 2998-3005.

Wilkinson, S.B., M.A. Tarnopolsky, M.J. Macdonald, J.R. Macdonald, D. Armstrong, and S.M. Phillips. 2007. Consumption of fluid skim milk promotes greater muscle protein accretion after resistance exercise than does consumption of an isonitrogenous and isoenergetic soy-protein beverage. *American Journal of Clinical Nutrition* 85(4): 1031-1040.

Willoughby, D.S., J.R. Stout, and C.D. Wilborn. 2007. Effects of resistance training and protein plus amino acid supplementation on muscle anabolism, mass, and strength. *Amino Acids* 32(4): 467-477.

Wright, D.A., W.M. Sherman, and A.R. Dernbach. 1991. Carbohydrate feedings before, during, or in combination improve cycling endurance performance. *Journal of Applied Physiology* 71(3): 1082-1088.

Yaspelkis, B.B., J.G. Patterson, P.A. Anderla, Z. Ding, and J.L. Ivy. 1993. Carbohydrate supplementation spares muscle glycogen during variable-intensity exercise. *Journal of Applied Physiology* 75(4): 1477-1485.

Zawadzki, K.M., B.B. Yaspelkis, and J.L. Ivy. 1992. Carbohydrate-protein complex increases the rate of muscle glycogen storage after exercise. *Journal of Applied Physiology* 72(5): 1854-1859.

Chapter 10

Andersen, L.L., G. Tufekovic, M.K. Zebis, R.M. Crameri, G. Verlaan, M. Kjaer, C. Suetta, P. Magnusson, and P. Aagaard. 2005. The effect of resistance training combined with timed ingestion of protein on muscle fiber size and muscle strength. *Metabolism* 54(2): 151-156.

Anderson, J.W., E.C. Konz, R.C. Frederich, and C.L. Wood. 2001. Long-term weight-loss maintenance: A meta-analysis of US studies. *American Journal of Clinical Nutrition* 74(5): 579-584.

Ball, S.D., K.R. Keller, L.J. Moyer-Mileur, Y.W. Ding, D. Donaldson, and W.D. Jackson. 2003. Prolongation of satiety after low versus moderately high glycemic index meals in obese adolescents. *Pediatrics* 111(3): 488-494.

Barkeling, B., S. Rossner, and H. Bjorvell. 1990. Effects of a high-protein meal (meat) and a high-carbohydrate meal (vegetarian) on satiety measured by automated computerized monitoring of subsequent food intake, motivation to eat and food preferences. *International Journal of Obesity* 14(9): 743-751.

Biolo, G., S.P. Maggi, B.D. Williams, K.D. Tipton, and R.R. Wolfe. 1995. Increased rates of muscle protein turnover and amino acid transport after resistance exercise in humans. *American Journal of Physiology* 268(3 Pt 1): E514-520.

Borsheim, E., A. Aarsland, and R.R. Wolfe. 2004. Effect of an amino acid, protein, and carbohydrate mixture on net muscle protein balance after resistance exercise. *International Journal of Sport Nutrition and Exercise Metabolism* 14(3): 255-271.

Borsheim, E., K.D. Tipton, S.E. Wolf, and R.R. Wolfe. 2002. Essential amino acids and muscle protein recovery from resistance exercise. *American Journal of Physiology: Endocrinology, and Metabolism* 283(4): E648-657.

Bouche, C., S.W. Rizkalla, J. Luo, H. Vidal, A. Veronese, N. Pacher, C. Fouquet, V. Lang, and G. Slama. 2002. Five-week, low-glycemic index diet decreases total fat mass and improves plasma lipid profile in moderately overweight nondiabetic men. *Diabetes Care* 25(5): 822-828.

Branch, J.D. 2003. Effect of creatine supplementation on body composition and performance: A meta-analysis. *International Journal of Sport Nutrition and Exercise Metabolism* 13(2): 198-226.

Bray, G.A. 2000. Afferent signals regulating food intake. *Proceedings of the Nutrition Society* 59(3): 373-384.

Bray, G.A. 2003. Risks of obesity. *Endocrinology and Metabolism Clinics of North America* 32(4): 787-804, viii.

Brehm, B.J., and D.A. D'Alessio. 2008. Benefits of high-protein weight loss diets: Enough evidence for practice? *Current Opinions in Endocrinology, Diabetes, and Obesity* 15(5): 416-421.

Brose, A., G. Parise, and M.A. Tarnopolsky. 2003. Creatine supplementation enhances isometric strength and body composition improvements following strength exercise training in older adults. *Journals of Gerontology: Series A, Biological Sciences and Medical Sciences* 58(1): 11-19.

Brynes, A.E., J. Adamson, A. Dornhorst, and G.S. Frost. 2005. The beneficial effect of a diet with low glycaemic index on 24 h glucose profiles in healthy young people as assessed by continuous glucose monitoring. *British Journal of Nutrition* 93(2): 179-182.

Campbell, B., R. Kreider, T. Ziegenfuss, P. La Bounty, M. Roberts, D. Burke, J. Landis, H. Lopez, and J. Antonio. 2007. International Society of Sports Nutrition position stand: Protein and exercise. *Journal of the International Society of Sports Nutrition* 4: 8.

Candow, D.G., N.C. Burke, T. Smith-Palmer, and D.G. Burke. 2006. Effect of whey and soy protein supplementation combined with resistance training in young adults. *International Journal of Sport Nutrition and Exercise Metabolism* 16(3): 233-244.

Chrusch, M.J., P.D. Chilibeck, K. Chad, K. Davison, and D.G. Burke. 2001. Creatine supplementation combined with resistance training in older men. *Medicine and Science in Sports and Exercise* 33(12): 2111-2117.

Cook, C.M., and M.D. Haub. 2007. Low-carbohydrate diets and performance. *Current Sports Medicine Reports* 6(4): 225-229.

Cox, K.L., V. Burke, A.R. Morton, L.J. Beilin, and I.B. Puddey. 2003. The independent and combined effects of 16 weeks of vigorous exercise and energy restriction on body mass and composition in free-living overweight men—a randomized controlled trial. *Metabolism: Clinical and Experimental* 52(1): 107-115.

Cribb, P.J., A.D. Williams, C.G. Stathis, M.F. Carey, and A. Hayes. 2007. Effects of whey isolate, creatine, and resistance training on muscle hypertrophy. *Medicine and Science in Sports and Exercise* 39(2): 298-307.

Das, S.K., C.H. Gilhooly, J.K. Golden, A.G. Pittas, P.J. Fuss, R.A. Cheatham, S. Tyler, M. Tsay, M.A. McCrory, A.H. Lichtenstein, G.E. Dallal, C. Dutta, M.V. Bhapkar, J.P. Delany, E. Saltzman, and S.B. Roberts. 2007. Long-term effects of 2 energy-restricted diets differing in glycemic load on dietary adherence, body composition, and metabolism in CALERIE: A 1-y randomized controlled trial. *American Journal of Clinical Nutrition* 85(4): 1023-1030.

Demling, R.H., and L. DeSanti. 2000. Effect of a hypocaloric diet, increased protein intake and resistance training on lean mass gains and fat mass loss in overweight police officers. *Annals of Nutrition and Metabolism* 44(1): 21-29.

Dengel, D.R., J.M. Hagberg, P.J. Coon, D.T. Drinkwater, and A.P. Goldberg. 1994a. Comparable effects of diet and exercise on body composition and lipoproteins in older men. *Medicine and Science in Sports and Exercise* 26(11): 1307-1315.

Dengel, D.R., J.M. Hagberg, P.J. Coon, D.T. Drinkwater, and A.P. Goldberg. 1994b. Effects of weight loss by diet alone or combined with aerobic exercise on body composition in older obese men. *Metabolism* 43(7): 867-871.

de Rougemont, A., S. Normand, J.A. Nazare, M.R. Skilton, M. Sothier, S. Vinoy, and M. Laville. 2007. Beneficial effects of a 5-week low-glycaemic index regimen on weight control and cardiovascular risk factors in overweight non-diabetic subjects. *British Journal of Nutrition* 98(6): 1288-1298.

Earnest, C.P., P.G. Snell, R. Rodriguez, A.L. Almada, and T.L. Mitchell. 1995. The effect of creatine monohydrate ingestion on anaerobic power indices, muscular strength and body composition. *Acta Physiologica Scandinavica* 153(2): 207-209.

Eston, R.G., S. Shephard, S. Kreitzman, A. Coxon, D.A. Brodie, K.L. Lamb, and V. Baltzopoulos. 1992. Effect of very low calorie diet on body composition and exercise response in sedentary women. *European Journal of Applied Physiology and Occupational Physiology* 65(5): 452-458.

Forbes, G.B. 2000. Body fat content influences the body composition response to nutrition and exercise. *Annals of the New York Academy of Sciences* 904: 359-365.

Frimel, T.N., D.R. Sinacore, and D.T. Villareal. 2008. Exercise attenuates the weight-loss-induced reduction in muscle mass in frail obese older adults. *Medicine and Science in Sports and Exercise* 40(7): 1213-1219.

Gilden Tsai, A., and T.A. Wadden. 2006. The evolution of very-low-calorie diets: An update and meta-analysis. *Obesity (Silver Spring)* 14(8): 1283-1293.

Gornall, J., and R.G. Villani. 1996. Short-term changes in body composition and metabolism with severe dieting and resistance exercise. *International Journal of Sport Nutrition* 6(3): 285-294.

Gotshalk, L.A., J.S. Volek, R.S. Staron, C.R. Denegar, E.C. Hagerman, and W.J. Kraemer. 2002. Creatine supplementation improves muscular performance in older men. *Medicine and Science in Sports and Exercise* 34(3): 537-543.

Halton, T.L., and F.B. Hu. 2004. The effects of high protein diets on thermogenesis, satiety and weight loss: A critical review. *Journal of the American College of Nutrition* 23(5): 373-385.

Horswill, C.A., R.C. Hickner, J.R. Scott, D.L. Costill, and D. Gould. 1990. Weight loss, dietary carbohydrate modifications, and high intensity, physical performance. *Medicine and Science in Sports and Exercise* 22(4): 470-476.

Hunter, G.R., N.M. Byrne, B. Sirikul, J.R. Fernandez, P.A. Zuckerman, B.E. Darnell, and B.A. Gower. 2008. Resistance training conserves fat-free mass and resting energy expenditure following weight loss. *Obesity* 16(5): 1045-1051.

Jeukendrup, A., and M. Gleeson. 2004. *Sport nutrition: An introduction to energy production and performance.* Champaign, IL: Human Kinetics.

Johnston, C.S., C.S. Day, and P.D. Swan. 2002. Postprandial thermogenesis is increased 100% on a high-protein, low-fat diet versus a high-carbohydrate, low-fat diet in healthy, young women. *Journal of the American College of Nutrition* 21(1): 55-61.

Kelly, V., and D. Jenkins. 1998. Effect of oral creatine supplementation on near-maximal strength and repeated sets of high intensity bench press exercise. *Journal of Strength and Conditioning Research* 12(2): 109-115.

Kerksick, C.M., C.J. Rasmussen, S.L. Lancaster, B. Magu, P. Smith, C. Melton, M. Greenwood, A.L. Almada, C.P. Earnest, and R.B. Kreider. 2006. The effects of protein and amino acid supplementation on performance and training adaptations during ten weeks of resistance training. *Journal of Strength and Conditioning Research* 20(3): 643-653.

Kraemer, W.J., J.S. Volek, K.L. Clark, S.E. Gordon, T. Incledon, S.M. Puhl, N.T. Triplett-McBride, J.M. McBride, M. Putukian, and W.J. Sebastianelli. 1997. Physiological adaptations to a weight-loss dietary regimen and exercise programs in women. *Journal of Applied Physiology* 83(1): 270-279.

Kreider, R.B., M. Ferreira, M. Wilson, P. Grindstaff, S. Plisk, J. Reinardy, E. Cantler, and A. Almada. 1998. Effects of creatine supplementation on body composition, strength, and sprint performance. *Medicine and Science in Sports and Exercise* 30(1): 73-82.

Kreider, R.B., R. Klesges, K. Harmon, P. Grindstaff, L. Ramsey, D. Bullen, L. Wood, Y. Li, and A. Almada. 1996. Effects of ingesting supplements designed to promote lean tissue accretion on body composition during resistance training. *International Journal of Sport Nutrition* 6(3): 234-246.

Krotkiewski, M., K. Landin, D. Mellstrom, and J. Tolli. 2000. Loss of total body potassium during rapid weight loss does not depend on the decrease of potassium concentration in muscles. Different methods to evaluate body composition during a low energy diet. *International Journal of Obesity and Related Metabolic Disorders* 24(1): 101-107.

Kushner, R.F., and B. Doerfler. 2008. Low-carbohydrate, high-protein diets revisited. *Current Opinion in Gastroenterology* 24(2): 198-203.

Lambert, C.P., L.L. Frank, and W.J. Evans. 2004. Macronutrient considerations for the sport of bodybuilding. *Sports Medicine* 34(5): 317-327.

Latner, J.D., and M. Schwartz. 1999. The effects of a high-carbohydrate, high-protein or balanced lunch upon later food intake and hunger ratings. *Appetite* 33(1): 119-128.

Layman, D.K., R.A. Boileau, D.J. Erickson, J.E. Painter, H. Shiue, C. Sather, and D.D. Christou. 2003. A reduced ratio of dietary carbohydrate to protein improves body composition and blood lipid profiles during weight loss in adult women. *Journal of Nutrition* 133(2): 411-417.

Livesey, G. 2001. A perspective on food energy standards for nutrition labelling. *British Journal of Nutrition* 85(3): 271-287.

Meredith, C.N., W.R. Frontera, K.P. O'Reilly, and W.J. Evans. 1992. Body composition in elderly men: Effect of dietary modification during strength training. *Journal of the American Geriatrics Society* 40(2): 155-162.

Moayyedi, P. 2008. The epidemiology of obesity and gastrointestinal and other diseases: An overview. *Digestive Diseases and Sciences* 53(9): 2293-2299.

Mourier, A., A.X. Bigard, E. de Kerviler, B. Roger, H. Legrand, and C.Y. Guezennec. 1997. Combined effects of caloric restriction and branched-chain amino acid supplementation on body composition and exercise performance in elite wrestlers. *International Journal of Sports Medicine* 18(1): 47-55.

National Task Force on the Prevention and Treatment of Obesity and National Institutes of Health. 1993. Very low-calorie diets. *Journal of the American Medical Association* 270(8): 967-974.

Nieman, D.C., D.W. Brock, D. Butterworth, A.C. Utter, and C.C. Nieman. 2002. Reducing diet and/or exercise training decreases the lipid and lipoprotein risk factors of moderately obese women. *Journal of the American College of Nutrition* 21(4): 344-350.

Noble, C.A., and R.F. Kushner. 2006. An update on low-carbohydrate, high-protein diets. *Current Opinion in Gastroenterology* 22(2): 153-159.

Rasmussen, B.B., K.D. Tipton, S.L. Miller, S.E. Wolf, and R.R. Wolfe. 2000. An oral essential amino acid-carbohydrate supplement enhances muscle protein anabolism after resistance exercise. *Journal of Applied Physiology* 88(2): 386-392.

Reaven, G.M. 2008. Insulin resistance: The link between obesity and cardiovascular disease. *Endocrinology and Metabolism Clinics of North America* 37(3): 581-601, vii-viii.

Redman, L.M., L.K. Heilbronn, C.K. Martin, A. Alfonso, S.R. Smith, and E. Ravussin. 2007. Effect of calorie restriction with or without exercise on body composition and fat distribution. *Journal of Clinical Endocrinology and Metabolism* 92(3): 865-872.

Rennie, M.J., and K.D. Tipton. 2000. Protein and amino acid metabolism during and after exercise and the effects of nutrition. *Annual Review of Nutrition* 20: 457-483.

Rodriguez, N.R., N.M. DiMarco, S. Langley; American Dietetic Association; and Dietitians of Canada; American College of Sports Medicine. 2009. Position of the American Dietetic Association, Dietitians of Canada, and the American College of Sports Medicine: Nutrition and athletic performance. *Journal of the American Dietetic Association* 109(3): 509-527.

Saris, W.H., A. Astrup, A.M. Prentice, H.J. Zunft, X. Formiguera, W.P. Verboeket-van de Venne, A. Raben, S.D. Poppitt, B. Seppelt, S. Johnston, T.H. Vasilaras, and G.F. Keogh. 2000. Randomized controlled trial of changes in dietary carbohydrate/fat ratio and simple vs complex carbohydrates on body weight and blood lipids: The CARMEN study. The Carbohydrate Ratio Management in European National diets. *International Journal of Obesity and Related Metabolic Disorders* 24(10): 1310-1318.

Sichieri, R., A.S. Moura, V. Genelhu, F. Hu, and W.C. Willett. 2007. An 18-mo randomized trial of a low-glycemic-index diet and weight change in Brazilian women. *American Journal of Clinical Nutrition* 86(3): 707-713.

Skov, A.R., S. Toubro, B. Ronn, L. Holm, and A. Astrup. 1999. Randomized trial on protein vs carbohydrate in ad libitum fat reduced diet for the treatment of obesity. *International Journal of Obesity and Related Metabolic Disorders* 23(5): 528-536.

Sloth, B., I. Krog-Mikkelsen, A. Flint, I. Tetens, I. Bjorck, S. Vinoy, H. Elmstahl, A. Astrup, V. Lang, and A. Raben. 2004. No difference in body weight decrease between a low-glycemic-index and a high-glycemic-index diet but reduced LDL cholesterol after 10-wk ad libitum intake of the low-glycemic-index diet. *American Journal of Clinical Nutrition* 80(2): 337-347.

Stevenson, E., C. Williams, M. Nute, P. Swaile, and M. Tsui. 2005. The effect of the glycemic index of an evening meal on the metabolic responses to a standard high glycemic index breakfast and subsequent exercise in men. *International Journal of Sport Nutrition and Exercise Metabolism* 15(3): 308-322.

Stiegler, P., and A. Cunliffe. 2006. The role of diet and exercise for the maintenance of fat-free mass and resting metabolic rate during weight loss. *Sports Medicine* 36(3): 239-262.

Stone, M.H., K. Sanborn, L.L. Smith, H.S. O'Bryant, T. Hoke, A.C. Utter, R.L. Johnson, R. Boros, J. Hruby, K.C. Pierce, M.E. Stone, and B. Garner. 1999. Effects of in-season (5 weeks) creatine and pyruvate supplementation on anaerobic performance and body composition in American football players. *International Journal of Sport Nutrition* 9(2): 146-165.

Stout, J., J. Eckerson, and D. Noonan. 1999. Effects of 8 weeks of creatine supplementation on exercise performance and fat-free weight in football players during training. *Nutrition Research* 19(2): 217-225.

Strasser, B., A. Spreitzer, and P. Haber. 2007. Fat loss depends on energy deficit only, independently of the method for weight loss. *Annals of Nutrition and Metabolism* 51(5): 428-432.

Strychar, I. 2006. Diet in the management of weight loss. *Canadian Medical Association Journal* 174(1): 56-63.

Tappy, L. 1996. Thermic effect of food and sympathetic nervous system activity in humans. *Reproduction, Nutrition, Development* 36(4): 391-397.

Terjung, R.L., P. Clarkson, E.R. Eichner, P.L. Greenhaff, P.J. Hespel, R.G. Israel, W.J. Kraemer, R.A. Meyer, L.L. Spriet, M.A. Tarnopolsky, A.J. Wagenmakers, and M.H. Williams. 2000. American College of Sports Medicine roundtable. The physiological and health effects of oral creatine supplementation. *Medicine and Science in Sports and Exercise* 32(3): 706-717.

Tipton, K.D., E. Borsheim, S.E. Wolf, A.P. Sanford, and R.R. Wolfe. 2003. Acute response of net muscle protein balance reflects 24-h balance after exercise and amino acid ingestion. *American Journal of Physiology: Endocrinology, and Metabolism* 284(1): E76-89.

Tipton, K.D., T.A. Elliott, M.G. Cree, A.A. Aarsland, A.P. Sanford, and R.R. Wolfe. 2007. Stimulation of net muscle protein synthesis by whey protein ingestion before and after exercise. *American Journal of Physiology: Endocrinology, and Metabolism* 292(1): E71-76.

Tipton, K.D., T.A. Elliott, M.G. Cree, S.E. Wolf, A.P. Sanford, and R.R. Wolfe. 2004. Ingestion of casein and whey proteins result in muscle anabolism after resistance exercise. *Medicine and Science in Sports and Exercise* 36(12): 2073-2081.

Tipton, K.D., A.A. Ferrando, S.M. Phillips, D. Doyle Jr., and R.R. Wolfe. 1999a. Postexercise net protein synthesis in human muscle from orally administered amino acids. *American Journal of Physiology* 276(4 Pt 1): E628-634.

Tipton, K.D., B.E. Gurkin, S. Matin, and R.R. Wolfe. 1999b. Nonessential amino acids are not necessary to stimulate net muscle protein synthesis in healthy volunteers. *Journal of Nutritional Biochemistry* 10(2): 89-95.

Tipton, K.D., B.B. Rasmussen, S.L. Miller, S.E. Wolf, S.K. Owens-Stovall, B.E. Petrini, and R. Wolfe. 2001. Timing of amino acid-carbohydrate ingestion alters anabolic response of muscle to resistance exercise. *American Journal of Physiology: Endocrinology, and Metabolism* 281(2): E197-206.

Valtuena, S., S. Blanch, M. Barenys, R. Sola, and J. Salas-Salvado. 1995. Changes in body composition and resting energy expenditure after rapid weight loss: Is there an energy-metabolism adaptation in obese patients? *International Journal of Obesity and Related Metabolic Disorders* 19(2): 119-125.

Vandenberghe, K., M. Goris, P. Van Hecke, M. Van Leemputte, L. Vangerven, and P. Hespel. 1997. Long-term creatine intake is beneficial to muscle performance during resistance training. *Journal of Applied Physiology* 83(6): 2055-2063.

van Loon, L.J., A.M. Oosterlaar, F. Hartgens, M.K. Hesselink, R.J. Snow, and A.J. Wagenmakers. 2003. Effects of creatine loading and prolonged creatine supplementation on body composition, fuel selection, sprint and endurance performance in humans. *Clinical Science (London)* 104(2): 153-162.

Vgontzas, A.N. 2008. Does obesity play a major role in the pathogenesis of sleep apnoea and its associated manifestations via inflammation, visceral adiposity, and insulin resistance? *Archives of Physiology and Biochemistry* 114(4): 211-223.

Volek, J.S., N.D. Duncan, S.A. Mazzetti, R.S. Staron, M. Putukian, A.L. Gomez, D.R. Pearson, W.J. Fink, and W.J. Kraemer. 1999. Performance and muscle fiber adaptations to creatine supplementation and heavy resistance training. *Medicine and Science in Sports and Exercise* 31(8): 1147-1156.

Wadden, T.A., and D.L. Frey. 1997. A multicenter evaluation of a proprietary weight loss program for the treatment of marked obesity: A five-year follow-up. *International Journal of Eating Disorders* 22(2): 203-212.

World Health Organization. 2000. Obesity: Preventing and managing the global epidemic. Report of a WHO consultation. *World Health Organization Technical Report Series* 894, i-xii: 1-253.

Willoughby, D.S., and J. Rosene. 2001. Effects of oral creatine and resistance training on myosin heavy chain expression. *Medicine and Science in Sports and Exercise* 33(10): 1674-1681.

Zahouani, A., A. Boulier, and J.P. Hespel. 2003. Short- and long-term evolution of body composition in 1389 obese outpatients following a very low calorie diet (Program 18 VLCD). *Acta Diabetologica* 40(Suppl 1): S149-150.

Chapter 11

Ball, S.D., and T.S. Altena. 2004. Comparison of the BOD POD and dual energy x-ray absorptiometry in men. *Physiological Measures* 25: 671-678.

Bentzur, K.M., L. Kravitz, and D.W. Lockner. 2008. Evaluation of the BOD POD for estimating percent body fat in collegiate track and field female athletes: A comparison of four methods. *Journal of Strength and Conditioning Research* 22: 1985-1991.

Chang, C.J., C.H. Wu, C.S. Chang, W.J. Yao, Y.C. Yang, J.S. Wu, and F.H. Lu. 2003. Low body mass index but high percent body fat in Taiwanese subjects: Implications of obesity cutoffs. *International Journal of Obesity* 27: 253-259.

Hollis, J.F., C.M. Gullion, V.J. Stevens, P.J. Brantley, L.J. Appel, J.D. Ard, C.M. Champagne, A. Dalcin, T.P. Erlinger, K. Funk, D. Laferriere, P. Lin, C.M. Loria, C. Samuel-Hodge, W.M. Vollmer, and L.P. Svetkey. 2008. Weight loss during the intensive intervention phase of the weight-loss maintenance trial. *American Journal of Preventive Medicine* 35: 118-126.

Jones, L.M., M. Legge, and A. Goulding. 2003. Healthy body mass index values often underestimate body fat in men with spinal cord injury. *Archives of Physical Medicine and Rehabilitation* 84: 1068-1071.

Lee, S.Y., and D. Gallagher. 2008. Assessment methods in human body composition. *Current Opinion in Nutrition and Metabolic Care* 11: 566-572.

Lukaski, H.C. 1993. Soft tissue composition and bone mineral status: Evaluation by dual energy x-ray absorptiometry. *Journal of Nutrition* 123: 438-443.

Lukaski, H.C., P.E. Johnson, W.W. Bolonchuk, and G.I. Lykken. 1985. Assessment of fat-free mass using bioelectrical impedance measurements of the human body. *American Journal of Clinical Nutrition* 41: 810.

McArdle, W.D., F.I. Katch, and V.L. Katch. 2005. *Essentials of exercise physiology.* Baltimore: Lippincott, Williams & Wilkins.

McCrory, M.A., P.A. Mole, T.D. Gomez, K.G. Dewey, and E.M. Bernauer. 1998. Body composition by air-displacement plethysmography by using predicted and measured thoracic gas volumes. *Journal of Applied Physiology* 84: 1475-1479.

Moon, J.R., A.E. Smith, K.L. Kendall, J.L. Graef, D.H. Fukuda, T.W. Beck, J.T. Cramer, M.L. Rea, and J.R. Stout. 2009. Concerns and limitations of dual-energy x-ray absorptiometry (DXA) for the evaluation of fat and fat-free mass in older men and women. NSCA Conference Abstracts.

Moon, J.R., S.E. Tobkin, P.B. Costa, M. Smalls, W.K. Mieding, J.A. O'Kroy, R.F. Zoeller, and J.R. Stout. 2008. Validity of the BOD POD for assessing body composition in athletic high school boys. *Journal of Strength and Conditioning Research* 22: 263-268.

Ortiz-Hernández, L., N.P. López Olmedo, M.T. Genis Gómez, D.P. Melchor López, and J. Valdés Flores. 2008. Application of body mass index to schoolchildren of Mexico City. *Annals of Nutrition and Metabolism* 53: 205-214.

Piers, L.S., M.J. Soares, S.L. Frandsen, and K. O'Dea. 2000. Indirect estimates of body composition are useful in groups but unreliable in individuals. *International Journal of Obesity* 24: 1145-1152.

Romero-Corral, A., V.K. Somers, J. Sierra-Johnson, R.J. Thomas, M.L. Collazo-Clavell, J. Korinek, T.G. Allison, J.A. Batsis, F.H. Sert-Kuniyoshi, and F. Lopez-Jimenez. 2008. Accuracy of body mass index in diagnosing obesity in the adult general population. *International Journal of Obesity* 32: 959-966.

Saunders, M.J., J.E. Blevins, and C. Broeder. 1998. Effects of hydration changes on bioelectrical impedance in endurance trained individuals. *Medicine and Science in Sports and Exercise* 30: 885-892.

Sinha, R., W.H. Chow, M. Kulldorff, J. Denobile, J. Butler, M. Garcia-Closas, R. Weil, R.N. Hoover, and N. Rothman. 1999. Well-done, grilled red meat increases the risk of colorectal adenomas. *Cancer Research* 59: 4320-4324.

Sun, G., C.R. French, G.R. Martin, B. Younghusband, R.C. Green, Y. Xie, M. Mathews, J.R. Barron, D.G. Fitzpatrick, W. Gulliver, and H. Zhang. 2005. Comparison of multifrequency bioelectrical impedance analysis with dual-energy X-ray absorptiometry for assessment of percentage body fat in a large, healthy population. *American Journal of Clinical Nutrition* 81: 74-78.

Tylavsky, F., T. Lohman, B.A. Blunt, D.A. Schoeller, T. Fuerst, J.A. Cauley, M.C. Nevitt, M. Visser, and T.B. Harris. 2008. QDR 4500A DXA overestimates fat-free mass compared with criterion methods. *Journal of Applied Physiology* 94: 959-965.

United States Department of Health and Human Services, and Centers for Disease Control and Prevention. 2009. Body mass index. www.cdc.gov/nccdphp/dnpa/healthyweight/assessing/bmi/index.htm.

United States Department of Health and Human Services, and Centers for Disease Control and Prevention. 2010. National Health and Nutrition Examination Survey. www.cdc.gov/nchs/nhanes/new_nhanes.htm.

Witt, K., and E. Bush. 2005. College athletes with an elevated body mass index often have a high upper arm muscle area, but not elevated triceps and subscapular skinfolds. *Journal of the American Dietetic Association* 105: 599-602.

World Health Organization. 2010. BMI classification. www.who.int/bmi/index.jsp?introPage=intro_3.html.

Chapter 12

American College of Sports Medicine, American Dietetic Association, and Dietitians of Canada. 2000. Joint position statement: Nutrition and athletic performance. *Medicine and Science in Sports and Exercise* 32(12): 2130-2145.

American Dietetic Association. n.d. Become a registered dietitian. www.eatright.org/students/education/starthere.aspx.

American Psychiatric Association. 1994. *Diagnostic and statistical manual of mental disorders, DSM-IV.* 4th ed. Washington, DC: American Psychiatric Association.

Antonio, J., M. Gann, D. Kalman, F. Katch, S. Kleiner, R. Kreider, and D. Willoughby. 2005. ISSN roundtable: FAQs about the ISSN. *Journal of the International Society of Sports Nutrition* 2(2): 1-3.

Baum, A. 2006. Eating disorders in male athletes. *Sports Medicine* 36(1): 1-6.

Becker, C.B., S. Bull, K. Schaumberg, A. Cauble, and A. Franco. 2008. Effectiveness of peer-led eating disorder prevention: A replication trial. *Journal of Consulting and Clinical Psychology* 76(2): 347-354.

Bonci, C.M., L.J. Bonci, L.R. Granger, C.L. Johnson, R.M. Malina, L.W. Miline, R.R. Ryan, and E.M. Vanderbunt. 2008. National Athletic Trainers' Association position statement:

Preventing, detecting and managing disordered eating in athletes. *Journal of Athletic Training* 43(1): 80-108.

Burke, L.M., G.R. Cox, N.K. Cummings, and B. Desbrow. 2001. Guidelines for daily carbohydrate intake: Do athletes achieve them? *Sports Medicine* 31: 267-299.

Campbell, B., R.B. Kreider, T. Ziegenfuss, P. La Bounty, M. Roberts, D. Burke, J. Landis, H. Lopez, and J. Antonio. 2007. International society of sports nutrition position stand: Protein and exercise. *Journal of the International Society of Sports Nutrition* 4: 8.

Casa, D.J., L.E. Armstrong, S.K. Hilllman, S.J. Montain, R.V. Reiff, B.S.E. Rich, W.O. Roberts, and J.A. Stone. 2000. National Athletic Trainers' Association position statement: Fluid replacement for athletes. *Journal of Athletic Training* 35(2): 212-224.

Dandoval, W., K. Heller, and W. Wiese. 1994. Stages of change model for nutritional counseling. *Topics in Clinical Nutrition* 9: 64-69.

Dionne, M.M., and F. Yeudall. 2005. Monitoring of weight in weight loss programs: A double-edged sword. *Journal of Nutrition Education Behavior* 37: 315-318.

Esmarck, B., J.L. Anderson, S. Olsen, E.A. Richter, M. Mizuno, and M. Kjaer. 2001. Timing of postexercise protein intake is important for muscle hypertrophy with resistance training in elderly humans. *Journal of Physiology* 535(Pt 1): 301-131.

Glazer, J.L. 2008. Eating disorders among male athletes. *Current Sports Medicine Reports* 7(6): 332-337.

Institute of Medicine. 2004. Dietary reference intakes: Water, potassium, sodium, chloride, and sulfate. www.nap.edu/catalog.php?record_id=10925#toc.

Jeukendrup, A.E., R. Jentjens, and L. Moseley. 2005. Nutritional considerations in triathlon. *Sports Medicine* 35: 163-181.

Karp, J.R., J.D. Johnston, S. Tecklenburg, T.D. Mickleborough, A.D. Fly, and J.M. Stager. 2006. Chocolate milk as a post-exercise recovery aid. *International Journal of Sport Nutrition and Exercise Metabolism* 16: 78-91.

Kerksick, C., J. Stout, B. Campbell, C. Wilborn, R. Kreider, D. Kalman, T. Ziegenfuss, H. Lopez, J. Landis, J. Ivy, and J. Antonio. 2008. International society of sports nutrition position stand: Nutrient timing. *Journal of the International Society of Sports Nutrition* 5: 17.

Lacey, K., and E. Pritchett. 2003. Nutrition care process model: ADA adopts roadmap to quality care and outcomes management. *Journal of the American Dietetic Association* 103: 1061-1072.

Louisiana Board of Examiners in Dietetics and Nutrition. 2009. Rules and regulations title 46, professional and occupational standards part LXX: Registered dieticians. www.lbedn.org/rules.pdf.

McArdle, W.D., F. Katch, and V. Katch. 2005. *Sports and exercise nutrition.* 3rd ed. Baltimore: Lippincott, Williams & Wilkins.

Michael, P., and E. Pritchett. 2002. Complying with Health Insurance Portability and Accountability Act: What it means to dietetic practitioners. *Journal of the American Dietetic Association* 102: 1402-1403.

Nattiv, A., A.B. Loucks, M.M. Manore, C.F. Sanborn, J. Sundgot-Borgen, and M.P. Warren. 2007. American College of Sports Medicine position stand: The female athlete triad. *Medicine Science Sports and Exercise* 39(10): 1867-1882.

Phillips, S. 2006. Dietary protein for athletes. *Applied Physiology, Nutrition, and Metabolism* 31: 647-654.

Prochaska, J.O., J.C. Norcross, and C.C. DiClemente. 1994. *Changing for good.* New York: William Morrow.

Rosenbloom, C. 2005. Sports nutrition: Applying ADA's nutrition care process and model to achieve quality care and outcomes for athletes. *SCAN Pulse* 24:10-17.

Rosenbloom, C. 2007. Sports nutrition: Applying the science. *Nutrition Today* 42: 248-254.

Santana, J.C., J. Dawes, J. Antonio, and D. Kalman. 2007. The role of the fitness professional in providing sports/exercise nutrition advice. *Strength and Conditioning Journal* 29(3): 69-71.

Sawka, M.N., L.M. Burke, E.R. Eichner, R.J. Maughan, S.J. Montain, and N.S. Stachenfeld. 2007. Exercise and fluid replacement position stand. *Medicine and Science in Sports and Exercise* 39(2): 377-389.

Sundgot-Borgen, J., and M.K. Tortsveit. 2004. Prevalence of eating disorders in elite athletes is higher than in the general population. *Clinical Journal of Sports Medicine* 14(1): 25-32.

Thiel, A. 1993. Subclinical eating disorders in male athletes: A study of the low weight category of rowers and wrestlers. *Acta Psychiatrica Scandinavica* 88: 259.

Tipton, K.D., T.A. Elliott, M.G. Cree, A. Aarsland, A.P. Sanford, and R.R. Wolfe. 2007. Stimulation of net muscle protein synthesis by whey protein ingestion before and after exercise. *American Journal of Physiology: Endocrinology and Metabolism* 292: E71-E76.

Tipton, K.D., B.B. Rasmussen, S.L. Miller, S.E. Wolf, S.K. Owens-Stovall, B.E. Petrini, and R.R. Wolfe. 2001. Timing of amino acid-carbohydrate ingestion alters anabolic response of muscle to resistance exercise. *American Journal of Physiology: Endocrinology and Metabolism* 281(2): E197-206.

Zawila, L.G., C. Steib, and B. Hoogenboom. 2003. The female collegiate cross country runner: Nutritional knowledge and attitudes. *Journal of Athletic Training* 38(1): 67-74.

Index

Note: The italicized *f* and *t* following page numbers refer to figures and tables, respectively.

About the Editors

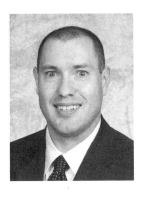

Bill I. Campbell, PhD, CSCS, FISSN, is assistant professor and director of the Exercise and Performance Nutrition Laboratory at the University of South Florida, a research laboratory dedicated to innovation in sport nutrition research. As a researcher and author, Campbell has published more than 100 scientific abstracts and papers related to sport nutrition and enhancement of sport performance. In addition, Campbell has published more than 50 articles for health and fitness magazines (print and electronic media). He is a paid consultant to professional sport team organizations and sport entertainment corporations and has lectured on various topics related to sport nutrition and exercise performance to audiences spanning five nations and four continents. He was the lead author on the International Society of Sports Nutrition's *Position Stand: Protein and Exercise,* which addresses some of the common questions and myths regarding protein intake and supplementation for athletes and physically active people.

Campbell is a member of the National Strength and Conditioning Association (NSCA), the American College of Sports Medicine (ACSM), and the International Society of Sports Nutrition (ISSN). Campbell is also a fellow of ISSN and serves on the organization's advisory board.

He received his PhD in exercise, nutrition, and preventive health from Baylor University in 2007. During that same year, he also received the Outstanding Doctoral Student Award for research and teaching. In 2009, Campbell received the Outstanding Undergraduate Teaching Award from the University of South Florida.

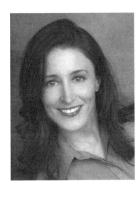

Marie A. Spano, MS, RD, LD, CSCS, CSSD, FISSN, is one of the country's leading sport nutritionists. She combines science with practical experience to help Olympic, professional, and recreational athletes implement customized nutrition plans to maximize athletic performance. Also a nutrition communications expert, Spano consults with leading food, beverage, and supplement companies regarding public relations and communications strategies.

Spano enjoys the challenge of communicating scientific information in an approachable, understandable format to a variety of audiences. She has appeared on NBC, ABC, Fox, and CBS affiliates. She has also authored hundreds of magazine articles, trade publication articles, book chapters, e-zines, and marketing materials.

A three-sport collegiate athlete, Spano earned her master's degree in nutrition from the University of Georgia and her bachelor's degree in exercise and sport science from the University of North Carolina at Greensboro (UNCG), where she also ran Division I cross country. Her experience as a college athlete gives her perspective on working with athletes of all levels, especially student-athletes. She has a firsthand understanding of how the demands of athletics and psychological aspects of injury, sleep, recovery, and sound nutrition can affect an athlete's overall well-being and performance.

Spano is a member of the National Strength and Conditioning Association (NSCA), the American Dietetic Association (ADA), the International Society of Sports Nutrition (ISSN), and Sports, Cardiovascular, and Wellness Nutrition (SCAN). She currently serves as vice president for the ISSN and is a member of the NSCA's Nutrition Special Interest Group.

Contributors

Jose Antonio, PhD, CSCS, FACSM, FISSN, FNSCA
Nova Southeastern University, Fort Lauderdale, Florida

Bill I. Campbell, PhD, CSCS, FISSN
University of South Florida, Tampa

Donovan L. Fogt, PhD
The University of Texas at San Antonio

Chad M. Kerksick, PhD; ATC; CSCS,*D; NSCA-CPT,*D
University of Oklahoma, Norman

Richard B. Kreider, PhD, FACSM, FISSN
Texas A&M University, College Station

Paul La Bounty, PhD, MPT, CSCS
Baylor University, Waco, Texas

Lonnie Lowery, PhD, RD, LD
Winona State University, Winona, Minnesota

Henry C. Lukaski, PhD, FACSM, FCASN
USDA, ARS Grand Forks Human Nutrition Research Center, Grand Forks, North Dakota

Amanda Carlson Phillips, MS, RD, CSSD
Athletes' Performance, Tempe, Arizona

Bob Seebohar, MS, RD, CSCS, CSSD
Fuel4mance, LLC, Littleton, Colorado

Marie A. Spano, MS, RD, LD, CSCS, CSSD, FISSN
Spano Sports Nutrition Consulting, Atlanta, Georgia

Colin Wilborn, PhD, ATC, CSCS, FISSN
University of Mary Hardin-Baylor, Belton, Texas

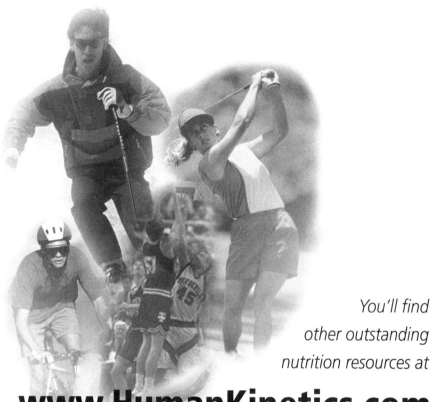